L m r p B A W
N a F E H C D s y z h n

# THE PSYCHOLOGY OF
# MEN AND
# MASCULINITIES

# THE PSYCHOLOGY OF
# MEN AND
# MASCULINITIES

EDITED BY
**RONALD F. LEVANT** AND **Y. JOEL WONG**

AMERICAN PSYCHOLOGICAL ASSOCIATION • *Washington, DC*

Published by
American Psychological Association
750 First Street, NE
Washington, DC 20002
www.apa.org

To order
APA Order Department
P.O. Box 92984
Washington, DC 20090-2984
Tel: (800) 374-2721; Direct: (202) 336-5510
Fax: (202) 336-5502; TDD/TTY: (202) 336-6123
Online: www.apa.org/pubs/books
E-mail: order@apa.org

In the U.K., Europe, Africa, and the Middle East, copies may be ordered from
American Psychological Association
3 Henrietta Street
Covent Garden, London
WC2E 8LU England

Typeset in Goudy by Circle Graphics, Inc., Columbia, MD

Printer: Edwards Brothers, Inc., Lillington, NC
Cover Designer: Naylor Design, Washington, DC

The opinions and statements published are the responsibility of the authors, and such opinions and statements do not necessarily represent the policies of the American Psychological Association.

**Library of Congress Cataloging-in-Publication Data**

Names: Levant, Ronald F., editor. | Wong, Y. Joel, editor.
Title: The psychology of men and masculinities / edited by Ronald F. Levant, Y. Joel Wong.
Description: Washington, D.C. : American Psychological Association, 2017. | Includes bibliographical references and index.
Identifiers: LCCN 2016036545 | ISBN 9781433826900 (hardback) | ISBN 1433826909 (paperback)
Subjects: LCSH: Men—Psychology. | Masculinity. | Sex role. | BISAC: PSYCHOLOGY / Social Psychology. | PSYCHOLOGY / Human Sexuality. | HEALTH & FITNESS / Men's Health.
Classification: LCC HQ1090 .P79 2017 | DDC 155.3/32—dc23 LC record available at https://lccn.loc.gov/2016036545

**British Library Cataloguing-in-Publication Data**
A CIP record is available from the British Library.

*Printed in the United States of America*
*First Edition*

http://dx.doi.org/10.1037/0000023-000

# CONTENTS

# CONTRIBUTORS

**Michael E. Addis, PhD,** Department of Psychology, Clark University, Worcester, MA

**Kate M. Bennett, PhD,** Department of Psychological Sciences, University of Liverpool, Liverpool, England

**Tyler C. Bradstreet, MS,** Department of Psychological Sciences, Texas Tech University, Lubbock

**Gary R. Brooks, PhD,** Department of Psychology and Neuroscience, Baylor University, Waco, TX

**Brendan Gough, PhD,** School of Social Sciences, Leeds Beckett University, Leeds, England

**Martin Heesacker, PhD,** Department of Psychology, University of Florida, Gainesville

**Christina Hermann, BS,** Department of Education and Human Services, Counseling Psychology Program, Lehigh University, Bethlehem, PA

**Ethan Hoffman, MA,** Department of Psychology, Clark University, Worcester, MA

**Anthony J. Isacco, PhD,** Graduate Psychology Programs, Chatham University, Pittsburgh, PA

**Bryan T. Karazsia, PhD,** Department of Psychology, The College of Wooster, Wooster, OH

**Elyssa M. Klann, BA,** Department of Counseling and Educational Psychology, Indiana University, Bloomington

**Ronald F. Levant, EdD, ABPP,** Department of Psychology, The University of Akron, Akron, OH

**Christopher T. H. Liang, PhD,** Department of Education and Human Services, Counseling Psychology Program, Lehigh University, Bethlehem, PA

**Tao Liu, MS, MA,** Department of Counseling and Educational Psychology, Indiana University, Bloomington

**Carin Molenaar, MEd,** Department of Education and Human Services, Counseling Psychology Program, Lehigh University, Bethlehem, PA

**Sarah K. Murnen, PhD,** Department of Psychology, Kenyon College, Gambier, OH

**James M. O'Neil, PhD,** Department of Educational Psychology, Neag School of Education, University of Connecticut, Storrs

**Mike C. Parent, PhD,** Department of Psychological Sciences, Texas Tech University, Lubbock

**Joseph H. Pleck, PhD,** Department of Human Development and Family Studies, University of Illinois at Urbana–Champaign

**Wizdom A. Powell, PhD,** Department of Health Behavior, Gillings School of Global Public Health, University of North Carolina, Chapel Hill

**Louis A. Rivera, MEd,** Department of Education and Human Services, Counseling Psychology Program, Lehigh University, Bethlehem, PA

**Steve Robertson, PhD,** Centre for Men's Health, Leeds Beckett University, Leeds, England

**Sarah Seymour-Smith, PhD,** Department of Psychology, Nottingham Trent University, Nottingham, England

**Steven J. Snowden, MS,** Department of Psychology, University of Florida, Gainesville

**Edward H. Thompson, Jr., PhD,** Department of Sociology and Anthropology, College of the Holy Cross, Worcester, MA

**Jay C. Wade, PhD,** private practice, Bali, Indonesia

**Stephen R. Wester, PhD,** Department of Educational Psychology, University of Wisconsin–Milwaukee

**Y. Joel Wong, PhD,** Department of Counseling and Educational Psychology, Indiana University, Bloomington

# FOREWORD: A BRIEF HISTORY OF THE PSYCHOLOGY OF MEN AND MASCULINITIES

JOSEPH H. PLECK

I first began working in the psychology of men and masculinities in the early 1970s, with Pleck (1973, 1974) and Pleck and Sawyer (1974) my first publications. I was honored when the editors invited me to contribute this Foreword and when they further encouraged me to make it a substantive one.

This book, *The Psychology of Men and Masculinities*, shows how far our field has advanced since the 1970s and identifies numerous new directions that our discipline is taking. To appreciate the long way our field has come, it is important to understand what it grew out of. When I started my career in the early 1970s, the new psychology of women was just emerging. At that time, many people thought that there was no psychology of men. But actually, there was. In fact, at that time U.S. psychology's understanding of gender and gender development was almost entirely a psychology of men. What was that psychology of men, and how did it come about?

# THE GENDER ROLE IDENTITY PARADIGM

Terman and Miles's (1936) *Sex and Personality* introduced the construct of *trait masculinity–femininity* (trait m-f) to academic psychology, conceptualized as a unitary, bipolar dimension of personality. Research using trait m-f measures took off in earnest in the late 1940s and focused almost entirely on males. Studies investigated such questions as the following: What is the effect of father absence on a son's masculinity? (The earliest of these trait m-f studies examined sons whose fathers were absent because of World War II military service.) How does a mother's employment affect a son's masculinity? What is the influence of birth order and sibling composition on sons' masculinity? What consequences does fathers' degree of marital power have on sons' masculinity? It was evident that researchers were greatly concerned about sons' masculinity!

These investigations continued for three more decades until the early 1970s, with countless new m-f measures proliferating and with the vast preponderance of research focusing on boys and men. Initially, psychologists viewed trait m-f as operationalizing the developmental construct of *sex-typing*. Then trait m-f was interpreted to reflect the more theoretically ambitious concept of *gender identity*.[1] Gender identity was not simply a descriptive construct; it was a profoundly prescriptive one, something that individuals *should* attain. Researchers viewed the development of male gender identity, however, as an inherently risky process, prone to failure because of high rates of father absence, domineering mothers, female elementary school teachers, the increasing acceptance of homosexuality, the broader cultural emasculation of men's roles, and so forth. Research on male gender identity, using trait m-f measures, grew to link it to a wide range of phenomena: male psychological adjustment, male homosexuality, male transsexuality, male delinquency and hypermasculinity, male initiation rites in non-Western cultures, boys' difficulties in the schools, and racial/ethnic and social class differences among men.

This traditional psychology of men was, at its core, an interpretation of the variations among males in trait masculinity–femininity. One direct legacy of this older psychology of men is that our discipline today is now generally termed the *psychology of men and masculinity*, whereas the corresponding study of women is called simply the *psychology of women*. The psychology of women has never been about variations in femininity in the way that the traditional psychology of men focused on the meaning of variations in masculinity.

My book *The Myth of Masculinity* (1981) drew on Thomas Kuhn's (1962) concept of scientific paradigms and how they change. I argued that

---

[1] It would be easy to assume that applying the "identity" frame to what trait m-f scales measured derived from psychoanalytic theory, but this is actually not the case. The gender identity construct is difficult to align with Anna Freud's and Erik Erikson's concept of "ego identity."

all the studies of trait m-f in men from the 1940s to the 1970s reflected an underlying *gender role identity paradigm* (GRIP),[2] comprising 11 major lines of research. The GRIP was in fact U.S. psychology's first psychology of men and masculinity.

This paradigm dominated developmental, personality, and clinical psychology through the 1970s. This psychology of masculinity also permeated clinical practice. The Minnesota Multiphasic Personality Inventory and other omnibus clinical and personality inventories prominently featured m-f scales. In my clinical psychology internship in 1970–1971, "weak passive father" was noted so frequently on male patients' intake histories as a source of insecure gender identity that it might as well have been preprinted on the intake form. In an article about my clinical training (Pleck, 1976), I described the clinical staff's contempt for gay men's inadequate male gender identities.[3] The GRIP took hold in popular culture as well. Growing up in the 1950s, I remember articles in Sunday newspaper magazine supplements inviting male readers to take an m-f questionnaire to determine how masculine they were.

My critical review of the 11 major lines of research within the GRIP (Pleck, 1981; see also Pleck, 1983) concluded that the findings widely viewed as conclusively supporting it (about trait m-f and psychological adjustment, father absence, homosexuality, and so forth) were actually weak and contradictory. A key issue arose in this research regarding one of the GRIP's most important propositions, concerning the effects of father absence on trait m-f. The GRIP predicts that father absence should be associated with low trait masculinity. However, in many studies, father-absent males actually score unusually high on masculinity. GRIP researchers argued that this finding confirms rather than disconfirms the GRIP because these father-absent males are actually exhibiting "hypermasculinity" as a "defense" against their underlying insecure gender identities. This interpretation is not inherently untenable. But using this hypermasculinity defense clause to explain away the finding made this GRIP proposition unfalsifiable and therefore unscientific.

## THE GENDER ROLE STRAIN PARADIGM

Research deriving from the GRIP died out by the early 1980s. The GRIP was gradually replaced by an alternative view of male gender development, in the same way that the Ptolemaic geocentric model of the solar system

---

[2]*Male sex role identity paradigm* in Pleck (1981).
[3]As described in Pleck (1976), in this psychoanalytically oriented hospital, women rape victims who kept obsessively thinking about the experience (what we now interpret as posttraumatic stress disorder) were told that they did this because "some part of them" was "gratified" by the experience.

in astronomy was discarded in favor of the Copernican heliocentric view. The concluding chapter of my book (Pleck, 1981) presented a formulation of this emerging alternative understanding of men and masculinities, termed the *gender role strain paradigm* (GRSP),[4] involving 10 major lines of research. The essential difference between the GRIP and the GRSP is that the GRIP views traditional norms for masculinity as valid, asserting that the only problem is that too many men fail to live up to them. By contrast, the GRSP views the problem as these traditional expectations themselves. I subsequently presented an updated formulation, distinguishing three major types of male gender role strain (discrepancy–strain, trauma–strain, and inherent–dysfunction-strain; Pleck, 1995). In addition, I also analyzed masculinity ideology as a key cofactor in male gender role strain (see also Pleck, Sonenstein, & Ku, 1993).

Turning to the present volume, *The Psychology of Men and Masculinities* reflects how the GRSP has been a dominant framework for our field for more than three decades. The book's three initial chapters ably review current research on the GRSP as a whole, on its central concept of masculinity ideology, and on the related construct of male gender role conflict. Isacco and Wade's subsequent chapter discusses a group of additional constructs or perspectives used in our research in recent years: male gender role stress, male reference group identity dependence, conformity to masculinity norms, precarious manhood, and masculinity contingency.[5] In my view, these are all processes that can be integrated within the broader GRSP. To borrow a term from particle physics, the GRSP has become our field's "standard model."[6]

Just as in particle physics, there are of course controversies, sometimes heated, about various constructs and dynamics within this standard model and the methodologies used to study them. Occasionally, adherents of some viewpoints and methodologies seem to argue that theirs is the only valid way to conceptualize and study men and masculinities. Nonetheless, I believe the range of constructs and methodologies in the wide range of contemporary GRSP research should be viewed as broadly compatible.

I offer two observations about how research on the psychology of men and masculinities, using the GRSP perspective, has evolved since the early 1980s. First, it is fascinating to see how some central GRSP constructs represent complete reversals—indeed, complete transvaluations—of GRIP-based ideas. The GRIP interpreted a male high in trait masculinity (only) as reflecting healthy male gender identity and therefore being highly desirable. But in

---

[4]Sex role strain paradigm in Pleck (1981).

[5]One further construct reviewed by Isacco and Wade, positive masculinity, represents a new direction that is not part of the GRSP, and is particularly important for that reason.

[6]In a content analysis of the 154 articles published in *Psychology of Men and Masculinity* during 2000–2008, 71% used the overall GRSP or theoretical concepts related to it (Wong et al., 2010, Table 1).

the GRSP perspective, it is interpreted quite differently as "conformity to masculine norms," which is likely disadvantageous.

As another example, *precarious manhood* is a term that could easily refer to the GRIP's view of male development: Acquiring male gender identity is inherently risky and highly prone to failure. But in GRSP research, precarious manhood refers instead to the negative consequences for males of the social construction of masculinity as something hard to achieve and easy to fail at.

Second, it is noteworthy how many of the topics highlighted in the psychology of men parallel topics emphasized in the psychology of women. For example, men's mental health, physical health, and body image, capably reviewed here (see, respectively, Chapters 6, 7, and 8, this volume), have been major areas of men and masculinities research (Wong, Steinfeldt, Speight, & Hickman, 2010). In the psychology of women, these were likewise among the first and most enduring research topics. Similarly, the study of racial minority men and of gay/bisexual men have been growing areas of research in the past decade or two (see Chapters 9 and 10, this volume), just as the corresponding topics in the psychology of women have been.

## FATHERHOOD AND THE PSYCHOLOGY
## OF MEN AND MASCULINITIES

The linkages between fatherhood, my own primary focus in recent years (Pleck, 1997, 2010b, 2012; Pleck & Masciadrelli, 2004), and the psychology of men and masculinities call for some special comment, especially because this volume does not include a chapter on fatherhood (but see McKelley & Rochlen, 2016). Fatherhood has become an enormous research area in its own right (see, e.g., Cabrera & Tamis-LeMonda, 2013; Lamb, 2010). The earliest writings in the 1970s presenting the emerging new perspective on masculinity identified fathering as one of the principal areas in which men's behavior needed to change, and was in fact changing, toward greater involvement in childrearing (e.g., Pleck & Sawyer, 1974). In the ensuing years, some practice-oriented (Oren & Chase Oren, 2010) and self-help (Levant & Kelly, 1991) writing on fatherhood further advanced the linkage between fatherhood and changing masculinity. But empirical research on fatherhood generally has not connected the two.

Fatherhood is now more situated in the disciplines of developmental psychology, family studies, and parenting than it is in the psychology of men and masculinities. To illustrate, of the 154 articles in *Psychology of Men and Masculinity* between 2000 and 2008, 14 concerned fatherhood (Wong et al., 2010). By contrast, between 2000 and 2006, in just two developmental psychology journals and three family studies journals, 30 to 45 articles focusing on fathering were published every year (Goldberg, Tan, & Thorsen, 2009). As a research topic, fatherhood has an obvious fit with developmental and family studies journals. In addition, many of those journals are long-established and prestigious, thus drawing fatherhood researchers to publish in them.[7]

But investigating fatherhood within developmental psychology and family studies frameworks has not pressed researchers to make plain the connections between fatherhood and masculinity. Even I and other researchers known for their contributions to the psychology of men and masculinities have, in our publications on fatherhood, not always made the role of masculinity explicit (e.g., Levant, Richmond, Cruickshank, Rankin, & Rummell, 2014; Pleck, 2012). In these publications, the notion that father involvement (in the sense of actual caregiving, rather than only rough-and-tumble play) is a nontraditional male behavior is only implicit.

The psychology of men and masculinities is beginning to make the connection between fatherhood and masculinity more explicit (McKelley & Rochlen, 2016; Pleck, 2010a; Silverstein, Auerbach, & Levant, 2002). The GRSP perspective is quite relevant to men's experience as fathers. A good recent illustration of explicit gender role strain in fathering comes from a Pew Research Center (2007) national survey. About three fifths of both men and women said that they think it is harder to be a father now than it was 20 or 30 years ago. How are today's fathers doing in the face of this "paternal challenge"? Of women in the survey, 56% said today's dads are doing as good a job or a better job raising their kids compared with fathers a generation ago. But among fathers themselves, there is a crisis of paternal self-confidence. Only 41% of men in the Pew survey thought contemporary fathers are doing better or even as well as fathers in the past. A majority of men (55%) said today's dads are actually doing a worse job. Levs's (2015) accounts of the workplace barriers and stigma encountered by fathers seeking parental leave at the birth of a child illustrate male gender role strain in another way.

There is a second reason why the psychology of men and masculinities field should address fatherhood to a greater extent than it has. Masculinity is central to what, in my view, is the single most widespread idea about fatherhood in American culture: That fathers are essential for good child development—the *essential father* (EF) hypothesis (Pleck, 2010a; Silverstein &

---

[7]However, just as fathering is not yet fully connected to the men and masculinities discipline, it is also not fully integrated in parenting research. To illustrate, I contributed an article on fatherhood (Pleck, 2012) to a special issue of *Parenting: Science and Practice* on new directions in parenting research (Fleming, Grusec, & Haley, 2012). Of the 18 articles in the issue, my article was placed next to last, between an article on the role of parenting in the development of the neural substrate of emotional behavior and one on the use of multilevel statistical modeling in parenting research. Fathers were nearly invisible in the issue's other 17 articles.

Auerbach, 1999).[8] The EF notion is so deeply ingrained that our society has what could be termed a *rhetoric of paternal essentiality*.[9]

Stated in formal terms, the EF hypothesis holds that (a) fathers make a contribution to child development that is *essential*, (b) fathers' contribution is essential because it is *unique*, and (c) fathers' contribution is essential and unique specifically because it is *uniquely masculine* (Pleck, 2010a). What is crucial to realize is that although the GRIP has been generally abandoned in social science research since the 1970s, it still lives on in the EF hypothesis. In fact, the EF hypothesis is in effect the surviving remnant of the GRIP, especially in popular discourse. Fatherhood and fathering are thus a problematic "special case" in the psychology of men and masculinities.

How should we regard the EF hypothesis? One important consideration is to understand that this view of fathering, like the GRIP itself, seems to be a uniquely American idea. When one examines research on fathering in cross-cultural perspective (Shwalb, Shwalb, & Lamb, 2013), the notion that fathering is "essential" to children's development seems to be a specifically American preoccupation (Pleck, 2013). To be sure, European and non-Western societies view fathers' roles as fundamental in gender relations and as central to how gender relations are reproduced (as well as change) from one generation to the next. But the ways that European and non-Western societies valorize the roles of fathers do not have the anxious undertone evident in U.S. discussions of fathers' "essential" and "unique" contributions. In U.S. discourse, many view boys and young men who do not receive good fathering as being "at risk" of everything from educational failure, delinquency and prison, and welfare dependency to homosexuality, drug addiction, and abusing women; there is simply no problem that absent or inadequate fathering cannot cause. In the United States, discussing the roles of fathers often seems close to pressing a panic button that is not so readily available in other countries.

Another important consideration: Is the EF hypothesis actually supported by empirical research? In Pleck (2010a; see also Pleck, 2007), I critically review six component lines of research entailed in the EF hypothesis: (a) gender differences in parenting behavior, (b) the association between father presence and child outcomes, (c) the mediation of this association specifically by paternal involvement, (d) the interpretation of the effects of fathers' presence to fathers' being male, (e) the uniqueness of fathering's

---

[8]It is noteworthy that Silverstein and Auerbach's (1999) first calling attention to "essential fatherhood" as a belief needing "deconstruction" evoked a firestorm of media as well as professional criticism. Notably, some APA members resigned in protest that *American Psychologist* had published the article.

[9]My Google search in June 2009 on the words *essential* and *father* together yielded five million hits; the same search in October 2015 yielded 144 million. Similar results were obtained for *unique* and *father*.

(compared with mothering's) effects on child outcomes, and (f) the association of paternal masculinity orientation to paternal involvement and to child outcomes. My review of these six areas reveals at best extremely modest support for any of these six lines of research.

If research support is so weak, why, then, do so many people believe so strongly that "fathers are essential"? It is simply because it is such a motivating, inspirational idea. This notion has been the underlying premise for many, perhaps most, programs promoting greater father involvement. The motivational power of the EF hypothesis occurs in this context: In many ways, our culture devalues fathering. Levs (2015) provided vivid accounts of the stigma fathers face for accommodations in the workplace to their being parents. He also shows how our society in effect "polices men out of the family" with workplace barriers, abetted by the "doofus Dad" stereotype. To many father activists, paternal essentiality seems to be the only narrative available that can counteract our cultural trivialization of fatherhood and thus justify their work with fathers.

In my experience, most fatherhood activists (and fathers) who say that "fathers are essential" are not actually using the word *essential* in its literal, dictionary meaning. Every dictionary I have seen uses the exact same example to illustrate the word's usage: "Water is *essential* to life." Clearly, fatherhood is not essential to good child development in this sense. (And motherhood is not essential, either.) In presentations about fathering, I sometimes ask audiences to imagine completing a two-item survey: (a) "Fathers are essential for good child development" (agree–disagree) and (b) "A child growing up with a single mother can develop just as well as a child growing up with a mother and father" (agree–disagree). Almost everyone agrees with Statement 1. But they also overwhelmingly agree with Statement 2. So I gently point out that if you agree with Statement 2, you must not really be agreeing with Statement 1 in its literal sense.

What most people actually mean by saying "fathers are essential" is that fathers are "important." In Pleck (2010a), I suggest that we can specify what "important" means by viewing father presence/good fathering as a protective factor, within the cumulative risk/protection perspective on development. In this perspective, no *single* risk/protective factor is necessary (or sufficient) for positive development. Rather, the effect of any particular factor is determined by the context of other risk and protective factors. Thus, if a child has other protective factors (e.g., family resources, good neighborhood, good schools, other supportive adults), father absence will not necessarily be associated with poor outcomes. But in the absence of other protective factors like these, father absence will often be associated with poor adjustment.

Understanding father presence/absence and fathering quality in this way helps us understand why research sometimes does, but sometimes does not, find linkages between father presence/parenting quality and child out-comes; it depends on levels of other risk or protective factors in the sample studied. In Pleck (2010a), I argued that seeing fathering as important in this way does not represent a demotion in fathers' significance. Rather, this view of fathering simply brings our understanding of fathering's effects in line with how contemporary research understands the effects of particular predictors on outcomes in most other research areas.[10]

## IN CLOSING

Over the last four decades, journalists have often asked me how much change there has really been in men's roles. I often reply that I like to collect items about men and masculinities from newspapers, magazines, TV news, and books. I then classify each item in one of three piles: (a) *things are getting worse* (e.g., "Murdered baby's father surrenders to police; details at 10," an actual TV headline from the 1980s); (b) *things are staying about the same*; and (c) *things are getting better*. I then track the three piles' relative sizes. Over the years, the balance has been shifting away from the first pile, and toward the third.

Our field, the psychology of men and masculinities, has made great progress over the past four decades. As well, it faces future challenges such as clarifying our thinking about fatherhood. This book, *The Psychology of Men and Masculinities*, belongs at the top of my third pile.

## REFERENCES

Cabrera, N. C., & Tamis-LeMonda, C. (Eds.). (2013). *The handbook of father involvement* (2nd ed.). New York, NY: Taylor & Francis.

Fleming, A., Grusec, J., & Haley, D. (Eds.). (2012). The arc of parenting from epigenomes to ethics [Special issue]. *Parenting: Science and Practice, 12*(2–3), 89–260.

Goldberg, W., Tan, E., & Thorsen, K. (2009). Trends in academic attention to fathers, 1930–2006. *Fathering, 7,* 159–179.

[10]For example, having cholesterol level in the normal range is widely recognized as a protective factor against heart attacks. However, it is not "essential" to have low cholesterol. After all, most people who lack this protective factor (i.e., who have high cholesterol) do not have heart attacks. Nonetheless, keeping cholesterol in the normal range is still important for cardiac health, particularly when other risk factors such as being male, being older, having high blood pressure, and family cardiac history are present.

Kuhn, T. (1962). *The structure of scientific revolutions*. Chicago, IL: University of Chicago Press.

Lamb, M. E. (Ed.). (2010). *The role of the father in child development* (5th ed.). New York, NY: Wiley.

Levant, R. F., & Kelly, J. (1991). *Between father and child: How to become the kind of father you want to be*. New York, NY: Penguin.

Levant, R. F., Richmond, K., Cruickshank, B., Rankin, T. J., & Rummell, C. M. (2014). Exploring the role of father involvement in the relationship between day care and children's behavior problems. *American Journal of Family Therapy, 42*, 193–204.

Levs, J. (2015). *All in: How our work-first culture fails dads, families, and businesses— and how we can fix it*. New York, NY: HarperOne.

McKelley, R. A., & Rochlen, A. B. (2016). Furthering fathering: What we know and what we need to know. In Y. J. Wong & S. R. Wester (Eds.), *APA handbook of men and masculinities* (pp. 525–550). Washington, DC: American Psychological Association.

Oren, C., & Chase Oren, D. (Eds.). (2010). *Counseling fathers*. New York, NY: Routledge.

Pew Research Center. (2007). *Being Dad may be tougher these days, but working moms are among their biggest fans*. Retrieved from http://pewsocialtrends.org/pubs/510/fathers-day

Pleck, J. H. (1973). Psychological frontiers for men. *Rough Times* [formerly *The Radical Therapist*], *3*(6), 14–15. Reprinted in S. Gordon & R. Libby (Eds.). (1976). *Sexuality today and beyond* (pp. 58–59). North Scituate, MA: Duxbury Press.

Pleck, J. H. (1974, April 18). My male sex role—and ours. *WIN Magazine*, 8–12. Reprinted in D. David & R. Brannon (Eds.). (1976). *The forty-nine percent majority: The male sex role* (pp. 54–58). Reading, MA: Addison-Wesley.

Pleck, J. H. (1976). Sex role issues in clinical training. *Psychotherapy: Theory, Research and Practice, 13*, 17–19.

Pleck, J. H. (1981). *The myth of masculinity*. Cambridge, MA: MIT Press.

Pleck, J. H. (1983). The theory of male sex role identity: Its rise and fall, 1936 to the present. In M. Lewin (Ed.), *In the shadow of the past: Psychology views the sexes* (pp. 205–225). New York, NY: Columbia University Press. Reprinted in H. Brod (Ed.). (1987). *The making of masculinities: The new men's studies* (pp. 21–38). Boston, MA: Allen and Unwin Hyman.

Pleck, J. H. (1995). The gender role strain paradigm: An update. In R. F. Levant & W. S. Pollack (Eds.), *A new psychology of men* (pp. 11–32). New York, NY: Basic Books.

Pleck, J. H. (1997). Paternal involvement: Levels, sources, and consequences. In M. E. Lamb (Ed.), *The role of the father in child development* (3rd ed., pp. 66–103). New York, NY: Wiley.

Pleck, J. H. (2007). Why could father involvement benefit children? Theoretical perspectives. *Applied Developmental Science, 11*(4), 1–7.

Pleck, J. H. (2010a). Fatherhood and masculinity. In M. E. Lamb (Ed.), *The role of the father in child development* (5th ed., pp. 32–66). New York, NY: Wiley.

Pleck, J. H. (2010b). Paternal involvement: Revised conceptualization and theoretical linkages with child outcomes. In M. E. Lamb (Ed.), *The role of the father in child development* (5th ed., pp. 67–107). New York, NY: Wiley.

Pleck, J. H. (2012). Integrating father involvement in parenting research. *Parenting: Science and Practice, 12*(2–3), 243–253. http://dx.doi.org/10.1080/15295192.2012.683365

Pleck, J. H. (2013). Foreword. In D. Shwalb, B. Shwalb, & M. E. Lamb (Eds.), *Fathers in cultural context* (pp. xii–xv). New York, NY: Wiley.

Pleck, J. H., & Masciadrelli, B. (2004). Paternal involvement in U.S. residential fathers: Levels, sources, and consequences. In M. E. Lamb (Ed.), *The role of the father in child development* (4th ed., pp. 222–271). New York, NY: Wiley.

Pleck, J. H., & Sawyer, J. (Eds.). (1974). *Men and masculinity.* Englewood Cliffs, NJ: Prentice-Hall.

Pleck, J. H., Sonenstein, F. L., & Ku, L. C. (1993). Masculinity ideology: Its impact on adolescent males' heterosexual relationships. *Journal of Social Issues, 49*(3), 11–29.

Shwalb, D., Shwalb, B., & Lamb, M. E. (Eds.). (2013). *Fathers in cultural context.* New York, NY: Wiley.

Silverstein, L. B., & Auerbach, C. F. (1999). Deconstructing the essential father. *American Psychologist, 54,* 397–407.

Silverstein, L. B., Auerbach, C. F., & Levant, R. F. (2002). Contemporary fathers reconstructing masculinity: Clinical implications of gender role strain. *Professional Psychology: Research and Practice, 33,* 361–369.

Terman, L., & Miles, C. (1936). *Sex and personality.* New York, NY: McGraw-Hill.

Wong, Y. J., Steinfeldt, J. A., Speight, Q. L., & Hickman, S. L. (2010). Content analysis of *Psychology of Men and Masculinity* (2000–2008). *Psychology of Men and Masculinity, 11,* 170–181.

# ACKNOWLEDGMENTS

The process of preparing this volume went amazingly smoothly. That can be attributed to the very high quality of our contributing authors; the support of the staff at APA Books, particularly our acquisitions editor, Christopher J. Kelaher, and our development editor, Beth Hatch; and to the fact that we as co-editors have a track record of collaboration on various projects that we were able to parlay into an outstanding working relationship for this volume.

We also acknowledge and thank our mentors, colleagues, and families. Ronald F. Levant wishes to acknowledge his primary mentors, John M. Shlien, Joseph H. Pleck, and Ralph Mosher; his long-term friends and collaborators, Gary R. Brooks and Louise B. Silverstein; his many friends and colleagues in the Society for the Psychological Study of Men and Masculinity; his more recent collaborators, Rosalie J. Hall, Ingrid K. Weigold, Y. Joel Wong, Mike C. Parent, Ryon McDermott, Ed Thompson, and Jennifer Stanley; and his many students over the past 40 years, who are too numerous to mention by name, but he wishes to name those who have become enduring colleagues, particularly Katherine Richmond and David J. Wimer. He also thanks the many students who have worked in the Gender Research Lab and its prior incarnations going back to the mid-1970s at Boston University, Rutgers University, Harvard Medical School, Nova Southeastern University, and The University of Akron. He thanks his family for their love, support, and forbearance on his endless projects: his wife, Carol L. Slatter; his daughter, Caren E. Levant; his daughter-in-law, Camille Veytia; his older grandson, Adrian Shanker; and his younger grandson, Jeremy Shanker. Finally, he wishes to honor the memories of his parents, Wilma I. Levant and Harry G. Levant, and his brother, the poet Lowell A. Levant.

Y. Joel Wong wishes to acknowledge his former advisor, Aaron Rochlen, for his mentorship and for introducing him to the psychology of men and masculinities. He appreciates his colleagues and students at Indiana University for providing a nourishing intellectual environment in which to work. He is also grateful to colleagues who have supported, broadened, and enriched his thinking on the psychology of men and masculinities, including Melissa Burkley, Hsiu-Lan Cheng, Ron Levant, Ryon McDermott, Jim O'Neil, Jesse Owen, Aaron Rochlen, Munyi Shea, Jesse Steinfeldt, Kim Tran, and Stephen Wester. Finally, he thanks his family—Angie, Kaitlyn, and Shawn—for their immense love, patience, and support, without which much of this work would be meaningless.

# THE PSYCHOLOGY OF
# MEN AND
# MASCULINITIES

# INTRODUCTION: MATURATION OF THE PSYCHOLOGY OF MEN AND MASCULINITIES

RONALD F. LEVANT AND Y. JOEL WONG

The psychology of men and masculinities is a dynamic young field that has come a long way in a relatively short time. It benefitted from the foundation laid by the psychology of women in conceptualizing, theorizing, and investigating the protean effects of gender. Not only has it contributed to the reconstruction of masculinity that is still evolving in response to the dramatic changes in women's roles that began 50 years ago, it has also addressed significant problems for men's physical and mental health (e.g., men's higher mortality rates, substance use, and stigma associated with help-seeking) and for society (e.g., men's gender-based and sexual violence).

When the first author first began to approach colleagues about starting a division in the American Psychological Association (APA) devoted to men's psychology, he was greeted with incredulous questions such as "Why do we need that? Isn't all psychology the psychology of men?" As noted in the Foreword, that statement had a certain truth to it, but the psychology they

http://dx.doi.org/10.1037/0000023-001
*The Psychology of Men and Masculinities*, R. F. Levant and Y. J. Wong (Editors)

were referring to took males as a proxy for the species and did not think it necessary to study females. This was challenged in the 1970s by feminist psychologists. By redefining sex and gender (Unger, 1979), the psychology of women upended the old order in psychology and paved the way for a critical analysis of gender. Therefore, there would not be a psychology of men and masculinities as we know it today had there not been a psychology of women. As a result, the mission statement of the Society for the Psychological Study of Men and Masculinity (Division 51 of the APA) states that the division "acknowledges its historical debt to feminist-inspired scholarship on gender, and commits itself to the support of groups such as women, gays, lesbians and people of color that have been uniquely oppressed by the gender/class/race system."

The critical study of men began in the 1970s (Pleck & Sawyer, 1974). It gained steam in the 1980s, when task forces on men's roles and special interest groups were formed in three APA divisions (17: Society of Counseling Psychology; 29: Psychopharmacology and Substance Abuse; and 43: Society for Couple and Family Psychology), which together presented symposia at the annual APA conventions on the emerging specialty of the psychology of men and masculinities and thus laid the foundation for the formation of Division 51 (Brooks & Elder, 2016). By 1995, the new psychology of men had arrived. In that year, the Society for the Psychological Study of Men and Masculinity entered the vestibule as a candidate to become APA's 51st division. In addition, A New Psychology of Men (Levant & Pollack, 1995) was published that year. This volume has been cited as "the most salient publication" in the new psychology of men (Cochran, 2010, p. 45) and has served as the standard graduate text and professional reference book for the fledgling field of the psychology of men and masculinity.

In the 20-plus years since the formation of Division 51 and the publication of A New Psychology of Men, the field has experienced tremendous growth and development. The original pioneers of this field have spawned several generations of scholars and practitioners, many of whom hold tenured and tenure-track positions in doctoral programs across the country and are now training the next generation of scholars and practitioners. A search in the PsycINFO database on December 28, 2015, for the terms masculinity or masculinities turned up 13,270 citations, compared with only 108 references in 1983 (Wong & Wester, 2016). As of this writing in 2016, the APA journal Psychology of Men and Masculinity (PMM) is in its 17th year of publication. PMM published two issues a year and 150 pages in the 7 × 10-inch trim size when it was launched in 2000; it now publishes four issues per year and 500 pages in the 8½ × 11-inch trim size, and has a 2015 Impact Factor of 2.947. As a result of these developments, the literature has grown and developed in many expected and unexpected ways, in terms of both the science and its applications. There is therefore a great need for a new resource that synthesizes and critically evaluates this evolved and expanded field, which is the aim of the present volume, The Psychology of Men *and Masculinities*. The very title of this volume, in referring to masculinities in the plural, alludes to some aspects of this development—in particular, the influence of social constructionism, multiculturalism, and intersectionality—that have led to a consensus among scholars that definitions of masculinity vary with time, place, culture, and circumstance.

There are five major parts to this volume. Part I, the lengthiest part, consisting of five chapters, covers the major theoretical perspectives and associated research in the psychology of men and masculinities. The first three chapters cover in depth the major theories that have been used in United States—namely, the gender role strain paradigm (GRSP), masculinity ideologies, and gender role conflict. These three theories (and related ones covered in Chapter 5—e.g., reference group identity dependence, conformity to masculine norms, masculine gender role stress, precarious manhood, and masculinity contingency) could be broadly defined as the GRSP and related approaches, which is the dominant research paradigm in the psychology of men and masculinities in the United States (Wong, Steinfeldt, Speight, & Hickman, 2010). Together they could be broadly described as empirical feminist and social constructionist approaches (Deaux, 1984), which are based primarily in psychology and rely largely (although by no means exclusively) on quantitative research. Meanwhile across the pond, another empirical feminist social constructionist approach took root and became the dominant approach in the United Kingdom, Europe, and in some of the Commonwealth countries (particularly Australia, New Zealand, and Canada). Going by several related names (discursive psychology, critical men's studies, critical discursive psychology), these approaches tend to be more interdisciplinary, focus on theoretical perspectives, and take a qualitative approach to empirical research. Recently *PMM* published a special section titled "Forum on the Intersection of Discursive Psychology and the Psychology of Men and Masculinity" to invite dialogue between these two perspectives on the psychology of men and masculinities originating in different parts of the world. In the hopes of continuing this dialogue, we have included Chapter 4 on critical discursive psychology, and a later chapter (Chapter 7) considers this perspective. Finally, Chapter 5 reviews in briefer form a selection of other theories and research used in the psychology of men and masculinities.

In Chapter 1, "The Gender Role Strain Paradigm," Ronald F. Levant and Wizdom A. Powell review and critically evaluate the GRSP. First fully formulated by Pleck (1981) in his landmark volume *The Myth of Masculinity*, the GRSP deconstructed and helped replace the earlier, biologically deterministic conceptualization of gender, the gender role identity paradigm (GRIP), that dominated research in the United States from about 1930 to 1980. In providing an alternative paradigm, the GRSP complicated and problematized the construct of masculinity. In much of this research, the focus has been on investigating the strains placed on men, women, children, and society as a result of socializing men for positions of dominance over women. The GRSP has been updated twice, most recently situating it in the framework of social psychology (Levant, 2011; Pleck, 1995). This chapter covers the development of the GRSP, types of masculine gender role strain (including discrepancy, dysfunction, and trauma types of strain), social contexts of masculine gender role strain, assessment of the GRSP, and directions for future research.

In Chapter 2, "Masculinity Ideologies," Edward H. Thompson, Jr. and Kate M. Bennett review the research on masculinity ideologies. This chapter begins with a discussion of the origin of the construct *masculinity ideologies*, considering both definitional and conceptual issues. Next the chapter considers the content of contemporary masculinity ideologies and provides a helpful table of "canons" used in the measurement of traditional (or, as the authors prefer) mainstream masculinity ideology, illustrated by items from the various scales. The chapter then reviews recent work in masculinity ideologies. This review is aimed at conveying how the construct is being studied and focuses on three areas in which masculinity ideologies have had negative implications for men and for society: health status and health behavior, health-related help-seeking, and the performance of marital status. Finally, avenues for new research are suggested.

In Chapter 3, "Masculinity as a Heuristic: Gender Role Conflict Theory, Superorganisms, and System-Level Thinking," James M. O'Neil, Stephen R. Wester, Martin Heesacker, and Steven J. Snowden present gender role conflict theory (GRC) in a new epistemological context to enable researchers to conceptualize gender roles as problem-solving strategies. Research questions would then investigate the ways in which men might use their masculinities to solve problems, evaluate the outcomes, and change as a result of experience. As such, this chapter does not provide a point-by-point review of the extant GRC literature, which is available elsewhere. Rather, this chapter first briefly summarizes the more recent empirical work. Next, similar to the direction taken in the GRSP, it offers a theoretical framework based in social psychology—specifically, social cognition, including heuristics and system-level thinking—within which GRC theory can continue to evolve.

In Chapter 4, "A Critical Discursive Approach to Studying Masculinities," Sarah Seymour-Smith provides a primer on the critical discursive psychological (CDP) approach to studying masculinities, which treats masculinity as a situated, fluid, and negotiated set of contingent actions and responses. CDP is a particular version of discursive psychology, focused on the performance of identity and using qualitative research to chart the ways in which men talk about themselves. This enables the investigation of the complex, dynamic way that masculinities are created, negotiated, and deployed and demonstrates how identity fluctuates within each participant. The chapter provides three illustrations of the CDP approach using processed transcripts of interviews: how medical personnel construct the identities of male patients, testicular cancer patients' views of self-help groups, and Afro Caribbean men's views on the digital rectal exam to screen for prostate cancer.

In Chapter 5, "A Review of Selected Theoretical Perspectives and Research in the Psychology of Men and Masculinities," Anthony J. Isacco and Jay C. Wade review six other theories and research in the psychology of men and masculinities, including masculine gender role stress, male reference group identity dependence, conformity to masculine norms, precarious manhood, positive psychology–positive masculinity, and masculinity contingency. The first three are more established approaches, whereas the latter three are emerging perspectives. Masculine gender role stress, which integrates stress and coping literature with the GRSP, is the oldest of these approaches; it was initially applied to cardiovascular health but has also been applied to aggression. Male reference group identity dependence is a theory of male identity based on psychodynamic ego identity development theory and reference group theory. Conformity to masculine norms is a theoretical model based in the social psychology literature on social norms, conformity, and compliance. As a relatively new approach, it has produced an impressive body of research.

Part II of this volume consists of three chapters on several of the major research topics in the psychology of men and masculinities. In Chapter 6, "Men's Depression and Help-Seeking Through the Lenses of Gender," Michael E. Addis and Ethan Hoffman focus on research on men's depression, stigma, and help-seeking. After critically reviewing the literature on sex differences in the epidemiology of major depression, they address issues related to the diagnosis of depression (e.g., do men tend to be underdiagnosed relative to women, and are the diagnostic criteria for depression gendered?) and to coping with depression. They then critically review research on masculinity and help-seeking in relation to mental health. They find evidence that the social construction and social learning of traditional masculine norms is associated with stigma in regard to both depression and help-seeking. A unique feature of this chapter is its insistence that we move away from generalizing (negatively) about all men and consider how, when, where, and why men might position themselves differently in regard to health issues (e.g., the contexts) so that more tailored interventions can be developed.

In Chapter 7, "A Review of Research on Men's Physical Health," Brendan Gough and Steve Robertson present a critical overview of psychological theory and research on men's health. This chapter is unique in that it covers both the quantitative work in the United States using the GRSP and the qualitative work in the United Kingdom and Europe in the interdisciplinary field of critical studies of men and masculinity (which overlaps with the CDP perspective discussed in Chapter 4). They examine the evidence linking aspects of masculinity to specific health behaviors. Recognizing that relationships between masculinity factors and health practices are complex and tied to race, social class, sexual orientation, and other social identities, they consider the importance of intersectionality and include literature on health disparities in the United States and on the health of men in non-Western regions of the world (e.g., the global South). Their concluding section evaluates recent approaches to men's health promotion (e.g., salutogenic masculinities) as well as policy initiatives in this area.

In Chapter 8, "A Review of Research on Men's Body Image and Drive for Muscularity," Sarah K. Murnen and Bryan T. Karazsia review research on men's body image and drive for muscularity. They emphasize recent research (after 2000) that seeks to understand male body image in its own right, rather than in comparison with female body concerns. They document the existence of a masculine muscular ideal in popular culture that is hypothesized to pressure men to adopt muscularity motives, and they review several scales designed to measure this phenomenon. Research conducted on subgroups of men with heightened body concerns is reviewed, as is research on several maladaptive and potentially serious body change behaviors, including the use of anabolic–androgenic steroids, unhealthy eating, excessive weight training, cosmetic surgery, and muscle dysmorphia.

Part III consists of two chapters on multicultural diversity. In Chapter 9, "The Intersection of Race, Ethnicity, and Masculinities: Progress, Problems, and Prospects," Y. Joel Wong, Tao Liu, and Elyssa M. Klann delineate three research paradigms for the application of intersectionality to the psychology of racial/ethnic minority men. The intergroup paradigm involves quantitative group comparisons based on individuals' social identities. The interconstruct paradigm investigates the relationships among constructs associated with individuals' social identities. The intersectional uniqueness paradigm assumes that social identities are inherently intertwined; thus, experiences associated with multiple identities cannot be separated, nor can they simply be added together to account for individuals' overall experiences. Although these three paradigms can be broadly applied, this chapter focuses in particular on the intersection of race, ethnicity, and gender as applied to men of color.

In Chapter 10, "Gay, Bisexual, and Transgender Masculinities," Mike C. Parent and Tyler C. Bradstreet provide a critical overview of empirical, theory-driven research on gay, bisexual, and transgender (GBT) men's masculinities and highlight areas for growth of the field. They focus on qualitative and quantitative work with GBT men that has been conducted within the frameworks of four paradigms: hegemonic masculinity, gender role strain or conflict, gender role ideology, and gender role conformity. They cover the following topics: heterosexuals' attitudes toward GBT masculinities, relationships, health, body image and eating disorders, mental health, and help-seeking. They highlight areas for future research and note that research has focused on cisgender gay men to the exclusion of bisexual and transgender men.

In Part IV of this volume, we have two chapters on the implications for practice of the psychology of men and masculinities. Gary R. Brooks contributed Chapter 11, "Counseling, Psychotherapy, and Psychological Interventions for Boys and Men." Because there are (happily) a lot of books on psychotherapies for men, this chapter restricts its focus to how established therapy approaches— psychodynamic, cognitive and cognitive behavioral, interpersonal, humanistic/ existential/experiential, and group therapies—can be adapted to fit the needs and styles of male populations and refers the reader to the available resources. Next the chapter highlights the expanding possibilities for interventions with boys and men. This is a surprisingly vast area and includes mental health consultation (such as Courtenay's HEALTH model, executive coaching, men's groups in religious organizations, gender-aware programs in the military and the U.S. Department of Veterans Affairs (VA), in jails and prisons, and in physical and alcohol rehabilitation programs), primary prevention (including psychoeducational programs and consciousness-raising activities such as the Gender Role Journey approach, the Boys' Forum, and Alexithymia Reduction Treatment), weekend retreats, adventure therapy, men's centers, public service announcements and use of digital media, and primary prevention programs for vulnerable boys and young men. Finally, this chapter discusses several ways that practitioners can welcome and treat reluctant male clients, including contextualizing the stages of change model, incorporating insights from research on the working alliance and multicultural competence, and offering an overall framework for male-friendly therapy.

Chapter 12, "Dysfunction Strain and Intervention Programs Aimed at Men's Violence, Substance Use, and Help-Seeking Behaviors," was contributed by Christopher T. H. Liang, Carin Molenaar, Christina Hermann, and Louis A. Rivera. *Dysfunction strain* refers to the type of strain resulting from conforming to traditional masculine norms. This type of masculine gender role strain often has a greater negative impact on others and society at large than on the men who experience it. This is the first attempt to identify dysfunction strain as a distinct focus for intervention and to catalogue such programs. The chapter covers interventions aimed at reducing gender-based and sexual violence, substance use, and stigma associated with help-seeking. This review covers both treatment and prevention efforts, focuses on several major types of problems associated with boys and men (e.g., violence, alcohol use), and includes programs with and without empirical support. Small effect sizes, in addition to the high levels of recidivism that are found in the literature, suggest that interventions for gender-based and sexual violence and substance use are at an early stage of development and can be strengthened.

The authors advocate a gender-transformative approach, in which men are encouraged to transform their gender roles and work toward more equitable gender relationships, as one way for programs to yield stronger effects.

Part V of the book is a conclusion by Y. Joel Wong and Ronald F. Levant. This final chapter examines a few unresolved and controversial issues concerning the nature of masculinities. We address criticisms of the construct of masculinities and explain why it remains useful and vital to the psychology of men. We also explore the debate on whether masculinities research reflects social constructionist or essentialist perspectives on gender. We argue that a continuum perspective acknowledging that masculinities research can reflect a hybrid of both perspectives is preferable to one that simply categorizes studies into one of two mutually exclusive paradigms. The chapter concludes by analyzing the evolving nature of masculine norms, noting that existing measures of masculinities developed over the past few decades might not adequately capture recent and rapidly shifting trends in masculine norms and ideologies. We then discuss several methodological strategies for identifying contemporary masculine norms and ideologies.

As Levant (2014) noted, "We have come a long way, baby." Benefitting from the insights of the psychology of women, we have built a new psychology of men and masculinities, one that we can pass on with pride to the next generations of scholars and practitioners. As scholars and practitioners, we have much to offer men in our society to help them find new ways to be men in 21st century. The current generation of boys holds promise for developing new ways to be men in their resistance to masculine norms (Way et al., 2014). The specialty seems to be coming together in certain ways, for example, the fact that several chapters point toward integration with social psychology and in the increased engagement between the U.S. and U.K. psychologies of men and masculinities. There are also points of tension and controversy, such as that between Chapters 1 and 6 on whether the individual differences approach taken in quantitative GRSP research is essentialistic or (framed less critically) acontextual. In the final analysis, we believe that gender can be conceptualized from many perspectives, and it has been our aim to promote a "big-tent," "both–and" approach to investigating masculinities. As noted earlier, this topic is discussed more fully in the Conclusion.

## REFERENCES

Brooks, G. R., & Elder, W. B. (2016). History and future of the psychology of men and masculinities. In Y. J. Wong & S. R. Wester (Eds.), APA handbook of men and masculinities (pp. 3–21). http://dx.doi.org/10.1037/14594-001

Cochran, S. V. (2010). Emergence and development of the psychology of men and masculinity. In J. C. Chrisler & D. R. McCreary (Eds.), *Handbook of gender research in psychology: Vol. 1. Gender research in general and experimental psychology* (pp. 43–58). http://dx.doi.org/10.1007/978-1-4419-1465-1_3

Deaux, K. (1984). From individual differences to social categories: Analysis of a decade's research on gender. *American Psychologist, 39,* 105–116. http://dx.doi.org/10.1037/0003-066X.39.2.105

Levant, R. F. (2011). Research in the psychology of men and masculinity using the gender role strain paradigm as a framework. *American Psychologist, 66,* 765–776. http://dx.doi.org/10.1037/a0025034

Levant, R. F. (2014). At 15 years we have come a long way, baby! *Psychology of Men & Masculinity, 15,* 1–3. http://dx.doi.org/10.1037/a0035319

Levant, R. F., & Pollack, W. S. (Eds.). (1995). *A new psychology of men.* New York, NY: Basic Books.

Pleck, J. H. (1981). *The myth of masculinity.* Cambridge, MA: MIT Press.

Pleck, J. H. (1995). The gender role strain paradigm: An update. In R. F. Levant & W. S. Pollack (Eds.), *A new psychology of men* (pp. 11–32). New York, NY: Basic Books.

Pleck, J. H., & Sawyer, J. (Eds.). (1974). *Men and masculinity.* Englewood Cliffs, NJ: Prentice-Hall.

Unger, R. K. (1979). Toward a redefinition of sex and gender. *American Psychologist, 34,* 1085–1094. http://dx.doi.org/10.1037/0003-066X.34.11.1085

Way, N., Cressen, J., Bodian, S., Preston, J., Nelson, J., & Hughes, D. (2014). "It might be nice to be a girl . . . then you wouldn't have to be emotionless": Boys' resistance to norms of masculinity during adolescence. *Psychology of Men & Masculinity, 15,* 241–252. http://dx.doi.org/10.1037/a0037262

Wong, Y. J., Steinfeldt, J. A., Speight, Q. L., & Hickman, S. L. (2010). Content analysis of psychology of men and masculinity (2000–2008). *Psychology of Men & Masculinity, 11,* 170–181. http://dx.doi.org/10.1037/a0019133

Wong, Y. J., & Wester, S. R. (2016). Introduction: The evolution, diversification, and expansion of the psychology of men and masculinities. In Y. J. Wong & S. R. Wester (Eds.), *APA handbook of men and masculinities* (pp. xvii–xxiv). http://dx.doi.org/10.1037/14594-000

# I

# GENDER ROLE STRAIN
# PARADIGM AND
# RELATED THEORIES

AMNPBIWUN
CUZD

# 1

# THE GENDER ROLE STRAIN PARADIGM

RONALD F. LEVANT AND WIZDOM A. POWELL

The gender role strain paradigm (GRSP) has been called the "standard model" for research in the psychology of men and masculinities (see Foreword, this volume). In this chapter, we discuss, in turn, the development of the GRSP, types of masculine gender role strain, social contexts of masculine gender role strain, assessment of the GRSP, and future research directions.

## DEVELOPMENT OF THE GRSP

Feminist scholarship on the psychology of women and gender redefined sex and gender (Unger, 1979), developing in the process a perspective that viewed gender roles as socially constructed by gender ideologies, rooted in power differences between men and women (Deaux, 1984; Gergen, 1985).

Parts of this chapter were adapted from Hammond, Fleming, and Villa-Torres (2016); Levant (2015); and Levant and Richmond (2016).

http://dx.doi.org/10.1037/0000023-002
*The Psychology of Men and Masculinities*, R. F. Levant and Y. J. Wong (Editors)

Pleck (1981) applied these insights to men in his seminal volume, *The Myth of Masculinity*. There, he formulated the sex role strain paradigm, later termed the GRSP (Pleck, 1995). The GRSP is regarded as the major theoretical paradigm in the field of the psychology of men and masculinity (Cochran, 2010; Wong, Steinfeldt, Speight, & Hickman, 2010; see also Foreword, this volume). It is an empirical feminist and social constructionist perspective that encompasses both quantitative and qualitative work.

The GRSP views gender roles not as biologically determined but rather as socially constructed entities that arise from, and serve to maintain and protect, the patriarchal social and economic order. Traditional gender roles, therefore, undergird power differences between men and women by defining masculinity as dominance and aggression and femininity as submissiveness and nurturance (Levant, 1996). According to the social constructionist perspective, gender roles of "masculinity" and "femininity" are thought of as "performances," independent of sex (Butler, 1990). Hence, women can perform masculinity, men can perform femininity, and both sexes can perform any combination and permutation of parts or all of these gender roles. Yet within a patriarchal society, there are tangible rewards associated with conforming to the sex-typed and socially sanctioned traditional gendered roles, as well as negative consequences associated with failure to conform (Pleck, 1981, 1995). Over time, traditional gendered performances become normative and compulsory, which in turn is encoded in everything from the neural pathways of individuals to social interactions (Fausto-Sterling, 2000).

Pleck (1995) proffered the GRSP as an alternative to the older approach that had dominated research on masculinity for 50 years (1930–1980), which he termed the *gender role identity paradigm* (GRIP).[1] The GRIP drew from early psychoanalytic theory (particularly drive and ego theories); it assumed that people have a powerful psychological need to form a gender role identity that corresponded to their biological sex and that optimal personality development hinged on its formation. The extent to which this "inherent" need was met was determined by how completely a person adopted his or her traditional gender role. From this perspective, the development of appropriate gender role identity was viewed as a failure-prone process, and failure for men to achieve a masculine gender role identity was thought to result in homosexuality, negative attitudes toward women, and/or defensive hypermasculinity (Pleck, 1981). This paradigm sprung from the same philosophical roots as the essentialist view of sex roles—the notion that (in the case of men) there is a clear masculine "essence" that is historically invariant—that is, that biological

---

[1]Pleck (1981) used the term *paradigm* to contrast these two overarching approaches, but after three decades of use, it would probably be more appropriate to refer to the GRSP as a theory. However, the name seems to have stuck, so it may be difficult to change.

sex determined gender. Pleck (1981) provided a convincing demonstration not only that the GRIP poorly accounted for the observed data in many foundational studies on personality development but also that such studies often arbitrarily reinterpreted the meaning of the data to adduce evidence for the GRIP. For example, after analyzing the study by Mussen (1961), one of the most important studies in the GRIP literature on the relationship between sex typing and adjustment, Pleck (1981) concluded that "if a measure ordinarily indicating good adjustment occurs in non-masculine males, it is arbitrarily reinterpreted to indicate poor adjustment" (p. 86).

In contrast to the essentialist perspective of the GRIP, Pleck (1981) put forth 10 propositions for the GRSP that reflected the view that gender roles arose from society: (a) contemporary gender roles are operationally defined by gender role stereotypes and norms, (b) gender roles are contradictory and inconsistent, (c) the proportion of persons who violate gender roles is high, (d) violation of gender roles leads to social condemnation, (e) violation of gender roles leads to negative psychological consequences, (f) actual or imagined violation of gender roles leads people to overconform to them, (g) violating gender roles has more severe consequences for males than for females, (h) certain prescribed gender role traits (e.g., male aggression) are often dysfunctional, (i) each sex experiences gender role strain in its paid work and family roles, and (j) historical change causes gender role strain. In essence, what the GRSP did was deconstruct and help topple the earlier conceptualization of gender, the GRIP, that had dominated research from ca. 1930 to 1980, in which the personality traits stereotypically associated with men and thought of as "masculine" were regarded as the standard for human behavior for both men and women; as a result, the GRSP problematized masculinity. In the GRSP, the focus is on investigating the strains placed on men, women, children, and society as a result of socializing men for positions of dominance over women.

## MAJOR CLARIFICATIONS OF THE GRSP

Since the original formulation of the GRSP, there have been four major clarifications. These pertain to gender ideologies, the social psychology of gender, the types of masculine gender role strain, and the social contexts of masculine gender role strain.

### Gender Ideologies

Pleck (1995) indicated that although they were not explicitly mentioned in the 10 original propositions, gender ideologies are considered to be "central" to the GRSP and a "vital co-factor in male role strain" (p. 19). The term *gender ideologies* refers to beliefs about the importance of men and women adhering to culturally defined standards for gendered behavior. The dominant gender ideologies in a given society thus define the norms for gender roles. Through social learning and social influence processes that occur over the lifespan, the dominant gender ideologies influence how parents, teachers, coaches, peers, and society at large socialize children and how individuals think, feel, and behave in regard to gender-salient matters (Levant, 1996, 2011; Pleck, 1995; Pleck, Sonenstein, & Ku, 1994; Thompson & Pleck, 1995). Hence, another proposition should be added to the GRSP, at the beginning of the list: The dominant gender ideologies in a given society define the norms for gender roles.

Despite the potential diversity in masculinity ideologies in the contemporary United States, Pleck (1995) pointed out that "there is a particular constellation of standards and expectations that individually and jointly have various kinds of negative concomitants" (p. 20). This is referred to as *traditional masculinity ideology* because it was the dominant view before the deconstruction of gender that took place beginning in the late 1960s driven by second wave feminism. Despite the gains of the women's movement, traditional masculinity ideology is still the dominant cultural script that organizes and informs the development and maintenance of the traditional masculine role (Levant, 2011; Pleck, 1995). The psychological construct of traditional masculinity ideology shares fundamental assumptions about patriarchy with the sociological construct of hegemonic masculinity (Connell & Messerschmidt, 2005). Whereas hegemonic masculinity refers to practices that promote the dominant social position of men and the subordinate social position of women, traditional masculinity ideology refers to the cultural beliefs regarding the norms for men's roles that sustain these practices. The first investigators to attempt to define traditional masculinity ideology were David and Brannon (1976), who identified four components: men should not be feminine ("no sissy stuff"); men should strive to be respected for successful achievement ("the big wheel"); men should never show weakness ("the sturdy oak"); and men should seek adventure and risk, even accepting violence if necessary ("give 'em hell").

Investigations of the endorsement of traditional masculinity ideology have supported a central tenet of the GRSP, namely, that the endorsement varies according to the cultural context and social location of the individual (Levant, 1996, 2011; Pleck, 1981, 1995). Greater endorsement of traditional masculinity ideology using the Male Role Norms Inventory (MRNI) was found to be associated with a host of demographic variables: sex (being male), age (being younger), marital status (being single), race and ethnicity (African Americans endorse traditional masculinity ideology to a greater extent than do Latino/a Americans, who in turn endorse traditional masculinity ideology to a greater extent than do European Americans), geographic region of residence in the United States (those living in the South endorse traditional masculinity ideology to a greater extent than do those living in the North), and nationality (Chinese and Russians endorse traditional masculinity ideology to a greater extent than do Americans). Further, traditional masculinity ideology was found to be related to a number of variables measuring social location: generational differences (sons scored less traditional than fathers), sexual orientation and social support (gay men scored less traditional than heterosexual men), relationship violence (batterers in treatment endorsed less traditional ideology), alcoholism (midlife alcoholics were less traditional), and head injury (mixed results). See Levant and Richmond (2007) for citations and more details on these results.

## Social Psychology of Gender

Although the main contributors to the theory were trained as clinical psychologists at Harvard University (Levant, 1996; Pleck, 1995), the original theory implied a social psychological (social learning theory) foundation for gender role socialization (Pleck, 1981). Later, Levant (2011) explicitly framed the GRSP in social psychological terms, using social cognitive and social influence theories, and the constructs of gender roles and social norms. Thus, in the current formulation, traditional masculinity ideology is posited to exert social influence through interactions resulting in reinforcement, punishment, and observational learning. Traditional masculinity ideology thus informs, encourages, and constrains boys and men to conform to, comply with, or obey the prevailing male role norms (both descriptive and injunctive) by adopting certain socially sanctioned (prescribed) masculine behaviors and avoiding certain forbidden (proscribed) behaviors (Levant, 2011).

## Types of Masculine Gender Role Strain

Pleck (1995), in his third clarification of the GRSP, pointed out that his original formulation of the paradigm stimulated research on three varieties of male gender role strain, discrepancy strain, dysfunction strain, and trauma strain.

### Discrepancy Strain

In this section, we discuss attempts to assess discrepancy strain and the masculine gender role stress approach to it. *Discrepancy strain* results when one fails to live up to one's internalized manhood ideal, which, in the case of men reared traditionally, may closely approximate traditional norms.

*Attempts to Assess Discrepancy Strain.* In formulating the GRSP, Pleck (1981, 1995) hypothesized that discrepancy strain leads to lower self-esteem and other negative psychological consequences; however, little research to date has empirically tested this hypothesis. The first method used a comparison between ratings of the self/ideal self-concept test and was not very useful (Pleck, 1995). According to Pleck (1995), masculine discrepancy strain can be operationalized by assessing a man's idealized gender role standards (or his perception of the "ideal" man) and his perception of his own gender role characteristics, and then seeing how the two compare. This can be done by calculating the discrepancy score between responses on measures of these constructs. Unfortunately, only one study using this method found a relationship between gender role discrepancy strain and self-esteem (Deutsch & Gilbert, 1976). According to Pleck (1995), "other research of this type is limited and has not produced strong confirmation" (p. 14).

Nabavi (2004) developed and assessed a measure of masculine discrepancy strain, called the Masculine Attitudes, Stress, and Conformity Questionnaire. Using the same question base, he varied the stems of the questions to reflect the person's endorsement of traditional attitudes about men in society (e.g., "A man should avoid crying in front of people"), whether the participant experiences said male role expectations as stressful (e.g., "It bothers me that men are expected to avoid crying in front of people"), and the participant's behavioral conformity to traditional male role norms (e.g., "I avoid crying in front of people"). This researcher theorized that gender role discrepancy could be calculated by the difference scores between the corresponding items from endorsement of traditional attitudes measure and the behavioral conformity measure. From this he derived scores that he referred to as *traditional strain* and *nontraditional strain*. However, the manner in which these scales are scored is unclear, and their relationship with self-esteem was not assessed.

Using a different approach, Liu, Rochlen, and Mohr (2005) investigated the relationship between real and ideal gender role conflict (GRC) and psychological distress. In their model, the relationships between real and ideal GRC consisted of four quadrants created by two axes: low-to-high ideal GRC and low-to-high real GRC. The four quadrants were thus: norm-favoring discrepancy (high ideal GRC and low real GRC), norm-rejecting discrepancy (low ideal GRC and high real GRC), norm-favoring consistency (high ideal GRC and high real GRC), and norm-rejecting consistency (low ideal GRC and low real GRC). They found that the vast majority of participants (80%–90% depending on the scale) exhibited the pattern of norm-rejecting discrepancy strain, whereas only 5% to 17% exhibited the pattern of norm-favoring discrepancy strain. This conceptualization broadens the research perspective on gender role discrepancy strain because it had heretofore been conceptualized only as norm-favoring discrepancy. Because (as discussed subsequently) research indicates that, on average, men and women reject most of the traditional masculine norms, the concept of norm-rejecting discrepancy could be of significant value to gender researchers. It would also be of interest to determine whether norm-rejecting discrepancy results in strain.

Rummell and Levant (2014) conducted two studies with college men, assessing the relationship between masculine gender role discrepancy strain and self-esteem, each operationalizing discrepancy strain differently. The first study used standardized difference scores between two existing measures, the revised MRNI (to assess idealized gender role standards), and Conformity to Masculine Norms Inventory (to assess actual gender role behavior). For the total discrepancy strain score and the scores for two specific norms (Self-Reliance and Importance of Sex), the higher the norm-favoring discrepancy strain, the higher the self-esteem, contrary to hypotheses. The norm-rejecting discrepancy strain for one norm, Disdain for Sexual Minorities, also had a positive relationship with self-esteem. The second study implemented three recommendations made by Pleck (1995). Here, measures of the endorsement of and conformity to masculine norms, self-esteem, and salience for specific norms were developed, and salience was assessed as a moderator of the discrepancy strain–self-esteem relationship. The total discrepancy strain score reflected norm-rejecting discrepancy and was not significantly correlated with the total self-esteem score; further, salience did not emerge as a moderator of the relationship between discrepancy strain and self-esteem. Although these studies had significant limitations, they failed to find support for the hypothesized negative relationship between masculine gender role discrepancy strain and self-esteem.

Recently, Reidy, Berke, Gentile, and Zeichner (2015) developed the Masculine Gender Role Discrepancy Scale, for which they have found links between high discrepancy stress and risky sexual behaviors, the contraction of sexually transmitted diseases, the perpetration of psychological, physical and sexual violence toward female intimate partners, assault with a weapon, and assault causing injury. This is promising new development, and it would be easy to study the relationship between masculine gender role discrepancy stress and self-esteem.

*Masculine Gender Role Stress.* The masculine gender role stress (MGRS) approach is a more promising way to assess discrepancy strain. Stemming from the GRSP and the cognitive stress model (Eisler, 1995), it inquires to what degree participants would experience particular situations that are discrepant with traditional male role norms as stressful. In accord with the cognitive stress model (Lazarus & Folkman, 1984), vulnerability depends on the extent to which a situation (a) threatens an individual's idiosyncratic commitments or goals and (b) elicits coping mechanisms that the individual is unable to perform adequately. Thus, a situation could promote masculine gender role stress if the situation is in direct conflict with the masculine norms that person endorses. MGRS has been associated with the endorsement of traditional masculinity ideology, adverse health habits, anger, anxiety, and cardiovascular reactivity to situation stress among men (Eisler & Blalock, 1991; Eisler & Skidmore, 1987; Lash, Eisler, & Schulman, 1990; Lash, Gillespie, Eisler, & Southard, 1991; Thompson, 1991).

### Dysfunction Strain

Dysfunction strain results when one fulfills the requirements of the masculine norms because many of the characteristics traditionally viewed as desirable in men can have negative side effects on the men themselves and on others, including those close to them. Brooks and Silverstein (1995, p. 281) further developed this proposition of the GRSP by theorizing a catalogue of the behaviors that characterize the "dark side of masculinity," arising from the "normative socialization of men." These behaviors include "various forms of violence, sexual dysfunctions, socially irresponsible behaviors, and relationship inadequacies." There is substantial empirical support for this tenet of the GRSP, coming from three lines of investigation influenced by the GRSP: the endorsement of traditional masculinity ideology, conformity to masculine norms, and GRC.

*Traditional Masculinity Ideology.* The endorsement of traditional masculinity ideology has been found to be associated with a range of problematic individual and relational variables, including reluctance to discuss condom use with partners, fear of intimacy, lower relationship satisfaction, more negative beliefs about the father's role and lower paternal participation in child care, negative attitudes toward racial diversity and women's equality, attitudes conducive to sexual harassment, self-reports of sexual aggression, racial group marginalization, ethnocentrism, lower forgiveness of racial discrimination, alexithymia and related constructs, and negative attitudes toward help-seeking (Levant & Richmond, 2007; see also Levant & Richmond, 2016; O'Neil, 2012).

*Conformity to Masculine Norms.* The Conformity to Masculine Norms Inventory (Mahalik et al., 2003), which measures the extent to which men conform to traditional masculine norms, has been associated with unhealthy alcohol use, substance use, marijuana use, binge drinking, not seeking help with emotional difficulties, negative attitudes about help-seeking, health risks, few health promotion behaviors, not going to health care appointments, getting into physical fights, difficulty managing anger, taking risks, risky behavior with automobiles and sexual practices, sexism, internalized homophobia, masculine body ideal distress, poor sexual functioning, lower self-esteem, and psychological distress (O'Neil, 2012).

*Gender Role Conflict.* O'Neil (2008) indicated that GRC related to all three types of gender role strain but commented that "Pleck's dysfunction strain has the most theoretical relevance to GRC because this subtype implies negative outcomes from endorsing restrictive gender role norms" (p. 366). After an extensive review of the literature, O'Neil (2008), concluded that "GRC is significantly related to men's psychological and interpersonal problems" (p. 358). These psychological and interpersonal problems include low self-esteem, anxiety, depression, stress, shame, negative help-seeking attitudes, alexithymia, alcohol and substance use, hopelessness, psychological strain, traditional gender role attitudes, machismo, homonegativity, self-silencing, body image, family problems and stress, conduct problems, problems with anger, health risk-taking, suicide, physical health problems, drive for muscularity, interpersonal problems, shyness, racial bias, abusive attitudes and behaviors, hostile sexism, hostility toward women, attitudes toward sexual harassment, rape myth attitudes, dating violence, sexual aggression and coercion, men's entitlement, victim blaming, and violence (O'Neil, 2012).

### Trauma Strain

The concept of trauma strain was originally applied to certain groups of men whose experiences with gender role strain were thought to be particularly harsh: men of color (Watkins, Walker, & Griffith, 2010), professional athletes (Messner, 1992), veterans (Brooks, 1990), and survivors of child abuse (Lisak, 1995). It was also recognized that gay and bisexual men are normatively traumatized by gender role strain by virtue of growing up in a heterosexist society (Connell & Messerschmidt, 2005; Sánchez, Westerfeld, Liu, & Vilain, 2010). Beyond the recognition that certain classes of men may experience trauma strain, a perspective on the male role socialization process emerged in the 1990s (Levant & Pollack, 1995) that viewed socialization under traditional masculinity ideology as inherently traumatic. Levant (1992) specifically proposed that mild-to-moderate alexithymia may result from the normative emotion socialization of boys to conform to the norm of restrictive emotionality. This is the normative male alexithymia (NMA) hypothesis, to which we now turn.

*The NMA Hypothesis.* Literally, *alexithymia* means "without words for emotions." Sifneos (1967) originally used the term to describe the extreme difficulty patients with psychosomatic, posttraumatic stress, substance use, and chronic pain disorders had in identifying and describing their feelings. In addition, variability along a continuum of alexithymia symptoms has also been observed in nonclinical populations (Levant, 1992). Levant (1992) proposed the NMA hypothesis to account for a socialized pattern of restrictive emotionality that he observed in many men. Working with both research participants in the Boston University Fatherhood Project and clients in his clinical practice, Levant observed that only with great difficulty and practice could many of the men find the words to describe their emotional states. He theorized that those men had been discouraged as boys from expressing and talking about their emotions by parents, peers, teachers, or coaches, and some were punished for doing so. Hence, they did not develop a vocabulary for nor an awareness of many of their emotions.

In particular, these men showed the greatest deficits in identifying and expressing emotions that reflect a sense of vulnerability (e.g., sadness, fear) or that express attachment (e.g., fondness, caring). Although restricted emotionality may be adaptive in some ways, particularly in highly competitive or aggressive environments, Levant's clients often reported significant difficulties in their personal lives and presented with a variety of problems, including marital difficulties, estrangement from their children, substance abuse, domestic violence, and sexual addiction (Levant & Kopecky, 1995).

Levant's clinical observations are consistent with a central tenet of the GRSP that societal forces differentially shape men according to the degree to which they have been reared as boys to adhere to the norms of traditional masculinity, one of which is the restriction of emotional expression (Levant, 1996, 2011). Levant (1992, 1996, 1998) drew on the GRSP to theorize that mild-to-moderate forms of alexithymia would occur more frequently among men whose socialization as boys was informed to greater degrees by traditional masculinity ideology. Indeed, empirical research found a relationship between the endorsement of traditional masculinity ideology and alexithymia in men (Levant, Richmond, et al., 2003).

The view that socialization plays a role in the development of restricted emotionality confronts the conventional view in our society that boys and men are essentially hard-wired to be less emotional and more logical than are girls and women. This more conventional view derives from presumed biologically based gender differences in the experience and expression of emotion (for a review, see Wester, Vogel, Pressly, & Heesacker, 2002). Levant's (1998) review of relevant developmental psychology research literature on the emotion socialization of boys concluded that the conventional perspective that men are, by nature, less emotional was not supported by the existing evidence. Indeed, evidence suggests that boys start life with greater emotional reactivity and expressiveness than girls and maintain this advantage until 1 year of age (Levant, 1998). However, they become less verbally expressive than girls at about age 2 years and less facially expressive by 6 years. This crossover in emotional expressivity suggests that socialization shapes emotional behavior by gender and may account for gender differences in emotional awareness and expressivity (Levant, 1998).

To assess the extent of gender differences in alexithymia, Levant et al. (2006) reviewed 45 published studies that examined such gender differences.

Although few of the 12 studies using clinical samples found gender differences, of the 32 studies using nonclinical samples, 17 found males more alexithymic than females, one found females more alexithymic than males, and 14 found no differences between males and females. The alexithymia literature was next meta-analyzed to determine whether there was empirical support for gender differences (Levant, Hall, Williams, & Hasan, 2009). An effect size estimate based on 41 existing samples found consistent, although expectedly small, differences in mean alexithymia between women and men (Hedges's $d = .22$). Men exhibited higher levels of alexithymia.

This line of investigation has led to the development of clinical assessment and intervention tools. Levant et al. (2006) developed the Normative Male Alexithymia Scale. Results of analyses of gender differences, relations with other instruments, and its incremental validity in predicting the endorsement of traditional masculinity ideology, provided evidence supporting the validity of the scale. Levant (1998, 2006) developed a psychoeducational program for treating NMA, which was recently manualized as Alexithymia Reduction Treatment (ART) and assessed in a pilot study (Levant, Halter, Hayden, & Williams, 2009).

## SOCIAL CONTEXTS OF MASCULINE GENDER ROLE STRAIN

The socialization of emotion and the ensuing gender role strains are context dependent. In addition, the social contexts where men live, work, and play often have different, and sometimes opposing, gender role expectations. For example, men may be expected to be aggressive at work but find that displaying this trait at home results in more familial conflict. Failing to meet gender role expectations in some contexts may also produce deeper threats to what Hammond, Fleming, and Villa-Torres (2016) called the "masculine social self" than others. Building largely on social self-preservation theory (Dickerson, Gruenewald, & Kemeny, 2004), Hammond and colleagues speculated that GRCs emerge most in contexts that threaten the masculine social self. According to Dickerson et al. (2004), threats to the social self occur most often in contexts that (a) require a public display of idealized values, traits, and abilities (*performance contexts*); (b) are characterized by the high possibility of social group rejection (*rejection-laden contexts*); and (c) make those unworthy or undesirable aspects of individual identity more salient (*stigmatizing contexts*). Specifying the gender role performance contexts (e.g., workplace, school, family, health care) that elicit the most significant threats to the masculine social self is a critical area warranting research expansion.

Hammond and colleagues (2016) speculated that threatening contexts elicit maladaptive psychological and behavioral responses that place certain men (specifically African American men) at greater risk for health problems. They posit shame-producing situations in those contexts as the primary catalysts for African American men's emotion restriction and negative behavioral responses. Although the authors theorize specifically about African American men, their work suggests the need to understand whether situational demands in threatening contexts potentiate different types of gender role strain (e.g., discrepancy, dysfunction, trauma) among other groups of men. This understanding is critical to advancing efforts to reduce health disparities among more marginalized men, who are more likely to be embedded in rejection-laden and stigmatizing contexts.

## Life-Course Developmental Differences in Gender Role Strain

In addition to the contexts in which gender role strain manifests, men's stage of life-course development also matters. Gender role strains are not static. Men confront different situational demands and threats to masculinity as they make role transitions. Biobehavioral and emotion regulation processes that can lead to gender role strain are also life-course variant. Sensitive life stages are rife with opportunities to experience gender role strain and conflict. For example, during the transition to adulthood, when identity is most in flux and risk-taking is heightened, men may be particularly vulnerable to discrepancy and dysfunction strain. Such strains may be exacerbated as men take on familial roles (e.g., as husbands or fathers). In later life, gender role strain stemming from declines in physical functioning may be especially pronounced. Emotion regulation and biobehavioral development also vary over men's life-course and shape how they respond to gender role strain. The influence of normative life-course development on gender role strain has been acknowledged by other masculinity scholars (Thompson & Bennett, 2015). These authors urge researchers to focus specifically on creating measures to assess men's internalization and endorsement of masculinity ideologies as they grapple with work and family-based roles.

Empirical investigations about life-course variations in socially constructed meanings of masculinity and gender role strain are somewhat scarce. However, there are some studies investigating life-course changes in masculinity using measures assessing trait or personality-based gender role orientations (Barrett & White, 2002; Caspi & Roberts, 1990, 2001; Feldman, Biringen, & Nash, 1981; Helson & Wink, 1992; Sinnott & Shifren, 2001). For example, Helson and Wink's (1992) longitudinal work detected increases in "masculine" personality characteristics (e.g., decisiveness) among women between the ages of 43 and 52. Similarly, in a longitudinal investigation among adolescents and young adults, Barrett and colleagues observed the steepest increase in masculine gender role orientation among 12- to 15-year-olds (Barrett & White,

2002). Rounding out the quantitative evidence-base are qualitative studies investigating masculine gender role meaning at pivotal life-course transitions (Ribeiro, Paúl, & Nogueira, 2007; Tannenbaum & Frank, 2011). Tannenbaum and Frank's (2011) qualitative work among late life men (those aged 55–97) suggests that men might develop less rigid masculine gender roles as they age. Moreover, researchers find that older male caregivers address potential strains and conflicts by renegotiating more dominant or hegemonic gender role proscriptions (Ribeiro et al., 2007). Other studies detect shifts in masculinity that occur in tandem with men's shifts in social roles (e.g., as fathers; Brannen & Nilsen, 2006; Roy, 2006, 2008). Taken together, extant evidence suggests that the manifestation of gender role strains are dependent on men's reflexivity as they move across the life course.

### Intersectionality and Gender Role Strain (What Race/Ethnicity, Class, and Sexual Orientation Might Add to Men's Experience With Gender Role Strain)

As already noted, the GRSP is rooted in social constructionism. Rather than privileging a particular type of masculinity, the GRSP posits the idea of multiple masculinities. A critical examination of the ways in which masculinity operates differently in the lives of individual men is an important next step (Bowleg, 2013; Coston & Kimmel, 2012; Veenstra, 2013) and would be considerably strengthened by integrating the theory of intersectionality (Crenshaw, 1991). Although the theory of intersectionality is rooted in the experiences of women of color (Collins, 2002; Crenshaw, 1991), several theoretical parallels would be useful to the study of men and masculinity. For example, an intersectional approach might highlight the ways in which individual men, particularly men of color, will construct distinctive masculinities because of their relationship to more than one social group (Richmond, Levant, & Ladhani, 2012; Rogers, Sperry, & Levant, 2015). The positions men occupy within other power structures can exacerbate or mitigate gender role strain. The gender structure is largely hierarchical but intersects with other axes of social stratification (race, socioeconomic status, ability status, and sexual orientation). Intersectionality theory is a useful framework to discuss how the inequitable distribution of male privilege and power affects how relatively subordinated men experience gender role strain.

Gender role strain may be especially felt by poor and minority men whose access to the male opportunity structure is disproportionately blocked (Courtenay, 2000; Williams, 2008). These more socially vulnerable groups of men may experience more pronounced discrepancy strain because they lack sufficient power and freedom to actualize idealized manhood (Muñoz Boudet,

Petesch, Turk, & Thumala, 2012). Poor and minority men are at increased risk for exposure to race and other identity-based microaggressions that work in tandem with traditional masculinity ideology to increase health risks. For example, Hammond (2012) found increased depressive symptomatology among African American men exposed to more frequent everyday racism when they endorsed norms encouraging emotion restriction.

Using an intersectional approach, Levant and Wong (2013) examined the role of race and gender as moderators of the relationship between the endorsement of traditional masculinity ideology and alexithymia. The moderating effect of race on the relationship between endorsement of traditional masculinity ideology and alexithymia was strongly affected by gender: In contrast to the findings of Hammond (2012), this study found that the endorsement of traditional masculinity ideology was more strongly related to alexithymia for White men than for racial minority men. On the other hand, the endorsement of traditional masculinity ideology was more strongly related to alexithymia for racial minority women than for White women.

Levant, Wong, Karakis, and Welsh (2015) found that emotional control mediated the relationship between restrictive emotionality and alexithymia. Additionally, race moderated the relationship between restrictive emotionality and alexithymia. That relationship was stronger for Latino American men versus men from other racial groups, but weaker for Asian American men versus men from other racial groups. Finally, the restrictive emotionality by race (Latinos vs. others) moderation effect on alexithymia was mediated through its association with emotional control, providing support for a mediated moderation effect. This suggests the utility of investigating hypothesized mediation and moderation of established relationships between variables as a means for furthering knowledge of cultural variations and social identity differences in the endorsement of traditional masculinity ideology and its consequences.

Taken together, research in this vein reminds us that we must above all be mindful of the ways in which variations (previously thought to be deviations) from traditional masculinity were once considered to reflect an individual's deficiencies. As a result of a growing body of evidence, we have a much more complex understanding of how men occupying different social positions, racial/ethnic groups, and sexual orientation statuses differentially define masculinity meaning (Casas, Wagenheim, Banchero, & Mendoza-Romero, 1994; Hammond & Mattis, 2005; Kimmel, 2004; Lang, 1998; Shek, 2007; Whitehead, Peterson, & Kaljee, 1994). Thus, any future gender role strain research must explicitly connect how context, including historical and structural inequalities, informs the construction, embodiment, and enactment of masculinity.

## ASSESSMENT OF THE GRSP

The literature on the psychology of men and masculinities influenced by the GRSP is now quite substantial, having developed over the 35 years since Pleck (1981) and has advanced our psychological understanding of men and masculinities. When considered broadly, to include research programs that have been influenced by the GRSP, such as GRC, masculine gender role stress, reference group identity, and conformity to masculine norms, it is the dominant research paradigm in the psychology of men and masculinities in the United States. As Wong et al. (2010) concluded in their content analysis of articles in the journal *Psychology of Men and Masculinity* (PMM), "most PMM articles were based on theories associated with the gender role strain paradigm" (p. 176). Specifically, research has strongly supported a central tenet of the GRSP: that the individual's endorsement of masculinity ideologies varies according to the cultural context and social location of the individual. In addition, there is strong empirical support for the dysfunction and trauma strain hypotheses, but the discrepancy strain hypothesis has received mixed support. However, the recent work by Reidy et al. (2015) using the Masculine Gender Role Discrepancy Scale shows great promise.

The field has thus accomplished quite a bit, but there is definitely room for improvement. Several critiques of this literature have emerged. First, there are critiques regarding measurement and sampling (Whorley & Addis, 2006). By and large, this domain of research has relied on self-report measures administered largely to White and heterosexual college students, in correlational studies, although studies using qualitative methods, more diverse samples, and more sophisticated designs and analyses have recently begun to appear. These latter developments should be encouraged.

There are also several substantive critiques. The first concerns the use of the term *traditional masculinity ideology* (Pleck, 1995) to refer to the dominant masculinity ideology in the United States. Because masculinity ideology varies by culture, there are many traditions that need to be accounted for. Hence, it would be more accurate to refer to this construct as *traditional White Western heterosexual masculinity ideology* to denote its association with the predominantly White Western heterosexual world.

Another critique, one that has been raised on the Society for the Psychological Study of Men and Masculinity's electronic mailing list (spsmm@lists.apa.org), concerns findings that on the average, men do not endorse most of the traditional norms, raising the question of their relevance. Studies reported over the 16-year period from 1997 to 2013 on the MRNI, MRNI—Revised, and MRNI—Short Form indicate that men (primarily White heterosexual

U.S. college students, as is typical of most studies of this kind[2]) "rejected" most of the norms, either four of seven or three of five norms, depending on the study. Norm rejection was defined as mean scores of less than 4 on a 7-point Likert scale, in which higher scores indicate greater endorsement (Levant, Cuthbert, et al., 2003; Levant et al., 2013; Levant & Majors, 1997; Levant, Rankin, Williams, Hasan, & Smalley, 2010). Furthermore, recall that Liu et al. (2005) found that 80% to 90% of participants exhibited the pattern of norm-rejecting discrepancy strain. Thus, it does not appear that most men endorse most of the traditional norms. Does this mean that the traditional norms are unimportant? We do not think so. First, these results are mean scores, and these data tend to be mildly nonnormally distributed (e.g., Levant et al., 2013, reported values of skew ranging from –.77 to 1.27). Hence, a substantial portion of men endorse traditional norms, and some do so strongly. But what about the majority of men who do not endorse these norms? Do they have another set of norms, a nontraditional set based on gender equality? A recent study suggests that they do not. Calton, Heesacker, and Perrin (2014) randomly assigned men and women college students to describe a time in which they had behaved either traditionally or progressively (i.e., flexible and egalitarian). Whereas more than 80% of men and women in the traditional condition and women in the progressive condition provided appropriate examples, only 17% of the men in the progressive condition did so. We think this opens up opportunities for scholars and practitioners in the psychology of men and masculinities to help young men develop progressive masculinities. Such interventions are more likely to be social marketing rather than therapy, such as the Mary Kay Foundation campaign against domestic violence, which attempts to reframe the gender policing exhortation "man up" (Zolla, 2015). Psychoeducational programs like the Gender Role Journey (O'Neil, 1996) may also be applicable.

Finally, an important critique concerns the way that constructs derived from the GRSP (including the central GRSP construct, masculinity ideologies, the closely related constructs of conformity to masculine norms, GRC and stress, male reference group identity dependence, among others) tend to be operationalized as self-report Likert-scaled instruments, which according to Addis, Mansfield, and Syzdek (2010) result in "individual difference" variables that function like "stable traits" (p. 80). If that were so, that would risk perpetuating the essentializing of gender, for as Bohan (1997) noted, "Essentialist views construe gender as resident within the individual, a quality or trait describing one's personality, cognitive processes . . . etc." (p. 32).

---

[2]One of the studies had a Black sample (Levant & Majors, 1997), and another had a Russian sample (Levant, Cuthbert, et al., 2003), but for the sake of consistency, we report only the data for White U.S. men.

Although the Addis et al. (2010) critique focused on the way that constructs derived from the GRSP tend to be operationalized, several papers beginning in the late 1980s have mislabeled the GRSP as a whole as non-social constructionist or even as essentialist. Kimmel (1987, p. 12) grouped the GRSP and GRIP together (failing to appreciate their fundamental differences as discussed earlier) as the "sex role model," which he contrasted with social constructionism. Pleck (1995) rebutted his position, highlighting work from his 1981 volume and asserting that "the gender role strain model for masculinity was, in the broad sense, a social constructionist perspective that simply predated the term" (p. 22). More recently, Wester and Vogel (2012) grouped the GRSP and related theories together as an "essentialist approach" because they took "the position that characteristics of a group are representative of global traits characteristic of hegemonic masculinity" (p. 377). Mahalik's (2014) rebuttal to a similar critique of GRSP research (Wetherell & Edley, 2014) applies equally well to Wester and Vogel (2012): "This is an important critique of quantitative research examining masculinity, although I do not see it as a critique of the gender role strain paradigm" (p. 365). The GRSP was originally based on social learning theory, which stressed the "contingent and contextual nature of gendered social learning" (Addis et al., 2010, pp. 77–78), thus positing some fluidity in masculinities constructs. Hence, the problem lies in the way that masculinities constructs are operationalized rather than in the GRSP itself. Our responses to this critique thus focus on the way that these masculinities constructs are operationalized. Although this critique applies to many of the masculinities constructs used in research, for the sake of simplicity, we focus here on only one of these constructs: masculinity ideologies. We have several points to make.

First, we acknowledge that measures of masculinity ideologies are to some extent stable, as reflected in the test–retest reliabilities, even if the construct is considered to be to some degree fluid. However, to describe them as "traits" is problematic because the word *traits* is strongly associated with personality traits. Because personality traits have a biological basis, this would take us back to the GRIP that Pleck (1981, 1995) so devastatingly critiqued. We do recognize that the word *traits* encompasses more than "personality traits" (e.g., life satisfaction, academic self-efficacy, and self-esteem are all traits). But given the baggage associated with the word in the field of the psychology of men and masculinities, we prefer the less loaded word *attributes*. Using this word, masculinity ideologies are best regarded as the attribute known as beliefs.

Further, the stability of endorsements of masculinity ideologies does not necessarily mean that they reside only within the individual. Although individuals may hold beliefs about masculine norms, it is also arguable that at least some of the stability seen in the test–retest reliabilities of the measures comes from the patriarchal culture that reproduces and maintains traditional gender ideologies. That being the case, we must (reluctantly and with some trepidation) argue for the qualification of Bohan's (1997) statement that social constructionism views "gender as not a trait of individuals at all, but simply a construct that identifies particular transactions that are understood to be appropriate to one sex" (p. 33). We would first make the distinction between gender and gender ideologies (or in this case, masculinity ideologies) and then note that the latter is in part a set of beliefs. Specifying masculinity ideologies as beliefs is necessary to account for that part of the person that enters into "particular transactions" with the environment. That is, people have views (i.e., beliefs) about the expectations (i.e., norms) for masculine behavior in specific transactions.

Likewise, as Fuss (1989) argued, it is a mistake to frame essentialism and constructionism as a binarism—an either–or proposition—because essentialistic elements are always embedded in constructionist arguments. Or in her words (italics added): "My position here is that the possibility of . . . constructionism can only be built on the foundations of a *hidden essentialism*" (Fuss, 1989, pp. 12–13). For example, when we inquire about "masculinities," the act of naming the object of inquiry "masculinities" presumes its ontological reality, and thus its existence. And if it exists, it has an essence. If we as a field were to agree that a quantitative social constructionist perspective on gender must completely eschew the notion that masculinity ideologies could in any way be beliefs, then we would devolve to something akin to the stimulus–response psychology of the early behaviorists (Skinner, 1953), who regarded the mind as "in the black box," before the cognitive revolution in psychology transformed social learning theory (Bandura, 1977) into social cognitive theory (Bandura, 2001).

Second, we noted earlier that we qualified Bohan (1997) "reluctantly and with some trepidation." There are two reasons for that. First, as psychologists, we are neither equipped nor inclined to enter into the philosophical debate on "essence" that goes back to Aristotle. However, as social justice–oriented psychologists, we are mindful that much of the tension about essentialism–social constructionism is connected to the historical legacy of psychologists (and other scientists) using essentialist ideas to justify oppressing and exploiting women (and other marginalized groups). It is possible that essentialism may not be oppressive if used in socially progressive ways. What those ways are is an important contemporary discussion that is just beginning. For example, Fine (2010) wrote about the *strategic essentialism* of the gay, lesbian, bisexual, and transgender movement, which has made great gains by defining sexual orientation and gender identity as inborn.

Third, although masculinity ideologies are probably to some degree dynamic and influenced by context, the patriarchal social order is nonetheless omnipresent and exerts continuous influence on individuals. The extent to which any boy (e.g., Way et al., 2014) or man is able to resist this pressure and ignore traditional masculine norms may be dependent on intersecting social identity variables because power is not solely determined by gender but is also influenced by these other variables, such as race, class, sexual orientation, gender identity, ability status, and age (Connell & Messerschmidt, 2005). The effects of these intersecting social identity variables on the relationships between masculinity ideologies and outcome variables (e.g., health behavior, help-seeking intentions) can be investigated using conditional process modeling, a set of new analytic techniques that encompass moderated mediation and mediated moderation, the goal of which "is to describe the conditional nature of the mechanism or mechanisms by which a variable transmits its effect on another and testing hypotheses about such contingent effects" (Hayes, 2013, p. 10).

Fourth, the masculinity constructs under discussion can be operationalized differently to assess the contingent and contextual nature of gendered social learning, thus enabling the assessment of their fluidity in response to context. Mahalik (2014) noted that fluidity in response to situational variables could be assessed by simply changing the directions for completing the scale, that is, by referencing specific situations. For example, Steinfeldt, Wong, Hagan, Hoag, and Steinfeldt (2011) addressed the contextual nature of masculinities by taking a domain-specific approach to conceptualizing GRC. They randomly assigned football players to two conditions; participants in both conditions completed the Gender Role Conflict Scale but with different instructions. In one condition, participants were told to focus on their life within the football environment, while those in the other condition were told to focus on their life outside of football. Further, Addis et al. (2010) provided examples of experimental research programs using semantic priming or manipulation of stereotype threat and longitudinal studies using diaries that operationalize masculinities constructs in ways that retain the contingent and contextual nature of gendered social learning. In addition, Wong et al. (2011) developed the subjective masculinity model that assesses men's subjective experience of what it means to be a man. Finally, Vandello and Bosson (2013) provided a review of their experimental social psychological research program on "precarious manhood," which also retains the contingent and contextual nature of gendered social learning. This research program demonstrates that the salience and influence of traditional masculinity ideology fluctuates across context (e.g., when a man's sense of meeting traditional masculine expectations is threatened, these expectations become more salient and influential).

Fifth, there is no robust alternative quantitative measurement approach to the GRSP masculinities constructs. Although there has been a recent call for a social constructionist measurement approach based on the assessment of group-level endorsement of dominant gender representations (the "gender [re] presentation" approach; Luyt, 2013), this approach has not yet developed usable scales and shares two thirds of its measurement assumptions with the GRSP.

Sixth, we note that Thompson and Bennett (2015; see also Chapter 2, this volume) distinguished between the culturally based and individually based parts of masculinity ideologies, referring to the former as masculinity ideologies and the latter as masculinity beliefs. Although we appreciate the authors' making room for viewing masculinity ideologies as in part beliefs, we are not sure that such a change in nomenclature is necessary. Pleck (1995) defined the individually based parts as the "individual's endorsement and internalization of cultural belief systems about masculinity" (p. 19). Would it not be sufficient to refer to the cultural part as "masculinity ideologies" and the individual part as "the individual's endorsement of masculinity ideologies"?

Finally, gender can be conceptualized from many perspectives, and it is our aim to promote a big-tent, both–and approach to investigating masculinities. Operationalizing masculinity ideologies as beliefs, as we do in quantitative GRSP research, has some advantages due to the methodological strengths of Likert-scale measures, and this approach can be improved to reflect their contingent and contextual nature, as we discussed earlier in the chapter. However, we acknowledge that this approach may not do full justice to their complexities of masculinities. Thus, we also support methods focused on moment-by-moment performance of gender that are not based on logical positivism, such as critical men's studies (Chapter 4, this volume), discursive psychology (Wetherell & Edley, 2014), grounded theory (Silverstein, Auerbach, & Levant, 2006), and phenomenological approaches.

## FUTURE DIRECTIONS

Recent reviews of the literature have highlighted the need to investigate healthy and egalitarian ways to be a man, to go beyond the study of the simple relationships between independent and dependent variables by including investigation of mediators and moderators (including contingent and contextual factors) of those relationships, to break our overreliance on college student samples and collect more diverse and representative samples, and to do experimental, longitudinal, and qualitative research (O'Neil, 2008, 2012; Smiler, 2004; Whorley & Addis 2006). We agree with all of those recommendations and offer as an illustration a recent example of the use of an experimental design. Wong et al. (2015) tested the effects of activating men's subjective masculinity experiences on state self-esteem by randomly assigning 183 men into either a masculinity priming condition or a control priming condition. Men who received masculinity priming completed the sentence "As a man . . ." 10 times, whereas control subjects completed the sentence "I am . . ." 10 times. Consistent with the social identity paradigm, participants who received masculinity priming reported higher state self-esteem than those in the control priming condition. A moderation effect showed that masculinity priming exerted the strongest effect on self-esteem among men with relatively negative self-perceptions. In addition, given the more explicit foundation of the GRSP in social psychology (Levant, 2011), greater use could be made of social cognitive and social influence theories, the constructs of gender roles and social norms, and the associated research methods and programs. Further, psychologists could incorporate into their research designs insights from the abundant literature on men and masculinity from other disciplines, such as sociology, history, anthropology, archaeology, primatology, and biology. For example, Vandello and Bosson's (2013) research program on "precarious manhood" was inspired by Gilmore's (1990) anthropological treatise on cultural concepts of masculinity, and Connell and Messerschmidt's (2005) sociological construct of hegemonic masculinity has been influential in the psychology of men and masculinities.

## REFERENCES

Addis, M. E., Mansfield, A. K., & Syzdek, M. R. (2010). Is masculinity a problem? Framing the effects of gendered social learning in men. *Psychology of Men & Masculinity, 11*, 77–90. http://dx.doi.org/10.1037/a0018602

Bandura, A. (1977). *Social learning theory*. Englewood Cliffs, NJ: Prentice Hall.

Bandura, A. (2001). Social cognitive theory: An agentic perspective. *Annual Review of Psychology, 52*, 1–26. http://dx.doi.org/10.1146/annurev.psych.52.1.1

Barrett, A. E., & White, H. R. (2002). Trajectories of gender role orientations in adolescence and early adulthood: A prospective study of the mental health effects of masculinity and femininity. *Journal of Health and Social Behavior, 43*, 451–468. http://dx.doi.org/10.2307/3090237

Bohan, J. S. (1997). Regarding gender: essentialism, constructionism, and feminist psychology. In M. M. Gergen & S. N. Davis (Eds.), *Toward a new psychology of gender* (pp. 31–47). New York, NY: Routledge.

Bowleg, L. (2013). "Once you've blended the cake, you can't take the parts back to the main ingredients": Black gay and bisexual men's descriptions and experiences of intersectionality. *Sex Roles, 68*, 754–767. http://dx.doi.org/10.1007/s11199-012-0152-4

Brannen, J., & Nilsen, A. (2006). From fatherhood to fathering: Transmission and change among British fathers in four-generation families. *Sociology, 40*, 335–352. http://dx.doi.org/10.1177/0038038506062036

Brooks, G. R. (1990). Post-Vietnam gender role strain: A needed concept? *Professional Psychology: Research and Practice, 21*, 18–25. http://dx.doi.org/10.1037/0735-7028.21.1.18

Brooks, G. R., & Silverstein, L. S. (1995). Understanding the dark side of masculinity: An interactive systems model. In R. F. Levant & W. S. Pollack (Eds.), *A new psychology of men* (pp. 280–333). New York, NY: Basic Books.

Butler, J. (1990). *Gender trouble.* New York, NY: Routledge.

Calton, J. M., Heesacker, M., & Perrin, P. B. (2014). The elusiveness of progressive masculinity: Gender differences in conceptualizations of nontraditional gender roles. *Journal of Gender and Power, 2*, 37–58.

Casas, J. M., Wagenheim, B. R., Banchero, R., & Mendoza-Romero, J. (1994). Hispanic masculinity: Myth or psychological schema meriting clinical consideration. *Hispanic Journal of Behavioral Sciences, 16*, 315–331. http://dx.doi.org/10.1177/07399863940163009

Caspi, A., & Roberts, B. W. (1990). Personality continuity and change across the life course. In L. A. Pervin (Ed.), *Handbook of personality: Theory and research* (pp. 300–326). New York, NY: Guilford Press.

Caspi, A., & Roberts, B. W. (2001). Personality development across the life course: The argument for change and continuity. *Psychological Inquiry, 12*, 49–66. http://dx.doi.org/10.1207/S15327965PLI1202_01

Cochran, S. V. (2010). Emergence and development of the psychology of men and masculinity. In J. C. Chrisler & D. R. McCreary (Eds.), *Handbook of gender research in psychology: Vol. 1. Gender research in general and experimental psychology* (pp. 43–58). http://dx.doi.org/10.1007/978-1-4419-1465-1_3

Collins, P. H. (2002). *Black feminist thought: Knowledge, consciousness, and the politics of empowerment.* New York, NY: Routledge.

Connell, R. W., & Messerschmidt, J. W. (2005). Hegemonic masculinity: Rethinking the concept. *Gender & Society, 19*, 829–859. http://dx.doi.org/10.1177/0891243205278639

Coston, B. M., & Kimmel, M. (2012). Seeing privilege where it isn't: Marginalized masculinities and the intersectionality of privilege. *Journal of Social Issues, 68*, 97–111. http://dx.doi.org/10.1111/j.1540-4560.2011.01738.x

Courtenay, W. H. (2000). Endangering health: A social constructionist examination of men's health beliefs and behaviors. *Psychology of Men & Masculinity, 1*, 4–15. http://dx.doi.org/10.1037/1524-9220.1.1.4

Crenshaw, K. (1991). Mapping the margins: Intersectionality, identity politics, and violence against women of color. *Stanford Law Review, 43*, 1241–1299. http://dx.doi.org/10.2307/1229039

David, D., & Brannon, R. (Eds.). (1976). *The forty-nine percent majority: The male sex role.* Reading, MA: Addison-Wesley.

Deaux, K. (1984). From individual differences to social categories: Analysis of a decade's research on gender. *American Psychologist, 39*, 105–116. http://dx.doi.org/10.1037/0003-066X.39.2.105

Deutsch, C. J., & Gilbert, L. A. (1976). Sex role stereotypes: Effect on perceptions of self and others and on personal adjustment. *Journal of Counseling Psychology, 23*, 373–379. http://dx.doi.org/10.1037/0022-0167.23.4.373

Dickerson, S. S., Gruenewald, T. L., & Kemeny, M. E. (2004). When the social self is threatened: Shame, physiology, and health. *Journal of Personality, 72*, 1191–1216. http://dx.doi.org/10.1111/j.1467-6494.2004.00295.x

Eisler, R. M. (1995). The relationship between masculine gender role stress and men's health risk: The validation of a construct. In R. F. Levant & W. S. Pollack (Eds.), *A new psychology of men* (pp. 207–225). New York, NY: Basic Books.

Eisler, R. M., & Blalock, J. A. (1991). Masculine gender role stress: Implications for the assessment of men. *Clinical Psychology Review, 11*, 45–60. http://dx.doi.org/10.1016/0272-7358(91)90137-J

Eisler, R. M., & Skidmore, J. R. (1987). Masculine gender role stress: Scale development and component factors in the appraisal of stressful situations. *Behavior Modification, 11*, 123–136.

Fausto-Sterling, A. (2000). *Sexing the body*. New York, NY: Basic Books.

Feldman, S. S., Biringen, Z. C., & Nash, S. C. (1981). Fluctuations of sex-related self-attributions as a function of stage of family life cycle. *Developmental Psychology, 17*, 24–35. http://dx.doi.org/10.1037/0012-1649.17.1.24

Fine, C. (2010). *Delusions of gender: How our minds, society, and neurosexism create difference*. New York, NY: Norton.

Fuss, D. (1989). *Essentially speaking: Feminism, nature and difference*. London, England: Routledge.

Gergen, K. J. (1985). The social constructionist movement in modern psychology. *American Psychologist, 40*, 266–275. http://dx.doi.org/10.1037/0003-066X.40.3.266

Gilmore, D. D. (1990). *Manhood in the making*. New Haven, CT: Yale University Press.

Hammond, W. P. (2012). Taking it like a man: Masculine role norms as moderators of the racial discrimination–depressive symptoms association among African American men. *American Journal of Public Health, 102*(Suppl. 2), S232–S241. http://dx.doi.org/10.2105/AJPH.2011.300485

Hammond, W. P., Fleming, P. F., & Villa-Torres, L. (2016). Everyday racism as a threat to the masculine social self: Framing investigations of African American male health disparities. In Y. J. Wong & S. R. Wester (Eds.), *APA handbook of men and masculinities* (pp. 259–283). http://dx.doi.org/10.1037/14594-012

Hammond, W. P., & Mattis, J. S. (2005). Being a man about it: Manhood meaning among African American men. *Psychology of Men & Masculinity, 6*, 114–126. http://dx.doi.org/10.1037/1524-9220.6.2.114

Hayes, A. F. (2013). *Introduction to mediation, moderation, and conditional process analysis: A regression-based approach*. New York, NY: Guilford Press.

Helson, R., & Wink, P. (1992). Personality change in women from the early 40s to the early 50s. *Psychology and Aging, 7*, 46–55. http://dx.doi.org/10.1037/0882-7974.7.1.46

Kimmel, M. S. (1987). Rethinking "masculinity": New directions in research. In M. S. Kimmel (Ed.), *Changing men: New directions in research on men and masculinity* (pp. 9–24). Newbury Park, CA: Sage.

Kimmel, M. S. (2004). Masculinity as homophobia: Fear, shame, and silence in the construction of gender identity. In P. S. Rothenberg (Ed.), *Race, class, and gender in the United States: An integrated study* (pp. 81–93). New York, NY: Worth.

Lang, S. (1998). *Men as women, women as men: Changing gender in Native American cultures*. Austin: University of Texas Press.

Lash, S. J., Eisler, R. M., & Schulman, R. S. (1990). Cardiovascular reactivity to stress in men. Effects of masculine gender role stress appraisal and masculine performance challenge. *Behavior Modification, 14*, 3–20. http://dx.doi.org/10.1177/01454455900141001

Lash, S. J., Gillespie, B. L., Eisler, R. M., & Southard, D. R. (1991). Sex differences in cardiovascular reactivity: Effects of the gender relevance of the stressor. *Health Psychology, 10*, 392–398. http://dx.doi.org/10.1037/0278-6133.10.6.392

Lazarus, R. S., & Folkman, S. (1984). *Stress, appraisal, and coping*. New York, NY: Springer.

Levant, R. F. (1992). Toward the reconstruction of masculinity. *Journal of Family Psychology, 5*, 379–402. http://dx.doi.org/10.1037/0893-3200.5.3-4.379

Levant, R. F. (1996). The new psychology of men. *Professional Psychology: Research and Practice, 27*, 259–265. http://dx.doi.org/10.1037/0735-7028.27.3.259

Levant, R. F. (1998). Desperately seeking language: understanding, assessing, and treating normative male alexithymia. In W. S. Pollack & R. F. Levant (Eds.), *New psychotherapy for men* (pp. 35–56). New York, NY: Wiley.

Levant, R. F. (2006). *Effective psychotherapy with men* [DVD and viewer's guide]. San Francisco, CA: Psychotherapy.net.

Levant, R. F. (2011). Research in the psychology of men and masculinity using the gender role strain paradigm as a framework. *American Psychologist, 66*, 765–776. http://dx.doi.org/10.1037/a0025034

Levant, R. F. (2015). The road goes ever on: An editorial. *Psychology of Men and Masculinity, 16*, 349–354.

Levant, R. F., Cuthbert, A. C., Richmond, K., Sellers, A., Matveev, A., Matina, O., & Soklovsky, M. (2003). Masculinity ideology among Russian and U.S. young men and women and its relationship to unhealthy lifestyle habits among young Russian men. *Psychology of Men & Masculinity, 4*, 26–36.

Levant, R. F., Good, G. E., Cook, S., O'Neil, J., Smalley, K. B., Owen, K. A., & Richmond, K. (2006). Validation of the Normative Male Alexithymia Scale: Measurement of a gender-linked syndrome. *Psychology of Men & Masculinity, 7*, 212–224. http://dx.doi.org/10.1037/1524-9220.7.4.212

Levant, R. F., Hall, R. J., & Rankin, T. J. (2013). Male Role Norms Inventory—Short Form (MRNI–SF): Development, confirmatory factor analytic investigation of structure, and measurement invariance across gender. *Journal of Counseling Psychology, 60*, 228–238. http://dx.doi.org/10.1037/a0031545

Levant, R. F., Hall, R. J., Williams, C., & Hasan, N. T. (2009). Gender differences in alexithymia: A meta-analysis. *Psychology of Men & Masculinity, 10,* 190–203. http://dx.doi.org/10.1037/a0015652

Levant, R. F., Halter, M. J., Hayden, E., & Williams, C. (2009). The efficacy of alexithymia reduction treatment: A pilot study. *The Journal of Men's Studies, 17,* 75–84. http://dx.doi.org/10.3149/jms.1701.75

Levant, R. F., & Kopecky, G. (1995). *Masculinity, reconstructed.* New York, NY: Dutton.

Levant, R. F., & Majors, R. (1997). An investigation into variations in the construction of the male gender role among young African-American and European-American women and men. *Journal of Gender, Culture, and Health, 2,* 33–43.

Levant, R. F., & Pollack, W. S. (Eds.). (1995). *A new psychology of men.* New York, NY: Basic Books.

Levant, R. F., Rankin, T. J., Williams, C., Hasan, N. T., & Smalley, K. B. (2010). Evaluation of the factor structure and construct validity of the Male Role Norms Inventory—Revised (MRNI–R). *Psychology of Men & Masculinity, 11,* 25–37. http://dx.doi.org/10.1037/a0017637

Levant, R. F., & Richmond, K. (2007). A review of research on masculinity ideologies using the Male Role Norms Inventory. *The Journal of Men's Studies, 15,* 130–146. http://dx.doi.org/10.3149/jms.1502.130

Levant, R. F., & Richmond, K. (2016). The gender role strain paradigm and masculinity ideologies. In Y. J. Wong & S. R. Wester (Eds.), *APA handbook of men and masculinities* (pp. 23–49). http://dx.doi.org/10.1037/14594-002

Levant, R. F., Richmond, K., Majors, R. G., Inclan, J. E., Rossello, J. M., Heesacker, M., . . . Sellers, A. (2003). A multicultural investigation of masculinity ideology and alexithymia. *Psychology of Men & Masculinity, 4,* 91–99. http://dx.doi.org/10.1037/1524-9220.4.2.91

Levant, R. F., & Wong, Y. J. (2013). Race and gender as moderators of the relationship between the endorsement of traditional masculinity ideology and alexithymia: An intersectional perspective. *Psychology of Men & Masculinity, 14,* 329–333. http://dx.doi.org/10.1037/a0029551

Levant, R. F., Wong, Y. J., Karakis, E. N., & Welsh, M. M. (2015). Mediated moderation of the relationship between the endorsement of restrictive emotionality and alexithymia. *Psychology of Men & Masculinity, 16,* 459–467. http://dx.doi.org/10.1037/a0039739

Lisak, D. (1995, August). *Integrating gender analysis in psychotherapy with male survivors of abuse.* Paper presented at the Convention of the American Psychological Association, New York, NY.

Liu, W. M., Rochlen, A. B., & Mohr, J. (2005). Real and ideal gender role conflict: Exploring psychological distress among men. *Psychology of Men & Masculinity, 6,* 137–148. http://dx.doi.org/10.1037/1524-9220.6.2.137

Luyt, R. (2013). Beyond traditional understanding of gender measurement: The gender (re)presentation approach. *Journal of Gender Studies, 24,* 207–226.

Mahalik, J. R. (2014). Both/and, not either/or: A call for methodological pluralism in research on masculinity. *Psychology of Men & Masculinity, 15,* 365–368. http://dx.doi.org/10.1037/a0037308

Mahalik, J. R., Locke, B. D., Ludlow, L. H., Diemer, M. A., Scott, R. P. J., Gottfried, M., & Frietas, G. (2003). Development of the Conformity to Masculine Norms Inventory. *Psychology of Men & Masculinity, 4,* 3–25. http://dx.doi.org/10.1037/1524-9220.4.1.3

Messner, M. A. (1992). *Power at play: Sports and the problem of masculinity.* Boston, MA: Beacon.

Muñoz Boudet, A., Petesch, P., Turk, C., & Thumala, A. (2012). *On norms and agency: Conversations about gender equality with women and men in 20 countries.* Washington, DC: World Bank.

Mussen, P. (1961). Some antecedents and consequents of masculine sex typing in adolescent boys. *Psychological Monographs: General and Applied, 75,* 1–24. http://dx.doi.org/10.1037/h0093767

Nabavi, R. (2004). The "Masculinity Attitudes, Stress, and Conformity questionnaire (MASC)": A new measure for studying psychology of men [Doctoral dissertation]. *Dissertation Abstracts International: Section B. The Sciences and Engineering, 65,* 2641.

O'Neil, J. M. (1996). The gender role journey workshop: Exploring sexism and gender role conflict in a co-educational setting. In M. A. Andronico (Ed.), *Men in groups: Insights, interventions, psychoeducational work* (pp. 193–213). http://dx.doi.org/10.1037/10284-013

O'Neil, J. M. (2008). Summarizing 25 years of research on men's gender role conflict using the Gender Role Conflict Scale. *The Counseling Psychologist, 36,* 358–445. http://dx.doi.org/10.1177/0011000008317057

O'Neil, J. M. (2012). The psychology of men. In E. M. Altmaier & J. C. Hansen (Eds.), *The Oxford handbook of counseling psychology* (pp. 375–408). New York, NY: Oxford University Press.

Pleck, J. H. (1981). *The myth of masculinity.* Cambridge, MA: MIT Press.

Pleck, J. H. (1995). The gender role strain paradigm: An update. In R. F. Levant & W. S. Pollack (Eds.), *A new psychology of men* (pp. 11–32). New York, NY: Basic Books.

Pleck, J. H., Sonenstein, F. L., & Ku, L. C. (1994). Problem behaviors and masculinity ideology in adolescent males. In R. D. Ketterlinus & M. E. Lamb (Eds.), *Adolescent problem behaviors: Issues and research* (pp. 165–186). Hillsdale, NJ: Erlbaum.

Reidy, D. E., Berke, D. S., Gentile, B., & Zeichner, A. (2015). Masculine discrepancy stress, substance use, assault and injury in a survey of U.S. men. *Injury Prevention.* Advance online publication. http://dx.doi.org/10.1136/injuryprev-2015-041599

Ribeiro, O., Paúl, C., & Nogueira, C. (2007). Real men, real husbands: Caregiving and masculinities in later life. *Journal of Aging Studies, 21,* 302–313. http://dx.doi.org/10.1016/j.jaging.2007.05.005

Richmond, K., Levant, R., & Ladhani, S. (2012). The varieties of the masculine experience. In R. Josselson & M. Harway (Eds.), *Navigating multiple identities: Race, gender, culture, nationality, and roles* (pp. 101–118). http://dx.doi.org/10.1093/acprof:oso/9780199732074.003.0004

Rogers, B. K., Sperry, H. S., & Levant, R. F. (2015). Masculinities among African American men: An intersectional perspective. *Psychology of Men & Masculinity, 16*, 416–425. http://dx.doi.org/10.1037/a0039082

Roy, K. M. (2006). Father stories: A life course examination of paternal identity among low-income African American men. *Journal of Family Issues, 27*, 31–54. http://dx.doi.org/10.1177/0192513X05275432

Roy, K. M. (2008). A life course perspective on fatherhood and family policies in the United States and South Africa. *Fathering: A Journal of Theory, Research, and Practice About Men as Fathers, 6*, 92–112.

Rummell, C., & Levant, R. F. (2014). Masculine gender role discrepancy strain and self-esteem. *Psychology of Men & Masculinity, 15*, 419–426. http://dx.doi.org/10.1037/a0035304

Sánchez, F. J., Westerfeld, J. S., Liu, W. M., & Vilain, E. (2010). Masculine gender role conflict and negative feelings about being gay. *Professional Psychology: Research and Practice, 41*, 104–111. http://dx.doi.org/10.1037/a0015805

Shek, Y. L. (2007). Asian American masculinity: A review of the literature. *The Journal of Men's Studies, 14*, 379–391. http://dx.doi.org/10.3149/jms.1403.379

Sifneos, P. E. (1967). Clinical observations on some patients suffering from a variety of psychosomatic diseases. *Proceedings of the Seventh European Conference on Psychosomatic Research.* Basel, Switzerland: Kargel.

Silverstein, L. B., Auerbach, C. F., & Levant, R. F. (2006). Using qualitative research to strengthen clinical practice. *Professional Psychology: Research and Practice, 37*, 351–358. http://dx.doi.org/10.1037/0735-7028.37.4.351

Sinnott, J. D., & Shifren, K. (2001). Gender and aging: Gender differences and gender roles. In J. E. Birren & K. W. Schaie (Eds.), *Handbook of psychology of aging* (5th ed., pp. 454–476). San Diego, CA: Academic Press.

Skinner, B. F. (1953). *Science and human behavior.* New York, NY: Simon & Schuster.

Smiler, A. P. (2004). Thirty years after the discovery of gender: Psychological concepts and measures of masculinity. *Sex Roles, 50*, 15–26. http://dx.doi.org/10.1023/B:SERS.0000011069.02279.4c

Steinfeldt, J. A., Wong, Y. J., Hagan, A. R., Hoag, J. M., & Steinfeldt, M. C. (2011). A contextual examination of gender role conflict among college football players. *Psychology of Men & Masculinity, 12*, 311–323. http://dx.doi.org/10.1037/a0023722

Tannenbaum, C., & Frank, B. (2011). Masculinity and health in late life men. *American Journal of Men's Health, 5*, 243–254. http://dx.doi.org/10.1177/1557988310384609

Thompson, E. H. (1991). Beneath the status characteristic: Gender variations in religiousness. *Journal for the Scientific Study of Religion, 30*, 381–394. http://dx.doi.org/10.2307/1387275

Thompson, E. H., & Bennett, K. M. (2015). Measurement of masculinity ideologies: A (critical) review. *Psychology of Men & Masculinity, 16*, 115–133. http://dx.doi.org/10.1037/a0038609

Thompson, E. H., & Pleck, J. H. (1995). Masculinity ideology: A review of research instrumentation on men and masculinities. In R. F. Levant & W. S. Pollack (Eds.), *A new psychology of men* (pp. 129–163). New York, NY: Basic Books.

Unger, R. K. (1979). Toward a redefinition of sex and gender. *American Psychologist, 34*, 1085–1094. http://dx.doi.org/10.1037/0003-066X.34.11.1085

Vandello, J. A., & Bosson, J. L. (2013). Hard won and easily lost: A review and synthesis of theory and research on precarious manhood. *Psychology of Men & Masculinity, 14*, 101–113. http://dx.doi.org/10.1037/a0029826

Veenstra, G. (2013). The gendered nature of discriminatory experiences by race, class, and sexuality: A comparison of intersectionality theory and the subordinate male target hypothesis. *Sex Roles, 68*, 646–659. http://dx.doi.org/10.1007/s11199-012-0243-2

Watkins, D. C., Walker, R. L., & Griffith, D. M. (2010). A meta-study of Black male mental health and well-being. *Journal of Black Psychology, 36*, 303–330. http://dx.doi.org/10.1177/0095798409353756

Way, N., Cressen, J., Bodian, S., Preston, J., Nelson, J., & Hughes, D. (2014). "It might be nice to be a girl . . . then you wouldn't have to be emotionless": Boys' resistance to norms of masculinity during adolescence. *Psychology of Men & Masculinity, 15*, 241–252. http://dx.doi.org/10.1037/a0037262

Wester, S. R., & Vogel, D. L. (2012). The psychology of men: Historical developments, current research, and future direction. In N. A. Fouad (Ed.), *APA handbook of counseling psychology: Vol. 1. Theories, research, and methods* (pp. 371–396). http://dx.doi.org/10.1037/13754-014

Wester, S. R., Vogel, D. L., Pressly, P. K., & Heesacker, M. (2002). Sex differences in emotion. *The Counseling Psychologist, 30*, 630–652. http://dx.doi.org/10.1177/0010000203000408

Wetherell, M., & Edley, N. (2014). A discursive psychological framework for analyzing men and masculinities. *Psychology of Men & Masculinity, 15*, 355–364. http://dx.doi.org/10.1037/a0037148

Whorley, M. R., & Addis, M. E. (2006). Ten years of psychological research on men and masculinity in the United States: Dominant methodological trends. *Sex Roles, 55*, 649–658. http://dx.doi.org/10.1007/s11199-006-9120-1

Whitehead, T. L., Peterson, J., & Kaljee, L. (1994). The "hustle": Socioeconomic deprivation, urban drug trafficking, and low-income, African-American male gender identity. *Pediatrics, 93*, 1050–1054.

Williams, D. R. (2008). The health of men: Structured inequalities and opportunities. *American Journal of Public Health, 98*(Suppl. 1), S150–S157. http://dx.doi.org/10.2105/AJPH.98.Supplement_1.S150

Wong, Y. J., Levant, R. F., Welsh, M. M., Zaitsoff, A., Garvin, M., King, D., & Aguilar, M. (2015). Priming masculinity: Testing the causal influence of subjective masculinity experiences on self-esteem. *The Journal of Men's Studies, 23,* 98–106.

Wong, Y. J., Shea, M., LaFollette, J. R., Hickman, S. J., Cruz, N., & Boghokian, T. (2011). The inventory of subjective masculinity experiences: Development and psychometric properties. *The Journal of Men's Studies, 19,* 236–255. http://dx.doi.org/10.3149/jms.1903.236

Wong, Y. J., Steinfeldt, J. A., Speight, Q. L., & Hickman, S. L. (2010). Content analysis of *Psychology of Men and Masculinity* (2000–2008). *Psychology of Men & Masculinity, 11,* 170–181. http://dx.doi.org/10.1037/a0019133

Zolla, A. (2015, June 22). Is it finally time to put down "man up"? *The Good Men Project.* Retrieved from http://www.goodmenproject.com/featured-content/is-it-finally-time-to-put-down-man-up-fiff/

# 2

# MASCULINITY IDEOLOGIES

EDWARD H. THOMPSON, JR. AND KATE M. BENNETT

Research and writing about men and masculinities has expanded rapidly in recent decades. This development reflects a great deal of popular interest in and the maturing scholarship on men's gendered lives, particularly their health, conduct, troubles, changing social responsibilities, and aging. There has been much discussion of men's likelihood not to seek health care during an illness or after an injury (Addis & Mahalik, 2003) and aging men's prostate and erectile health (Oliffe, 2009). Increasing debate on the "valorization" (Segal, 1990) of contemporary fathers and a nascent culture of "new fatherhood" (Cabrera & Tamis-LeMonda, 2013; Hearn, 2002) is mirrored in the discussion on sons and husbands who become caregivers to mothers and wives (Campbell & Carroll, 2007; Russell, 2007). Public agonizing about men's violence toward women is intensely voiced; these actions might unmask "aggrieved entitlement" (Kimmel, 2013), yet they are always the dark side of how our culture and its masculinity ideologies reward men's aggression—on the sports field, in the military, in the marketplace, through religious scripture.

http://dx.doi.org/10.1037/0000023-003
*The Psychology of Men and Masculinities*, R. F. Levant and Y. J. Wong (Editors)

A common thread running through these debates is how masculinity ideologies perpetuate varied actions. Critical men's studies view masculinities as dynamic patterns of ideologies and practices constructed in interaction. Paraphrasing Kimmel (1996, p. 6ff), men perform their gender in synch with respected, local traditions. This is the same argument as Olsen's (2000) analysis of why violence was associated with some early Southern masculinities, or Goffman's (1967) insight that "men must be prepared to put up their lives to save faces" (p. 257) in social worlds where honor is valued. Their collective voice underscores the importance of analyzing the values and beliefs that buttress patterns of gendered behavior.

By investigating the ideological underpinnings, a far greater scientific understanding of men's lives has become available. The first comprehensive synthesis, a handbook of research on men and masculinities (Kimmel, Hearn, & Connell, 2005), is already a decade old. The present chapter contributes to the American Psychological Association's updated synopsis of the distinctive scholarship within the psychology of men and masculinities over the past 20 years. In Europe, there have been large-scale comparative studies of EU countries on men's violence and health (Hearn et al., 2002) and why older men's nutrition and health habits differ across EU nations (e.g., Davidson, Arber, & Marshall, 2008). Social constructions of masculinities have been documented in societies as diverse as Sweden (Hearn et al., 2012), contemporary Russia (Janey et al., 2013) and the Cossack traditions in Ukraine (Bureychak, 2013), Mexico (Irwin, 2003; Wentzell, 2013), and Peru (Fuller, 2001). This widening scholarship on men and boys is rooted in feminist scholarship and the paradigm shift where psychological theories about "masculinity" and "femininity" as internalized, subjective identities were superseded by the constructionist view that masculinity and femininity are institutionalized patterns of ideologies and gender practices that contribute to the production of identities (Edley & Wetherell, 1995) and to social order (Connell, 1987).

Our primary aim in this chapter is to examine writing and research on "masculinity ideologies" through a gendered, critical lens, which acknowledges that "mainstream" gendered ideologies are integral to safeguarding a status quo and to the ongoing legitimation of (social) institutions such as heterosexuality, marriage, and law. Many types of gender inequality are preserved by the mainstream ideologies that are embedded in the structure of relationships between women and men and among men. Our analysis takes as given that mainstream masculinity ideologies are not benign; rather, they persist in pressuring men and boys to (un)wittingly engage in conduct that reproduces the social inequalities sited in economic arrangements, culture, the state, and everyday interpersonal relationships.

At the onset, we focus on the origin of the concept of "masculinity ideologies" and address several definitional and conceptual issues that warrant discussion. We next consider the content or "properties" of mainstream masculinity ideologies. Our scope does not allow a thorough review of recent work employing the concept of masculinity ideologies, yet we identify how the concept is being studied. We conclude by suggesting avenues for new research that would advance psychological studies of men and masculinities from a position that appreciates social structure as the context for the formation and practice of masculinity ideologies.

## ORIGIN OF THE CONCEPT

*Ideologies* are systems of values, expectations, beliefs, or ideas shared by a social group and often presumed to be natural or innately true. *Masculinity ideologies*, then, are a body of socially constructed ideas and beliefs about what it means to be a man and against which men are appraised within their communities. The concept of masculinity ideology emerged in the early 1990s (Thompson, Pleck, & Ferrera, 1992) and was derived from two constructionist traditions.

The first of these is Mannheim's (1936) writings on the meaning of *ideology*, later amplified by Berger and Luckmann's (1967) seminal analysis of the foundations of knowledge in everyday life. Although separated by generations, they studied how social organizations and relationships influence "mind" and "self" and analyzed how our biographies and *Weltanschauung* (worldview) reflect histories and societies. Mannheim theorized that everyone's knowledge and beliefs were products of the contexts in which they were created, and he argued that class, geographies, and generations were the greatest determinants of "mind." A key insight was that what each person understands, sees, and says is "not immune to ideological influences" (Berger & Luckmann, 1967, p. 21). Lorber's (1993) "believing is seeing" maxim recaps his thesis that ideologies shape perceptions and expectations. Here are two examples: "Believing" that masculinities are biologically determined led eugenicists to "know" certain national traits are superior/inferior (Nelkin & Michaels, 1998) and led early physicians to "see" differences between men's and women's bodies that do not in fact exist (cf. E. Martin, 1991). Travel to another geography; engage in intergenerational conversations; listen to a legislative debate on covenant marriage; and we readily understand that norms and values—ideologies—are culturally and social rooted and never absolute "facts."

Second are the writings on masculinity that originated within early social constructionist and feminist-inspired analyses of gender (e.g., Carrigan, Connell, & Lee, 1985; Gergen, 1985; West & Zimmerman, 2009). In this tradition, masculinity is viewed as distinctive gendered practices; it is a property of the collectivities and institutions that have the effect of subordinating women and some men, not a fixed quality that is a psychologically or biologically rooted property within the individual. Because masculinity is viewed as a dimension of gender as an institution (P. Y. Martin, 2004) and of social order (Lorber, 1994), constructionist discourses on masculinities address the production of gendered hierarchies and their inequalities.

This framework questioned pre-1980s role theories not least for presuming sex-based roles were necessary and complementary, but largely for ignoring the unequal power relations between men and women. Mirroring discourses within the literatures and philosophies of antiquity and scripture (cf. Moore & Anderson, 1998), personality psychology (e.g., Terman & Miles, 1936) and sex-role scholarship (e.g., Bem, 1974) had theorized masculinity and maleness only oppositionally as what is neither femininity and femaleness nor effeminate. Healthy lives were said to depend on heterosexuality and acquisition of a "sex-role identity." Constructionist theorizing debunked the thesis that people acquire an immutable sex-typed masculine (or feminine) sex role identity, or gendered self. Also disputed was the reasoning that characterized masculinity as an essential dimension of a healthy personality and said to be measured by the trait-based self-descriptions within the Minnesota Multiphasic Personality Inventory (H. Martin & Finn, 2010) or Bem Sex Role Inventory (Bem, 1974).

Emergent thinking about gender-related behavior as context dependent (e.g., Deaux & Major, 1987; Goffman, 1967), about the intersection of gender with other systems of oppression yielding gendered age-, class-, or body wholeness-based privilege (Baca Zinn & Thornton Dill, 1996; Gerschick & Miller, 1995; Pyke, 1996), and about the nexus of gender and sexuality (e.g., Garfinkel, 1967, pp. 118–140) helped strengthen Carrigan et al.'s (1985) core principle. Masculinities (and femininities) are situated ways of performing gender that change across time—both history and life course, geographies, cultures, and audience. There is not one masculinity but many, and these masculinities are about power relations among men, not only between women and men. What's more, they are infused with ideologies. Paraphrasing P. Y. Martin (2004, p. 1256ff), ideologies organize masculinities (and femininities); have histories; underpin the norm-governed practices that reproduce themselves; enable and constrain group members' choices and actions; and are in flux yet linger across time. These gendered ideologies are not universal across social institutions. The military, sports, and fundamentalist religions may espouse a similar ideology that noticeably privileges men, but the blueprints are not exactly the same.

## CONCEPTUAL TURNS

Commonplace during a paradigm shift, the lack of conceptual clarity among sociologists and psychologists studying masculinities during the mid-1980s led Thompson and Pleck (Thompson et al., 1992) to propose the construct *masculinity ideologies*. It named the societal-wide cultural values, beliefs, and norms scripting men's lives. The construct derived most directly from scholarly work on what "manliness" had meant over time and the research on what was generally called "attitudes toward masculinity." The construct intended to distinguish cultural ideologies from the dramaturgical metaphor of a "male role" and constructs associated with the metaphor, such as gender-role stress.

The construct also intended to distinguish masculinity ideologies from gender and femininity ideologies. Before a discussion of masculinity ideologies, there had been much consideration of the more global construct *gender ideology* in the 1960s and 1970s. Davis and Greenstein (2009) advised that the discussions of gender ideology address the values, beliefs, and cultural scripts supporting patriarchal families, principally the division of paid work and family responsibilities based on gendered separate spheres.[1] Gender ideologies— traditional, transitional, egalitarian (Hochschild, 1989)—communicate women's and men's work and family responsibilities as defined by the separate-spheres ideal. National population-based surveys interested in determining people's attitudes toward the traditionalist gender ideology were initiated in the mid-1960s and use items such as "A man's job is to earn money; a woman's job is to look after the home and family" (cf. Davis & Greenstein, 2009, p. 90). As might be illustrated in a Venn diagram, traditional masculinity ideologies predictably overlap with traditional gender ideology, yet are discrete (cf. Thompson, Grisanti, & Pleck, 1985).

Also preceding the explicit discussion of the masculinity ideologies evident in the works of O'Neil (1981), Baca Zinn (1982), Franklin (1994), and Connell (1995) was much debate on femininity ideologies. Friedan (1963) characterized the *feminine mystique* as an ideological stranglehold that advocated how women would find fulfillment in sexual passivity, motherhood, and surrendering themselves to domesticity. The linchpin of this conventional feminine ideology is its emphasis on self-sacrifice and deference. Tolman and Porche (2000) also discussed how conventional femininity ideology is not benign. It perpetuates body objectification and women reinforcing their own subordination. It complements the tenets of traditional masculinity ideologies that privilege men vis-à-vis women and unsurprisingly is interwoven with racial- and class-based ideologies that preserve other gender-related inequalities.

Another conceptual turn occurred when Pleck, Sonenstein, and Ku (1993) proposed that quantitative research addressing attitudes toward

---

[1] Davis and Greenstein (2009, p. 88) flagged how researchers use a mixture of constructs similar to *gender ideology* to describe people's support for the sexist, separate-spheres arrangement that resonates with patriarchal culture, including gender role attitudes, attitudes about gender, gender-related attitudes, and attitudes toward women and men.

masculinities requires a concept that describes the "individual male's acceptance or internalization of his society's definition of masculinity" (p. 15), and
masculinity ideology was the linking concept. At the opening of their article,
they defined masculinity ideology as "beliefs about the importance of men
adhering to culturally defined standards for male behavior" (p. 12). Later,
Pleck (1995) acknowledged that the construct masculinity ideology connotes
the "superordinate, organizing nature of beliefs" (p. 19), yet he continued
to locate those beliefs "at both the individual level and the social-structural
level" (p. 19). The theoretical footing for this line of reasoning was his gender
role strain theory (Pleck, 1981, 1995). Because he characterized masculinity ideology as an individual-level belief system and the existing measures of
masculinity ideologies as means to chart those personal beliefs, this proved
confusing. Quantitative researchers began to discuss masculinity ideologies
only as internalized belief systems (cf. Chu, Porche, & Tolman, 2005), not
as they are—cultural ideologies that individuals may or may not agree with,
endorse, enact, conform to, or view as normative. Thompson and Bennett
(2015b) cautioned that the discourse on internalized beliefs loses sight of
the sources of those acquired beliefs—the (forever changing, often competing) masculinity ideologies embedded within cultural traditions and social
practices:

> We remain unwavering in our concern that whenever a discourse about
> individual men's personal norms or level of acceptance of societal norms
> is equated with masculinity ideologies, the error of misplaced concrete-
> ness looms. The mistake is to liken self-defined conformity to, attitudes
> toward, or beliefs about an ideology with the ideology. (p. 146)

## CONTENT OF MASCULINITY IDEOLOGIES

Masculinity practices, not their ideologies, are usually the foci of public and scholarly discussion. These conversations regularly address trait-based
archetypes of manhood and esteemed behaviors. Shortly after World War II,
one archetype was the solid, self-confident, elegant, decisive patriarch sym-
bolized in Hollywood's Rock Hudson; another was the John Wayne single-
mindedness moral code, which venerated using fists and guns to make things
right. Film emerged as an instruction manual, providing audiences through
example a summary of what men should be. Similarly, the "3-minute word
movies" (Hartford, as cited in Lewis, 1984, p. 7) in country music lyrics help ossify
the archetype of the resilient, gristly, working-class Southern man (McCusker
& Pecknold, 2004) as much as rap lyrics affirm the hypermasculine hipster
(Neal, 1999). But what actually is the content of the masculinity ideologies
sustaining the archetypes of manhood within Anglophone societies?

First, the array of beliefs, expectations, and ideas composing dominant ideologies do not make up a single, orderly set. Nor is the content of masculinity ideologies limited to the work/family domain. The broad, gendered expectations men commonly face can appear demanding yet, except on a few features, not very specific. Some expectations also are contradictory, and some are inconsistent across different situations. There is no single ideal of masculinity, but many. Individual men surely encounter the reified mainstream standards in places of religious worship and many workplaces. But there are also distinctive "tributaries" that emphasize other dominant masculinities in families and workplaces or defend the variant archetypes of manhood found within, for example, working-class, white masculinities (Embrick, Walther, & Wickens, 2007; Farough, 2006), Southern traditions (Cohen, Nisbett, Bowdle, & Schwarz, 1996; Friend, 2009), or gay masculinities (Connell, 1992; Hennen, 2005; Nardi, 2000).

It is arguable that there is a "mainstream" ideology that is likely hegemonic and likely traditional, yet it need not be the commonest or most powerful pattern of masculinity. Connell (1987, 1995) originally conceptualized *hegemonic masculinity* as the form of masculinity evident in a society-wide setting that structured the hierarchal relations between men and women, and among men. Its cultural ascendancy, and thus its relational character to femininities and to other masculinities, were central to her analysis (Messerschmidt, 2012, p. 58).[2]

Brannon (1976) theorized that this blueprint for American culture's mainstream masculinity ideology involved four conceptually distinct canons:

1. *No Sissy Stuff*: Boys and men must avoid anything seen as even vaguely feminine.
2. *The Big Wheel*: Men and boys must strive to be respected and admired. To gain this needed status, they must distinguish themselves through achievement and embody the expectations to be successful in all they undertake, especially as breadwinners.
3. *The Sturdy Oak*: Best captured by the phrase "the strong silent type," not only is the expectation to remain calm in the most hectic and frightening situations, boys and men are expected to handle difficult problems on their own.
4. *Give 'Em Hell*: This canon underscores the virtues of risk-taking, adventure, and, when necessary, use of violence.

---

[2]This original formulation was revised (Connell & Messerschmidt, 2005) to recognize and urge scholars to empirically assess what hegemonic masculinities exist locally, as within families and immediate communities, and regionally, not just society-wide. As well, Coles (2009) maintained that there are a variety of dominant masculinity ideologies that coexist, contest one another, and must be continually renewed, recreated, defended, and modified.

As much as his model envisions one axis of masculinity in commonsense terms as the inverse to femininity, it also details the patriarchal family precept that men should be providers and protectors, the "enlightenment" model of manhood as reasoned and rational, the frontier tradition of risk-taking, and the ubiquitous guideline to be unendingly successful. And like Connell, Brannon (1976, p. 11ff) cautioned that definitions of masculinity are relationally constructed, and there seem to be many specific "strands" of masculinity ideology at the local level that men and boys can draw on to perform normative masculinity.

An excellent example of this is Barrett's (1996) qualitative study of U.S. Navy officers. Barrett used life history interviews with active duty officers. He detected that the hegemonic masculinity blueprint at the societal level permitted naval officers within different occupational communities— aviation, surface warfare, and supply—to draw on a number of aspects of masculinity ideology to confirm who and what they are as men. He noted that the structure of work facilitated aviators more opportunities for risk-taking, compared with supply officers' opportunities to perform as confident, decisive problem solvers. He further commented that there were variations within the three groups, yet masculinity practices within and across these local-level communities of naval officers routinely positioned women as subordinates.

Doss and Hopkins (1998) also challenged the universalizing Anglo American conceptions of mainstream masculinity. Using Chilean, African American, and European American undergraduates, they assessed the central tenets of masculinity ideologies in one or more cultures and to differentiate the cultural groups. They revealed *etic* (common) dimensions applicable to all groups and one to three *emic* (distinctive) components for each cultural group.

Second, recognition that numerous masculinities coexist does not mean that masculinity practices and ideologies can be readily categorized in terms of their ancestries in, for example, culture, generation, class, or ethnicity. As Schrock and Schwalbe (2009) noted, to invoke "the existence of Black masculinity, Latino masculinity, gay masculinity, Jewish masculinity, working-class masculinity, and so on is to imply that there is an overriding similarity in the gender arrangements" (p. 280) of the men who are Jewish, working class, or Black. This is a kind of categorical essentialism, and it loses sight of the pronounced variations within categories. One definitive example for the need to avoid categorical reductionism was made clear in Duneier's (1992) study of the class- and age-based African American masculinities in Chicago. The "respectable" citizenry of the older working-class men shared one ideology, and the young men within the South Side underclass shared another. Although the ideologies and resulting masculinity practices differed sharply at times, they also communicated the commonalities of being Black in White America.

Third, as the concept of hegemonic masculinit*ies* succeeds both the dramaturgical metaphor the "male role" and the falsely universalizing concept of hegemonic masculinity, analyses of men's lives have broadened to acknowledge men's agency and the way differing ideologies coexist. Here are two first-rate examples. According to Alexander (2003), mainstream masculinity "is no longer defined by what a man produces . . . but instead what he consumes" (p. 551). She argued that the hegemonic masculinity of one or two generations back has changed for urban-based, middle-class men living under the new economy and "a new social structure in which consumption is more important than production" (p. 535). This newly constituted consumer-oriented masculinity ideology appears to reject some aspects of traditional masculinity practices, but not all aspects, such as occupational achievement and heterosexuality. The ideological value of men and women partnering in work and family matters has replaced familial patriarchy and its separate spheres arrangement, and the value of physical perfection has replaced the importance of sheer physicality.

A very different masculinity context can be found within the social world of homeless heroin injectors. What Bourgois and Schonberg (2007) uncovered through a decade of participant-observation fieldwork was the differing masculinity ideologies and manhood acts between Whites and African Americans who shared indigent poverty and daily encampments. The men willfully constructed different income-generation strategies that were rooted in both traditional and "outlaw" masculinities. The African American heroin injectors refused to produce income by passive begging along highway access ramps for small change or by accepting off-the-books, "boy" labor jobs such as sweeping sidewalks or unloading trucks, as the White men did. The African Americans saw passive begging as "stooping down"; Bourgois and Schonberg (2007) noted that these men strongly "criticize the relationships that the whites develop with employers as being akin to slavery" and characterized odd-job working conditions as "demeaning, exploitative and feminizing" (p. 15). Presenting themselves as streetwise outlaws, and not socially marginal homeless men, they espoused an ideology that married traditional masculinity's emphasis on being successful (through theft) and maintaining family ties with an "outlaw" masculinity that valued daring, risk, rebelliousness, ingenuity, and sacrifice. The White men valued the "hard work" of recycling cans and bottles and humbly begging as their self-reliance strategies.

These few examples of the content within local or regional hegemonic masculinities draw almost exclusively on qualitative studies. There are too few quantitative studies analogous to Doss and Hopkins (1998) that examine the hegemonic masculinities established within local settings or other communities (two exceptions: Arciniega, Anderson, Tovar-Blank, & Tracey, 2008; Wong et al., 2011). Instead, most quantitative investigations of masculinity ideologies used standardized measures to assess the extent to which traditional, society-wide ideologies within Anglophone societies predict the expected gendered practices in terms of help-seeking, aggression, risk-taking, relationship satisfaction, and so on. From such studies, broad generalizations on men have often been made, with relatively small-scale data on specifically aged, classed, and racialized men.

## MEASURES OF MASCULINITY IDEOLOGIES

Quantitative investigations of masculinity ideologies typically use psychometrically reliable measures of attitudes toward traditional masculinity ideology, or other self-report measures designed to register people's experiences living with the society-wide "masculine mystique." All measures were developed using a deductive scale construction strategy in which an original pool of items was assembled by the scale developers to operationalize the perceived negative and positive aspects of the ideological canons. Typically, the measures assess the degree to which individuals agree or disagree with gender-related values tapped by the scale (e.g., "Men should be strong," "Nobody likes a man who cries in public").

When Thompson et al. (1992) critically reviewed the 18 measures of "attitudes toward men and masculinities" that existed at the time, they separated the scales designed to chart individuals' opinions of masculinity ideologies from the instruments that charted how the ideologies affected men's experiences. The content of the two classes of measures is quite similar. However, the instruments revealing how ideologies shape experience emphasize first-person statements of conformity to or distress aroused by masculinity standards (e.g., "Moving up the career ladder is important to me"). Instruments intending to assess the behavioral or cognitive dimensions of masculinity ideologies typically ask respondents to report whether they agree or disagree with a series of statements about men's gender practices (e.g., "The best way for a young man to get the respect of other people is to get a good job, take it very seriously, and do well at it"). Nonetheless, the latter scales often mixed together these third-person statements with some first-person statements, thus shifting the evaluative focus from the perceived "normativeness" of the ideological statement (e.g., "A *man* should never back down in the face of trouble") to a personal value (e.g., "It disgusts *me* when a man comes across as weak" or "*I* think a young man should try to become physically tough, even if he's not big"). It is no wonder, therefore, that because most measures have operationalized the construct to include reports of personal values, more than a few quantitative researchers agree with Pleck's line of reasoning that "masculinity ideology" conveys individuals' endorsement, and perhaps internalization of, the society-wide cultural mandate (cf. Levant & Richmond, 2007, p. 131).

Thompson and Bennett (2015a) restricted their critical review to the 16 measures of masculinity ideologies used in empirical studies during 1995–2014. Nearly all of the measures developed since 1995 continue to blend third-person and first-person statements and to chart respondents' opinions about cultural guidelines as operationalized by the pool of scale items. In each case, the instruments determined the extent to which individuals agreed with, endorsed, conformed to, or viewed as normative the cultural ideologies, particularly a society-wide "mainstream" masculinity, whether Russian, South African, or U.S./Canadian. Exactly what is being measured is not invariant. Assessment of the masculinity ideology could serve as evidence that certain normative standards are perceived as desirable (or important), reveal that these norms are personal values guiding decisions and actions, and/or disclose individuals' (dis)agreement that the behavioral norms exist locally.

Table 2.1 identifies the primary ideological canons that recur across measures of traditional masculinity ideologies. The table is organized to note example items used to operationalize each masculinity standard; we have organized the overall pool of items into 10 categories: relational power, importance of work/breadwinning, being respected, primacy of avoiding femininity, control of emotionality, toughness/self-reliance, physical toughness/violence, risk-taking, (hetero)sexuality, and heterosexism. Examining the content and factor structure of each measure, least often integrated into a measure were items assessing attitudes toward sexuality, heterosexism, and relational power; most often tapped were people's views about the masculinity standards calling for emotional toughness, control of emotionality, physical toughness, and employment. Consequently, the relational inequalities among men and between men and women are overshadowed by an emphasis on trait-related standards such as stoicism or self-sufficiency. Nor are most measures designed to assess adult men's family-based masculinities beyond earning respect for being a breadwinner or head of the household. As the field of measuring attitudes goes forward, new measures are necessary to determine adult men's views on fatherhood, coparenting, marital negotiation, retirement and generative mentoring, care work in later life, and recoupling after a wife's death.

Men's attitudes toward "nontraditional" masculinity practices also deserve research attention. Masculinity practices are context related, local, and not easily operationalized by simple spoken rules such as "A man should be willing to take risks." For example, standing out from other bystanders to intervene and stop one of his teammates from sexually touching an intoxicated woman risks a man's being ridiculed as not being a loyal "mate." Not intervening can equally risk punishing ridicule. The man in the situation is subject to being shamed by his girlfriend and her friends who heard about his

## TABLE 2.1
### Canons Used to Measure "Mainstream" Masculinity Ideology

| Characteristic item | Instrument(s) |
|---|---|
| **Relational power** | |
| Things tend to be better when men are in charge. | CMNI |
| In a family, a father's wish is law. | MM |
| Being smarter or physically stronger than other men is important to me. | GRCS |
| A real man should be a support to his wife. | RMNI |
| It's important for a guy to go after what he wants, even if it means hurting other people's feelings. | AMIRS |
| **Importance of work/breadwinning** | |
| A man owes it to his family to work at the best-paying job he can get. | BMS, MRNS, MIS–21, MMIS |
| If necessary, a man should sacrifice personal relationships for career advancement. | MRNI, MRNI–A |
| A job is more important for a man than family. | RMNI |
| My work is the most important part of my life. | CMNI |
| **Being respected** | |
| It's essential for a man to always have the respect and admiration of everyone who knows him. | BMS, MRNS, MIS–21 |
| A man always deserves the respect of his wife and children. | MRAS, MANI |
| A man should do whatever it takes to be admire and respected. | MRNI |
| A man who advocates his opinion is worth being respected. | RMNI |
| It feels good to be important. | CMNI |
| **Primacy of avoiding femininity** | |
| A man should avoid holding his wife's purse at all times. | MRNI, MRNI–A |
| It bothers me when a man does something that I consider "feminine." | BMS, MRNS, MIS–21 |
| As a man, how important is it not to engage in activities that you think others might consider feminine? | TAAM |
| It bothers me when a guy acts like a girl. | MRAS |
| **Control of emotionality** | |
| A man should never admit when others hurt his feelings. | MRNI–R, MRNI–A |
| It is best to keep your emotions hidden. | CMNI |
| Most men in this group believe that real men keep their feelings to themselves. | M2PIN |
| It would be shameful for a man to cry in front of his children. | MM |
| Men who cry in public are weak. | MANI |
| **Toughness/self-reliance** | |
| A man should never count on someone else to get the job done. | MRNI, MRNI–R, MRNI–A |
| A man should always try to project an air of confidence even if he doesn't really feel confident inside. | MRNS, BMS, MIS–21 |
| It's in man's nature to be cool-blooded and take decisions based on intellect, not emotions. | RMNI |
| Asking for help is a sign of failure. | CMNI |
| It's important for a guy to act like nothing is wrong, even when something is bothering him. | AMIRS |

TABLE 2.1

Canons Used to Measure "Mainstream" Masculinity Ideology    *(Continued)*

| Characteristic item | Instrument(s) |
|---|---|
| **Physical toughness/violence** | |
| I think a young man should try to become physically tough, even if he's not big. | BMS, MRNS, MIS–21, MRNI–SF, MRAS |
| If a man is assaulted, he should fight back. | RMNI |
| As a man, how important is it for you to be physically strong and tough? | TAAM |
| Fists are sometimes the only way to get out of a bad situation. | BMS, MRNS, MIS-21 |
| Sometimes violent action is necessary. | CMNI |
| It is necessary to fight when challenged. | MM |
| **Risk-taking** | |
| A real man enjoys a bit of danger now and then. | BMS, MRNS |
| It is important for a man to take risks, even if he might get hurt. | MRNI, MRNI–R, MRNI–A |
| Taking dangerous risks helps me to prove myself. | CMNI |
| Do you believe that taking risks that are sometimes dangerous is part of what it means to be a man? | TAAM |
| **(Hetero)sexuality** | |
| Men should always take the initiative when it comes to sex. | MRNI, MRNI–R |
| It's a shame for a man to be sexually inexperienced. | RMNI |
| If I could, I would frequently change sexual partners. | CMNI |
| A guy should prove his masculinity by having sex with a lot of people. | MMIS |
| If a man has a lot of girlfriends, he is seen as more of a man than if he sticks with one woman. | MS |
| I think it is important for a guy to act like he is sexually active even if he is not. | AMIRS |
| **Heterosexism** | |
| It is important to me that people think I am heterosexual. | CMNI |
| Men who touch other men make me uncomfortable. | GRCS |
| It is disappointing to learn that a famous athlete is gay. | MRNI–R |
| Being thought of as gay makes a guy seem like less of a man. | MAMS |
| A father should be embarrassed if his son is gay. | MANI |

*Note.* AMIRS = Adolescent Masculinity Ideology in Relationships Scale (Chu et al., 2005); BMS = Brannon Masculinity Scale (Brannon & Juni, 1984); CMNI = Conformity to Masculinity Norms Inventory (Mahalik et al., 2003); GRCS = Gender Role Conflict Scale (O'Neil, Helms, Gable, David, & Wrightsman, 1986); MAMS = Meanings of Adolescent Masculinity Scale (Oransky & Fisher, 2009); MANI = Male Attitudes Norms Inventory (Luyt, 2005); MIS–21 = Masculinity Ideology Scale—21 (Fischer, Tokar, Good, & Snell, 1998); MM = Machismo Measure (Arciniega et al., 2008); MRNI and MRNI–R = Male Role Norms Inventory and its revision (Levant, Hirsch, et al., 1992; Levant, Smalley, et al., 2007); MRNI–A = Male Role Norms Inventory—Adolescent (Levant, Graef, Smalley, Williams, & McMillan, 2008); MMIS = Multicultural Masculinity Ideology Scale (Doss & Hopkins, 1998); MRAS = Male Role Attitudes Scale (Pleck et al., 1993); MRNS = Male Role Norms Scale (Thompson & Pleck, 1986); MS = Macho Scale (Anderson, 2012); M2PIN = Measure of Men's Perceived Inexpressiveness Norms (Wong, Horn, Gomory, & Ramos, 2013); RMNI = Russian Male Norms Inventory (Janey et al., 2013); TAAM (Traditional Attitudes About Men; McCreary, Saucier, & Courtenay, 2005).

(poor) decision to do nothing to protect their friend. There are currently no measures of attitudes toward masculinity ideologies that include such context-specific actions, probably because nuance is harder to judge as verifiable evidence of someone complying with the masculinity rule "A man should be willing to take risks." The risk-taking canon has been imagined too conventionally as being adventurous or being financially aggressive with investments and almost exclusively measured with agree–disagree Likert scales.

## IMPLICATIONS OF MASCULINITY IDEOLOGIES

Feminist scholars directed attention to how the seemingly benign construct of "gender ideology" overlooked the consequences of the inequalities embedded in the normalcy of traditions. In *Second Shift*, for example, Hochschild (1989) identified the "leisure gap" between men and women at home since women annually worked an extra month of 24-hour days caring for both house and children. She urged scholars to recognize that people use behavioral and cognitive "gender strategies" to maintain or renegotiate traditional gender ideology's inegalitarian arrangements. To illustrate: When the husband nightly cleans up after dinner but the wife does all the planning, shopping, and food preparation, his kitchen labor is consistent with his "on top" situational ideology (Hochschild, 1990, p. 127) to share familial labor, yet this behavior preserves the supremacy of his "underneath" traditionalist ideology that makes it her responsibility to do most of the work at home. National studies reveal this fictive couple's kitchen labor is not atypical and that people's attitudes toward gender equality remain ambivalent (cf. Grubbs, Exline, & Twenge, 2014).

We focus on three areas where masculinity ideologies have noxious implications for men and for society: health status and health behavior, health-related help-seeking, and the performance of marital status.[3] Of these three, the most attention has been paid to individuals' health and health behaviors. This emphasis is driven by the epidemiological evidence that men die sooner and more often from preventable diseases and accidental deaths. The cumulative evidence reveals that endorsement of traditional masculinity ideals is a core cause of poorer health because men who adhere to the traditional ideological canons are the men more likely to engage in risky behaviors and hypermasculine practices, such as heavy drinking, womanizing,

---

[3]Many other implications of masculinity ideologies have been investigated: ones that safeguard the status quo in terms of hegemonic masculinities' relational power and remain noxious to social equality (see Chapters 11 and 12 in this volume) and ones that thwart individuals' quality of life (see Chapters 6–10 in this volume).

driving fast cars, and avoiding preventive health practices (Connell, 1995; Courtenay, 2000a).

## Health

A substantial body of research documents a robust relationship between men's efforts to acquire masculine capital and their health beliefs and health behavior. This research has aimed to understand why certain men, across the lifespan, have higher levels of mortality and preventable disease in comparison with other men (Courtenay, 2000b; Sabo, 2005; see also Chapters 6 and 7, this volume). This work has focused primarily on men from North America, the United Kingdom, Australia, and New Zealand; on either Caucasian or African American men (e.g., Emslie, Ridge, Ziebland, & Hunt, 2006; Gibbs, 2005; Levant, Parent, McCurdy, & Bradstreet, 2015); and on relatively few aspects of men's health: diet including drink-related behavior (Gough & Conner, 2006; Wimer & Levant, 2013), mental health (Emslie et al., 2006; Magovcevic & Addis, 2008), prostate cancer (Chapple & Ziebland, 2002; Harvey & Alston, 2011), and bodily aging (Calasanti, Pietilä, Ojala, & King, 2013; Evans, Frank, Oliffe, & Gregory, 2011). In the early work, conformity to hegemonic masculinity was advanced as an explanation for men's poorer health (Harrison, 1978). The majority of the research is now more nuanced.

Masculinity ideologies in the context of health behavior pivot on notions of power and control (Calasanti et al., 2013; Sloan, Gough, & Conner, 2010). In their study of older men and ill health, McVittie and Willock (2006) found that men's explanations of their health emphasized being in control. When discussing their ill health, these men referred to their powerlessness. Harvey and Alston (2011) found that men experiencing prostate cancer screening spoke to the masculinity ideals of illness as weakness and a pride in maintaining health without doctors. O'Brien, Hunt, and Hart (2005, 2009) called attention to the interaction of age and masculinities. They found that it was younger men more than older men who experienced illness as a threat to their masculine capital and performance of masculine identities. The older men in the study treated their illness as a problem to be solved and viewed physicians as providers of needed information. There is other evidence that there are age differences in relation to masculinity ideologies and health (Wenger & Oliffe, 2014), but this matter remains understudied.

There is also increasing evidence of men's navigation of local and societal masculinity ideologies to reflect their social and personal context. Robertson (2006) identified relationships between control of bodily regimes (e.g., diet and exercise) and release from those disciplines (e.g., drinking, smoking); and between don't care–should care (men acknowledging that they should care about their health but don't always do so) in relationship to health and how health discourses are mobilized at different times to achieve or reject hegemonic ideals. Noone and Stephens (2008) presented men with scenarios that facilitated frank focus group discussions of health. They found that although traditional masculinity ideologies were espoused (ill health seen as weakness), by evoking a biomedical discourse, men justified being a user of health services as a "legitimate" strategy to remain in control. In Emslie et al.'s (2006) study of depression, although the majority of men incorporated hegemonic masculinities into their narratives, a minority of men found ways of renegotiating masculinity outside of those discourses by arguing that they did not want to be normal anyway (see Nolan, 2013). Gibbs (2005) found that men with severe arthritis self-identified with traditional masculinity beliefs but recognized themselves that there were multiple masculinity ideologies. They were also aware that they reassessed their responses to hegemonic masculinity as their disease progressed.

Notable in many studies is the lack of differentiation among men in terms of social class, age, culture, and other contextual factors. Also notable is the qualitative methodologies used in the majority of studies. Relatively few studies are quantitative, exceptions being those that come from Levant's group (Levant et al., 2015; Levant & Wimer, 2014; Wimer & Levant, 2013) or from Wade (2008, 2009) that examine correlations between men's support for traditional ideologies and health status or risk-taking. One excellent exception is Springer and Mouzon's (2011) study, which used the Wisconsin Longitudinal Study and found, unexpectedly, that higher levels of wealth and education lowered the likelihood that older men with strong hegemonic masculinity beliefs would participate in preventive health care. They concluded, "our interaction results indicate that if we only looked at the main effects of masculinity or only the main effects of SES [socioeconomic status], we would have misspecified the causes of men's lower preventive health care" (p. 222). This study exposed not only how strong beliefs in traditional masculinity ideologies are linked to poor health behaviors but, ironically, how they interact with SES such that higher SES older men enact masculinity by exercising independence and not obtaining a preventive physical exam, a prostate screening, or a flu shot.

### Health-Related Help-Seeking

Masculinity ideologies influence men's health status not only directly but also indirectly via how those ideologies affect health-related help-seeking behavior (Addis & Mahalik, 2003). Influenced by ideological canons of "no sissy stuff" and "real men don't visit the doctor" (Brannon, 1976; Tannenbaum & Frank, 2011), men can be reluctant to seek help for both physical and mental health problems. Thus, when men's health is compromised, masculinity ideologies are theorized as barriers to men's seeking health care at an early enough stage to prevent their health from worsening.

The majority of research focuses primarily on American men, with some from the United Kingdom and Australia. The majority of the research presents correlational evidence that attitudes toward traditional ideologies and toward help-seeking are related, often using the Male Role Norms Inventory (and its variants; Levant et al., 1992). In all of these studies, authors find a direct relationship between endorsing traditional masculinity ideologies and negative attitudes to professional help-seeking. However, the picture is not straightforward. Levant et al. (2013) found evidence that self-efficacy did not moderate the already-mediated relationship between endorsing traditional masculinity ideology and help-seeking attitudes for mental health problems; there was, however, evidence of how self-stigma mediated the ideology and help-seeking relationship. They argued that it was important to take into account the social and personal context of men and thus how local hegemonic masculinities affect men's acceptance of, or refusal to, engage with help. Using the theory of planned behavior (Ajzen, 1991), J. P. Smith, Tran, and Thompson (2008) found that attitudes toward help-seeking mediated the relationship between masculinity and help-seeking intention. Positive attitudes toward help-seeking increased the intention to seek help in the face of traditional masculinity norms. However, often missing from research is an examination of the relations among attitudes to help-seeking, intention to seek help, and actual consultation.

The cumulative evidence suggests that the relationships between masculinity ideologies and help-seeking are not straightforward. Although there is evidence of the relationship between intention, or attitudes to seek help, and masculinity ideologies, there appears to be little research that examines how ideologies affect actual help-seeking. One exception is the Galdas and Cheater (2010) study of U.K. Asian men's accounts of help-seeking for cardiac chest pain. They found these men sought help promptly and distanced themselves from Western masculinity stereotypes. Another exception is Farrimond's (2012) study of higher SES men who interpreted their help-seeking in terms of being responsible, problem solving, and in control: "Neanderthal man" became "action man." If studies of men are to improve men's health, then researchers need to examine what men actually do, how different illnesses and severity affect decisions, in addition to their attitudes. Already noted is how older men can reconstruct help-seeking to manage a chronic or life-threatening illness as what "men" must do to remain in control. Further, as Levant et al. (2013) suggested, barriers for psychological help-seeking affect some men more than others, but we do not know whether it is the same for physical health problems. Chapple and Ziebland (2002) examined men's experience of prostate cancer and its treatment. They found that men were reluctant to consult doctors and, once in treatment, found the loss of the breadwinner role to be problematic.

An Australian study considered help-seeking more generally (J. A. Smith, Braunack-Mayer, Wittert, & Warin, 2007, 2008). They found that men were not disinterested in their health; rather, they engaged in self-monitoring and made conscious decisions about when, and when not, to seek help (2008). In their earlier paper, they focused on a subsample of older men who reported the avoidance of help-seeking as a means of maintaining independence and control in the face of increased age (and often in opposition to their wives' insistence that they seek help). In sum, the research on masculinity ideologies sheds light on why men resist help-seeking and on their attitudes toward help-seeking, but it tells us little about when men do seek help and how their masculine identities are renegotiated in the light of that help-seeking. But as Wenger (2011) summarized, as much as we know how masculinity is a determinant of the decision to seek medical help, too little is known about how men experience seeking help over the course of responding to the challenges of illness.

**Performance of Marital Status**

The performance of marital status is influenced by masculinity ideologies and proves challenging, whether it be widower, married, divorced, or never married. Much of the research that explicitly relates marital status to masculinity focuses on older men, whether in midlife or in later life. However, Kimmel (2009) discussed how young, never-married men live in accord with a peer-regulated masculinity ideology that shuns adult men's social worlds and, instead, endorses perilous risk-taking. Bandini and Thompson (2013–2014) examined how young widowers (median age 38) in the mid-1960s struggled with the care work their wives needed before they died, then with the challenges of their single-father status in light of the hegemonic masculinity canon to put work before family. Given their age and the era, some moved hurriedly toward remarriage to rebalance their preferred "separate-spheres" lives. In a study of suddenly unemployed middle-aged men, McDaniel (2003) found that they deeply felt the shifts from work to family and its impact on their identities as men. The men found the loss of their breadwinner opportunities challenging. They felt too hidden in the household and felt the loss of their public role.

A compelling body of work examines masculinity ideologies in the light of husbands' caregiving. Kirsi, Hervonen, and Jylhä (2000) asked men to write about the experiences of caring for their wives, a task that one might anticipate would challenge masculinity ideologies. They found that men used four masculinity scripts: factual, agentic, familistic, and destiny. Russell (2007), in his study of older men caring for their wives with dementia, found that the husbands felt their masculine capital was challenged by their necessary change from public careers to food preparer and nurse. Most challenging was the need to undertake intimate bodily care for their wives. It was also a task that they had never expected to undertake. However, in discursive masculinity terms, these men focused on care work as instrumental tasks. Ribeiro, Paúl, and Nogueira (2007), in a study of Portuguese caregivers, found that being in this traditional feminine domain was threatening to the husbands' masculine identities, so they reframed care work in terms of duty and responsibility and derived worth and social standing by "stepping up" to marital obligations.

There is also a small body of work that focuses on widowerhood among older men in relationship to masculinity and exposes how masculinities are not benign. Utilizing Kirsi et al.'s (2000) masculinity scripts, van den Hoonaard, Bennett, and Evans (2014), in a study of Canadian, American, and British widowers, found that when narrating the events that led up to the deaths of their wives, the men used self-blame and medical negligence to maintain a sense of continuity with core values of manhood that advocate taking action, accepting family responsibility, and exercising judgment. This research suggests that men were adhering to masculinity ideologies, while at the same time responding to the expectations of normative bereavement. Bennett (2007) had earlier identified that widowers faced the clashing challenges imposed by masculinity ideals and by the normative expectations of bereavement, after the death. Most widowers do reconstruct their disrupted marital identities to synch with masculinity ideologies. Contrary to expectations, she found that even when admitting to having been shaken and depressed, the widowers recounted how they rebounded and reclaimed masculine capital by being "sturdy oaks." This observation is not isolated (cf. Lund & Caserta, 2001). More recently, Bennett (2014) also pointed to the ways in which men not only behave in respect to traditional masculinity ideals but how they speak about the "rightness" of manhood ideals. The men may be doing traditionally female tasks while caring for wives, but they reconstruct them, using speech, into masculine tasks; as Moore and Stratton (2003) reported for one their widowers, he *built* a meal. These were older men, brought up with traditional notions of masculinity. Through necessity and masculinized speech, they transform their new (traditionally feminine) responsibilities into tasks for widowers.


## CONCLUSION

The past quarter century has seen tremendous advances in the study of masculinity ideologies. This progress was prompted by recognition that hegemonic masculinities exist and remained understudied, by consideration of the toxicity of patriarchal masculinities to relations among men and between women and men, and by determined efforts to empirically chart the effects of compliance with masculinities on men's bodies and personal well-being, including unacknowledged privilege. In using qualitative methodologies, and less so quantitative methodologies, to address these concerns, researchers across the social and medical science disciplines have prodded and encouraged greater attention to the society-wide, regional, and local hegemonic ideologies that coexist and codetermine interpersonal relations and individuals' actions.

Much more is known about the character and correlates of masculinities, the similarities and differences among ideologies across different demographic groups, the suspected pathways that lead from ideologies to observable actions, and the implications of masculinity ideologies for society, communities, and individuals. We know more about the mechanisms that link factors such as class, ethnicity, group memberships, and age to masculinity practices and capital. In the process, we have learned about the difficulties of measuring masculinity ideologies, the complexities of charting which coexisting ideologies steer decisions and actions, and the importance of mixed-method studies that supplement survey data with rich ethnographic or narrative-based understandings of the masculinity ideologies underpinning men's (and women's) lives, at the moment.

Despite these advances, much work remains. One problem is that the construct *masculinity ideology* was temporarily hijacked by a logic that the ideology resides inside the minds of individuals. Thompson and Bennett (2015a) proposed the importance of distinguishing masculinity ideologies from beliefs about or attitudes toward an ideology and prefer calling the latter *masculinity beliefs*. Their concern (Thompson & Bennett, 2015b) is that an individual-level of analysis can blind us to the contextual influences on men's lives as well as mask matters of inequality:

> Sorely needed is a broadening of perspectives to help determine how the relational character of masculinities and thus gender inequalities are influential as well as lived. How birth cohort, age, class, skin color, ethnicity, and one's "home" community (re)produce similar and different masculinity ideologies is a difficult question, but a critically important one as our social worlds become more global and thus less "mainstream" in normative structure. (p. 147)

Another matter warranting great attention are how the taxonomies of masculinity ideologies have used folk categories—"traditional," "nontraditional"—that are no longer sociologically or psychologically useful, given familiarity with the premise of hegemonic masculinities coexisting. Third, the study of the consequences, or implications, of masculinity ideologies has only just begun. Well charted are many ill effects that individuals experience and live with but understudied are matters of relational power and the intersections of masculinities with other systems of oppression yielding privilege based on gendered age, class, marital status, or body wholeness. The limited research on "intersectionality" is full of promise, but it has been largely confined to demographic categories. More studies are needed on variations within categories, such as how older men with and without life-threatening illnesses live in synch with what masculinity ideologies.

## REFERENCES

Addis, M. E., & Mahalik, J. R. (2003). Men, masculinity, and the contexts of help seeking. *American Psychologist, 58*, 5–14. http://dx.doi.org/10.1037/0003-066X.58.1.5

Ajzen, I. (1991). The theory of planned behavior. *Organizational Behavior and Human Decision Processes, 50*, 179–211. http://dx.doi.org/10.1016/0749-5978(91)90020-T

Alexander, S. M. (2003). Stylish hard bodies: Branded masculinity in *Men's Health* magazine. *Sociological Perspectives, 46*, 535–554. http://dx.doi.org/10.1525/sop.2003.46.4.535

Anderson, P. (2012). Measuring masculinity in an Afro-Caribbean context. *Social and Economic Studies, 61*, 49–93.

Arciniega, G. M., Anderson, T. C., Tovar-Blank, Z. G., & Tracey, T. J. G. (2008). Toward a fuller conception of machismo: Development of a traditional machismo and caballerismo scale. *Journal of Counseling Psychology, 55*, 19–33. http://dx.doi.org/10.1037/0022-0167.55.1.19

Baca Zinn, M. (1982). Chicano men and masculinity. *The Journal of Ethnic Studies, 10*, 29–44.

Baca Zinn, M., & Thornton Dill, B. (1996). Theorizing difference from multiracial feminism. *Feminist Studies, 22*, 321–331. http://dx.doi.org/10.2307/3178416

Bandini, J., & Thompson, E. H., Jr. (2013–2014). "Widowerhood": Masculinities and spousal loss in the late-1960s. *Omega: Journal of Death and Dying, 68*, 123–141. http://dx.doi.org/10.2190/OM.68.2.c

Barrett, F. J. (1996). The organizational construction of hegemonic masculinity: The case of the U.S. Navy. *Gender, Work and Organization, 3*, 129–142. http://dx.doi.org/10.1111/j.1468-0432.1996.tb00054.x

Bem, S. L. (1974). The measurement of psychological androgyny. *Journal of Consulting and Clinical Psychology, 42*, 155–162. http://dx.doi.org/10.1037/h0036215

Bennett, K. M. (2007). "No sissy stuff": Towards a theory of masculinity and emotional expression in older widowed men. *Journal of Aging Studies, 21*, 347–356. http://dx.doi.org/10.1016/j.jaging.2007.05.002

Bennett, K. M. (2014). "I thought I could look after her as good as anybody": How older widowers' reconstruct their masculinity. In A. Tarrant & J. Watts (Eds.), *Ageing masculinities* (pp. 20–37). Maidenhead, England: Open University Press.

Berger, P. L., & Luckmann, T. (1967). *The social construction of reality: A treatise in the sociology of knowledge*. New York, NY: Penguin Books.

Bourgois, P., & Schonberg, J. (2007). Ethnic dimensions of habitus among homeless heroin injectors. *Ethnography, 8,* 7–31. http://dx.doi.org/10.1177/1466138107076109

Brannon, R. (1976). The male sex role: Our culture's blueprint for manhood and what it's done for us lately. In D. David & R. Brannon (Eds.), *The forty-nine percent majority: The male sex role* (pp. 1–49). Reading, MA: Addison-Wesley.

Brannon, R., & Juni, S. (1984). A scale for measuring attitudes about masculinity. *Psychological Documents, 14,* 67 (Doc. #2612).

Bureychak, T. (2013). Zooming in and out: Historical icons of masculinity within and across nations. In J. Hearn, M. Blagojevic, & K. Harrison (Eds.), *Rethinking transnational men: Beyond, between and within nations* (pp. 219–237). London, England: Routledge.

Cabrera, N. J., & Tamis-LeMonda, C. S. (Eds.). (2013). *Handbook of father involvement: Multidisciplinary perspectives*. New York, NY: Routledge.

Calasanti, T., Pietilä, I., Ojala, H., & King, N. (2013). Men, bodily control, and health behaviors: The importance of age. *Health Psychology, 32,* 15–23. http://dx.doi.org/10.1037/a0029300

Campbell, L. D., & Carroll, M. P. (2007). The incomplete revolution: Theorizing gender when studying men who provide care to aging parents. *Men and Masculinities, 9,* 491–508. http://dx.doi.org/10.1177/1097184X05284222

Carrigan, T., Connell, B., & Lee, J. (1985). Towards a new sociology of masculinity. *Theory and Society, 14,* 551–604. http://dx.doi.org/10.1007/BF00160017

Chapple, A., & Ziebland, S. (2002). Prostate cancer: Embodied experience and perceptions of masculinity. *Sociology of Health & Illness, 24,* 820–841. http://dx.doi.org/10.1111/1467-9566.00320

Chu, J. Y., Porche, M. V., & Tolman, D. L. (2005). The Adolescent Masculinity Ideology in Relationships Scale: Development and validation of a new measure for boys. *Men and Masculinities, 8,* 93–115. http://dx.doi.org/10.1177/1097184X03257453

Cohen, D., Nisbett, R. E., Bowdle, B. F., & Schwarz, N. (1996). Insult, aggression, and the Southern culture of honor: An "experimental ethnography." *Journal of Personality and Social Psychology, 70,* 945–959. http://dx.doi.org/10.1037/0022-3514.70.5.945

Coles, T. (2009). Negotiating the field of masculinity: The production and reproduction of multiple dominant masculinities. *Men and Masculinities, 12,* 30–44. http://dx.doi.org/10.1177/1097184X07309502

Connell, R. W. (1987). *Gender and power*. Stanford, CA: Stanford University Press.

Connell, R. W. (1992). A very straight gay: Masculinity, homosexual experience, and the dynamics of gender. *American Sociological Review, 57*, 735–751. http://dx.doi.org/10.2307/2096120

Connell, R. W. (1995). *Masculinities*. Berkeley: University of California Press.

Connell, R. W., & Messerschmidt, J. W. (2005). Hegemonic masculinity: Rethinking the concept. *Gender & Society, 19*, 829–859. http://dx.doi.org/10.1177/0891243205278639

Courtenay, W. H. (2000a). Constructions of masculinity and their influence on men's well-being: A theory of gender and health. *Social Science & Medicine, 50*, 1385–1401. http://dx.doi.org/10.1016/S0277-9536(99)00390-1

Courtenay, W. H. (2000b). Engendering health: A social constructionist examination of men's health beliefs and behaviors. *Psychology of Men & Masculinity, 1*, 4–15. http://dx.doi.org/10.1037/1524-9220.1.1.4

Davidson, K., Arber, S., & Marshall, H. (2008). Gender and food in later life: Shifting roles and relationships. In M. M. Raats, C. P. G. M. de Groot, & W. A. van Staveren (Eds.), *Food for the ageing population* (pp. 110–127). Cambridge, England: Woodhead.

Davis, S. N., & Greenstein, T. N. (2009). Gender ideology: Components, predictors, and consequences. *Annual Review of Sociology, 35*, 87–105. http://dx.doi.org/10.1146/annurev-soc-070308-115920

Deaux, K., & Major, B. (1987). Putting gender into context: An interactive model of gender-related behavior. *Psychological Review, 94*, 369–389. http://dx.doi.org/10.1037/0033-295X.94.3.369

Doss, B. D., & Hopkins, J. R. (1998). The multicultural masculinity ideology scale: Validation from three cultural perspectives. *Sex Roles, 38*, 719–741. http://dx.doi.org/10.1023/A:1018816929544

Duneier, M. (1992). *Slim's table: Race, respectability, and masculinity*. Chicago, IL: University of Chicago Press.

Edley, N., & Wetherell, M. (1995). *Men in perspective: Practice, power and identity*. New York, NY: Prentice Hall.

Embrick, D. G., Walther, C. S., & Wickens, C. M. (2007). Working class masculinity: Keeping gay men and lesbians out of the workplace. *Sex Roles, 56*, 757–766. http://dx.doi.org/10.1007/s11199-007-9234-0

Emslie, C., Ridge, D., Ziebland, S., & Hunt, K. (2006). Men's accounts of depression: Reconstructing or resisting hegemonic masculinity? *Social Science & Medicine, 62*, 2246–2257. http://dx.doi.org/10.1016/j.socscimed.2005.10.017

Evans, J., Frank, B., Oliffe, J. L., & Gregory, D. (2011). Health, illness, men and masculinities (HIMM): A theoretical framework for understanding men and their health. *Journal of Men's Health, 8*, 7–15. http://dx.doi.org/10.1016/j.jomh.2010.09.227

Farough, S. D. (2006). Believing is seeing: The matrix of vision and white masculinities. *Journal of Contemporary Ethnography, 35*, 51–83. http://dx.doi.org/10.1177/0891241605280494

Farrimond, H. (2012). Beyond the cavemen: Rethinking masculinity in relation to men's help-seeking. *Health, 16,* 208–225. http://dx.doi.org/10.1177/1363459311403943

Fischer, A. R., Tokar, D. M., Good, G. E., & Snell, A. F. (1998). More on the structure of male role norms. *Psychology of Women Quarterly, 22,* 135–155. http://dx.doi.org/10.1111/j.1471-6402.1998.tb00147.x

Franklin, C. W., II. (1994). Ain't I a man? The efficacy of Black masculinities for men's studies in the 1990s. In R. Majors & J. U. Gordon (Eds.), *The American Black male: His present status and his future* (pp. 271–283). Chicago, IL: Nelson-Hall.

Friedan, B. (1963). *The feminine mystique.* New York, NY: Norton.

Friend, C. T. (2009). From Southern manhood to Southern masculinities: An introduction. In C. T. Friend (Ed.), *Southern masculinity: Perspectives on manhood in the South since Reconstruction* (pp. vii–xxvi). Athens: University of Georgia Press.

Fuller, N. (2001). The social construction of gender identity among Peruvian men. *Men and Masculinities, 3,* 316–331. http://dx.doi.org/10.1177/1097184X01003003006

Galdas, P. M., & Cheater, F. M. (2010). Indian and Pakistani men's accounts of seeking medical help for cardiac chest pain in the United Kingdom: Constructions of marginalised masculinity or another version of hegemonic masculinity? *Qualitative Research in Psychology, 7,* 122–139. http://dx.doi.org/10.1080/14780880802571168

Garfinkel, H. (1967). *Studies in ethnomethodology.* Englewood Cliffs, NJ: Prentice-Hall.

Gergen, K. J. (1985). The social constructionist movement in modern psychology. *American Psychologist, 40,* 266–275. http://dx.doi.org/10.1037/0003-066X.40.3.266

Gerschick, T. J., & Miller, A. S. (1995). Coming to terms: Masculinity and physical disability. In D. F. Sabo & D. F. Gordon (Eds.), *Men's health and illness: Gender, power, and the body* (pp. 183–204). http://dx.doi.org/10.4135/9781452243757.n9

Gibbs, L. (2005). Applications of masculinity theories in a chronic illness context. *International Journal of Men's Health, 4,* 287–300. http://dx.doi.org/10.3149/jmh.0403.287

Goffman, E. (1967). *Interaction ritual: Essays in face-to-face behavior.* New Brunswick, NJ: Transaction.

Gough, B., & Conner, M. T. (2006). Barriers to healthy eating amongst men: A qualitative analysis. *Social Science & Medicine, 62,* 387–395. http://dx.doi.org/10.1016/j.socscimed.2005.05.032

Grubbs, J. B., Exline, J. J., & Twenge, J. M. (2014). Psychological entitlement and ambivalent sexism: Understanding the role of entitlement in predicting two forms of sexism. *Sex Roles, 70,* 209–220. http://dx.doi.org/10.1007/s11199-014-0360-1

Harrison, J. (1978). Warning: The male sex role may be dangerous to your health. *Journal of Social Issues, 34,* 65–86. http://dx.doi.org/10.1111/j.1540-4560.1978.tb02541.x

Harvey, I. S., & Alston, R. J. (2011). Understanding preventive behaviors among mid-Western African-American men: A pilot qualitative study of prostate screening. *Journal of Men's Health, 8,* 140–151. http://dx.doi.org/10.1016/j.jomh.2011.03.005

Hearn, J. (2002). Men, fathers and the state: National and global relations. In B. Hobson (Ed.), *Making men into fathers: Men, masculinities and the social politics of fatherhood* (pp. 245–272). http://dx.doi.org/10.1017/CBO9780511489440.011

Hearn, J., Nordberg, M., Andersson, K., Balkmar, D., Gottzén, L., Klinth, P., . . . Sandberg, L. (2012). Hegemonic masculinity and beyond: 40 years of research in Sweden. *Men and Masculinities, 15,* 31–55.

Hearn, J., Pringle, K., Muller, U., Oleksy, E., Lattu, E., Chernova, J., . . . Tallberg, T. (2002). Critical studies of men in ten European countries: 1. The state of academic research. *Men and Masculinities, 4,* 380–408. http://dx.doi.org/10.1177/1097184X02004004007

Hennen, P. (2005). Bear bodies, bear masculinity: Recuperation, resistance, or retreat? *Gender & Society, 19,* 25–43. http://dx.doi.org/10.1177/0891243204269408

Hochschild, A. R. (1990). Ideology and emotion management. In T. D. Kemper (Ed.), *Research agendas in the sociology of emotions* (pp. 117–142). Albany: State University of New York Press.

Hochschild, A. R. (with Machung, A.). (1989). *The second shift.* New York, NY: Viking.

Irwin, R. M. (2003). *Mexican masculinities.* Minneapolis: University of Minnesota Press.

Janey, B. A., Kim, T., Jampolskaja, T., Khuda, A., Larionov, A., Maksimenko, A., . . . Shipilova, A. (2013). Development of the Russian Male Norms Inventory. *Psychology of Men & Masculinity, 14,* 138–147. http://dx.doi.org/10.1037/a0028159

Kimmel, M. S. (1996). *Manhood in America: A cultural history.* New York, NY: Free Press.

Kimmel, M. S. (2009). *Guyland: The perilous world where boys become men.* New York, NY: Harper Perennial.

Kimmel, M. S. (2013). *Angry White men: American masculinity at the end of an era.* New York, NY: Nation Books.

Kimmel, M. S., Hearn, J., & Connell, R. W. (2005). *Handbook of studies on men and masculinities.* Thousand Oaks, CA: Sage.

Kirsi, T., Hervonen, A., & Jylhä, M. (2000). A man's gotta do what a man's gotta do: Husbands as caregivers to their demented wives: A discourse analytic approach. *Journal of Aging Studies, 14,* 153–169. http://dx.doi.org/10.1016/S0890-4065(00)80009-2

Levant, R. F., & Richmond, K. (2007). A review of research on masculinity ideologies using the Male Role Norms Inventory. *The Journal of Men's Studies, 15,* 130–146. http://dx.doi.org/10.3149/jms.1502.130

Levant, R. F., & Wimer, D. J. (2014). Masculinity constructs as protective buffers and risk factors for men's health. *American Journal of Men's Health, 8,* 110–120. http://dx.doi.org/10.1177/1557988313494408

Levant, R. F., Graef, S. T., Smalley, K. B., Williams, C., & McMillan, N. (2008). Evaluation of the psychometric properties of the Male Role Norms Inventory—Adolescent (MRNI–A). *Thymos: Journal of Boyhood Studies, 2,* 46–59.

Levant, R. F., Hirsch, L. S., Celentano, E., Cozza, T. M., Hill, S., MacEachern, M., ... Schnedeker, J. (1992). The male role: An investigation of contemporary norms. *Journal of Mental Health Counseling, 14,* 325–337.

Levant, R. F., Parent, M. C., McCurdy, E. R., & Bradstreet, T. C. (2015). Moderated mediation of the relationships between masculinity ideology, outcome expectations, and energy drink use. *Health Psychology, 34,* 1100–1106. http://dx.doi.org/10.1037/hea0000214

Levant, R. F., Smalley, K. B., Aupont, M., House, A., Richmond, K., & Noronha, D. (2007). Initial validation of the Male Role Norms Inventory—Revised (MRNI–R). *The Journal of Men's Studies, 15,* 83–100. http://dx.doi.org/10.3149/jms.1501.83

Levant, R. F., Stefanov, D. G., Rankin, T. J., Halter, M. J., Mellinger, C., & Williams, C. M. (2013). Moderated path analysis of the relationships between masculinity and men's attitudes toward seeking psychological help. *Journal of Counseling Psychology, 60,* 392–406. http://dx.doi.org/10.1037/a0033014

Lewis, G. H. (1984). Mapping the fault lines: The core values trap in country music. *Popular Music and Society, 9,* 7–16. http://dx.doi.org/10.1080/03007768408591226

Lorber, J. (1993). Believing is seeing: Biology as ideology. *Gender & Society, 7,* 568–581. http://dx.doi.org/10.1177/089124393007004006

Lorber, J. (1994). *Paradoxes of gender.* New Haven, CT: Yale University Press.

Lund, D., & Caserta, M. (2001). When the unexpected happens: Husbands coping with the death of their wives. In D. Lund (Ed.), *Men coping with grief* (pp. 147–167). Amityville, NY: Baywood.

Luyt, R. (2005). The Male Attitude Norms Inventory—II: A measure of masculinity ideology in South Africa. *Men and Masculinities, 8,* 208–229. http://dx.doi.org/10.1177/1097184X04264631

Magovcevic, M., & Addis, M. E. (2008). The Masculine Depression Scale: Development and psychometric evaluation. *Psychology of Men & Masculinity, 9,* 117–132. http://dx.doi.org/10.1037/1524-9220.9.3.117

Mahalik, J. R., Locke, B. D., Ludlow, L. H., Diemer, M. A., Scott, R. P. J., Gottfried, M., & Freitas, G. (2003). Development of the Conformity to Masculine Norms Inventory. *Psychology of Men & Masculinity, 4,* 3–25.

Mannheim, K. (1936). *Ideology and utopia: An introduction to the sociology of knowledge.* London, England: Routledge.

Martin, E. (1991). The egg and the sperm: How science has constructed a romance based on stereotypical male–female roles. *Signs: Journal of Women in Culture and Society, 16*, 485–501. http://dx.doi.org/10.1086/494680

Martin, H., & Finn, S. E. (2010). *Masculinity and femininity in the MMPI–2 and MMPI–A*. Minneapolis: University of Minnesota Press.

Martin, P. Y. (2004). Gender as social institution. *Social Forces, 82*, 1249–1273. http://dx.doi.org/10.1353/sof.2004.0081

McCreary, D. R., Saucier, D. M., & Courtenay, W. H. (2005). The drive for muscularity and masculinity: Testing the associations among gender-role traits, behaviors, attitudes, and conflict. *Psychology of Men & Masculinity, 6*, 83–94. http://dx.doi.org/10.1037/1524-9220.6.2.83

McCusker, K. M., & Pecknold, D. (2004). *A boy named Sue: Gender and country music*. Jackson: University Press of Mississippi.

McDaniel, S. A. (2003). Hidden in the household: Now it's men in mid-life. *Ageing International, 28*, 326–344. http://dx.doi.org/10.1007/s12126-003-1007-7

McVittie, C., & Willock, J. (2006). "You can't fight windmills": How older men do health, ill health, and masculinities. *Qualitative Health Research, 16*, 788–801. http://dx.doi.org/10.1177/1049732306288453

Messerschmidt, J. W. (2012). Engendering gendered knowledge: Assessing the academic appropriation of hegemonic masculinity. *Men and Masculinities, 15*, 56–76. http://dx.doi.org/10.1177/1097184X11428384

Moore, A. J., & Stratton, D. C. (2003). *Resilient widowers: Older men adjusting to a new life*. New York, NY: Prometheus Books.

Moore, S. D., & Anderson, J. C. (1998). Taking it like a man: Masculinity in 4 Maccabees. *Journal of Biblical Literature, 117*, 249–273. http://dx.doi.org/10.2307/3266982

Nardi, P. M. (2000). *Gay masculinities*. Thousand Oaks, CA: Sage.

Neal, M. A. (1999). *What the music said: Black popular music and Black public culture*. New York, NY: Routledge.

Nelkin, D., & Michaels, M. (1998). Biological categories and border controls: The revival of eugenics in anti-immigration rhetoric. *The International Journal of Sociology and Social Policy, 18*(5–6), 35–63. http://dx.doi.org/10.1108/01443339810788425

Nolan, M. (2013). Masculinity lost: A systematic review of qualitative research on men with spinal cord injury. *Spinal Cord, 51*, 588–595. http://dx.doi.org/10.1038/sc.2013.22

Noone, J. H., & Stephens, C. (2008). Men, masculine identities, and health care utilisation. *Sociology of Health & Illness, 30*, 711–725. http://dx.doi.org/10.1111/j.1467-9566.2008.01095.x

O'Brien, R., Hunt, K., & Hart, G. (2005). "It's caveman stuff, but that is to a certain extent how guys still operate": Men's accounts of masculinity and help seeking. *Social Science & Medicine, 61,* 503–516. http://dx.doi.org/10.1016/j.socscimed.2004.12.008

O'Brien, R., Hunt, K., & Hart, G. (2009). "The average Scottish man has a cigarette hanging out of his mouth, lying there with a portion of chips": Prospects for change in Scottish men's constructions of masculinity and their health-related beliefs and behaviours. *Critical Public Health, 19,* 363–381. http://dx.doi.org/10.1080/09581590902939774

Oliffe, J. L. (2009). Health behaviors, prostate cancer and masculinities: A life course perspective. *Men and Masculinities, 11,* 346–366. http://dx.doi.org/10.1177/1097184X06298777

Olsen, C. J. (2000). *Secession in Mississippi: Masculinity, honor, and the antiparty tradition, 1830–1860.* New York, NY: Oxford University Press.

O'Neil, J. M. (1981). Patterns of gender role conflict and strain: Sexism and fear of femininity in men's lives. *Personnel & Guidance Journal, 60,* 203–210. http://dx.doi.org/10.1002/j.2164-4918.1981.tb00282.x

O'Neil, J. M., Helms, B. J., Gable, R. K., David, L., & Wrightsman, L. S. (1986). Gender Role Conflict Scale: College men's fear of femininity. *Sex Roles, 14,* 335–350.

Oransky, M., & Fisher, C. (2009). The development and validation of the Meanings of Adolescent Masculinity Scale. *Psychology of Men & Masculinity, 10,* 57–72. http://dx.doi.org/10.1037/a0013612

Pleck, J. H. (1981). *The myth of masculinity.* Cambridge, MA: MIT Press.

Pleck, J. H. (1995). The gender role strain paradigm: An update. In R. F. Levant & W. S. Pollack (Eds.), *A new psychology of men* (pp. 11–32). New York, NY: Basic Books.

Pleck, J. H., Sonenstein, F. L., & Ku, L. C. (1993). Masculinity ideology: Its impact on adolescent males' heterosexual relationships. *Journal of Social Issues, 49,* 11–29. http://dx.doi.org/10.1111/j.1540-4560.1993.tb01166.x

Pyke, K. D. (1996). Class-based masculinities: The interdependence of gender, class, and interpersonal power. *Gender & Society, 10,* 527–549. http://dx.doi.org/10.1177/089124396010005003

Ribeiro, O., Paúl, C., & Nogueira, C. (2007). Real men, real husbands: Caregiving and masculinities in later life. *Journal of Aging Studies, 21,* 302–313. http://dx.doi.org/10.1016/j.jaging.2007.05.005

Robertson, S. (2006). 'Not living life in too much of an excess': Lay men understanding health and well-being. *Health, 10,* 175–189. http://dx.doi.org/10.1177/1363459306061787

Russell, R. (2007). The work of elderly men caregiver: From public careers to an unseen world. *Men and Masculinities, 9,* 298–314. http://dx.doi.org/10.1177/1097184X05277712

Sabo, D. (2005). The study of masculinities and men's health. In M. Kimmel, J. Hearn, & R. Connell (Eds.), *Handbook of studies on men and masculinities* (pp. 326–352). http://dx.doi.org/10.4135/9781452233833.n19

Schrock, D., & Schwalbe, M. (2009). Men, masculinity, and manhood acts. *Annual Review of Sociology*, *35*, 277–295. http://dx.doi.org/10.1146/annurev-soc-070308-115933

Segal, L. (1990). *Slow motion: Changing masculinities, changing men.* Newark, NJ: Rutgers University Press.

Sloan, C., Gough, B., & Conner, M. (2010). Healthy masculinities? How ostensibly healthy men talk about lifestyle, health and gender. *Psychology & Health*, *25*, 783–803. http://dx.doi.org/10.1080/08870440902883204

Smith, J. A., Braunack-Mayer, A., Wittert, G., & Warin, M. (2007). "I've been independent for so damn long!" Independence, masculinity and aging in a help seeking context. *Journal of Aging Studies*, *21*, 325–335. http://dx.doi.org/10.1016/j.jaging.2007.05.004

Smith, J. A., Braunack-Mayer, A., Wittert, G., & Warin, M. (2008). "It's sort of like being a detective": Understanding how Australian men self-monitor their health prior to seeking help. *BMC Health Services Research*, *8*(1), 56. http://dx.doi.org/10.1186/1472-6963-8-56

Smith, J. P., Tran, G. Q., & Thompson, R. D. (2008). Can the theory of planned behavior help explain men's psychological help-seeking? Evidence for a mediation effect and clinical implications. *Psychology of Men & Masculinity*, *9*, 179–192. http://dx.doi.org/10.1037/a0012158

Springer, K. W., & Mouzon, D. M. (2011). "Macho men" and preventive health care: Implications for older men in different social classes. *Journal of Health and Social Behavior*, *52*, 212–227. http://dx.doi.org/10.1177/0022146510393972

Tannenbaum, C., & Frank, B. (2011). Masculinity and health in late life men. *American Journal of Men's Health*, *5*, 243–254. http://dx.doi.org/10.1177/1557988310384609

Terman, L. M., & Miles, C. C. (1936). *Sex and personality: Studies in masculinity and femininity.* http://dx.doi.org/10.1037/13514-000

Thompson, E. H., Jr., & Bennett, K. M. (2015a). Measurement of masculinity ideologies: A (critical) review. *Psychology of Men & Masculinity*, *16*, 115–133. http://dx.doi.org/10.1037/a0038609

Thompson, E. H., Jr., & Bennett, K. M. (2015b). Response to commentaries on masculinity ideologies. *Psychology of Men & Masculinity*, *16*, 145–148. http://dx.doi.org/10.1037/a0039083

Thompson, E. H., Jr., Grisanti, C., & Pleck, J. H. (1985). Attitudes toward the male role and their correlates. *Sex Roles*, *13*, 413–427. http://dx.doi.org/10.1007/BF00287952

Thompson, E. H., Jr., & Pleck, J. H. (1986). The structure of male role norms. *American Behavioral Scientist*, *29*, 531–543. http://dx.doi.org/10.1177/000276486029005003

Thompson, E. H., Jr., Pleck, J. H., & Ferrera, D. L. (1992). Men and masculinities: Scales for masculinity ideology and masculinity-related constructs. *Sex Roles*, *27*, 573–607. http://dx.doi.org/10.1007/BF02651094

Tolman, D. L., & Porche, M. V. (2000). The Adolescent Femininity Ideology Scale: Development and validation of a new measure for girls. *Psychology of Women Quarterly, 24*, 365–376. http://dx.doi.org/10.1111/j.1471-6402.2000.tb00219.x

van den Hoonaard, D. K., Bennett, K. M., & Evans, E. (2014). "I was there when she passed away": Older widowers' narratives of the death of their wife. *Ageing & Society, 34*, 974–991. http://dx.doi.org/10.1017/S0144686X12001353

Wade, J. C. (2008). Masculinity ideology, male reference group identity dependence, and African American men's health-related attitudes and behaviors. *Psychology of Men & Masculinity, 9*, 5–16. http://dx.doi.org/10.1037/1524-9220.9.1.5

Wade, J. C. (2009). Traditional masculinity and African American men's health-related attitudes and behaviors. *American Journal of Men's Health, 3*, 165–172. http://dx.doi.org/10.1177/1557988308320180

Wenger, L. M. (2011). Beyond ballistics: Expanding our conceptualization of men's health-related help seeking. *American Journal of Men's Health, 5*, 488–499. http://dx.doi.org/10.1177/1557988311409022

Wenger, L. M., & Oliffe, J. L. (2014). Men managing cancer: A gender analysis. *Sociology of Health & Illness, 36*, 108–122. http://dx.doi.org/10.1111/1467-9566.12045

Wentzell, E. A. (2013). *Maturing masculinities: Aging, chronic illness, and Viagra in Mexico.* http://dx.doi.org/10.1215/9780822377528

West, C., & Zimmerman, D. H. (2009). Accounting for doing gender. *Gender & Society, 23*, 112–122. http://dx.doi.org/10.1177/0891243208326529

Wimer, D. J., & Levant, R. F. (2013). Energy drink use and its relationship to masculinity, jock identity, and fraternity membership among men. *American Journal of Men's Health, 7*, 317–328. http://dx.doi.org/10.1177/1557988312474034

Wong, Y. J., Horn, A. J., Gomory, A. M. G., & Ramos, E. (2013). Measure of Men's Perceived Inexpressiveness Norms (M2PIN): Scale development and psychometric properties. *Psychology of Men & Masculinity, 14*, 288–299. http://dx.doi.org/10.1037/a0029244

Wong, Y. J., Shea, M., LaFollette, J. R., Hickman, S. J., Cruz, N., & Boghokian, T. (2011). The inventory of subjective masculinity experiences: Development and psychometric properties. *The Journal of Men's Studies, 19*, 236–255. http://dx.doi.org/10.3149/jms.1903.236

# 3

# MASCULINITY AS A HEURISTIC: GENDER ROLE CONFLICT THEORY, SUPERORGANISMS, AND SYSTEM-LEVEL THINKING

JAMES M. O'NEIL, STEPHEN R. WESTER, MARTIN HEESACKER, AND STEVEN J. SNOWDEN

*Gender role conflict* (GRC; O'Neil, Helms, Gable, David, & Wrightsman, 1986) is a psychological state in which socialized gender roles have negative consequences for individuals. It occurs when rigid, sexist, or restrictive gender roles result in personal restrictions, deviations, or violations of others or oneself. The ultimate outcome of this conflict is a restriction of the human potential of either the person experiencing it or those around that person. This definition has evolved from a series of theoretical and research manuscripts produced over the past 35 years (O'Neil, 1981, 2008, 2012, 2015; O'Neil & Denke, 2016), and a more detailed explanation of GRC theory is found in earlier publications (see http://web.uconn.edu/joneil), but it is important to note that GRC is distinct from theories about (and the measurement of) masculinity ideologies (e.g., Levant & Richmond, 2016) or hegemonic masculinity (Connell & Messerschmidt, 2005). Masculinity ideologies are beliefs and attitudes about masculine norms, and the idea of masculinity as a hegemony

http://dx.doi.org/10.1037/0000023-004
*The Psychology of Men and Masculinities*, R. F. Levant and Y. J. Wong (Editors)

refers to the dominant position of those ideologies. GRC, conversely, is a consequence of adherence to those beliefs and attitudes in situations where the contextual demands might require a different behavioral approach (e.g., Wester & Vogel, 2012). In essence, GRC results when the socialized gender role expectations do not allow individual men the behavioral flexibility to adaptively respond to specific situational demands (e.g., Wester, 2008).

GRC theory (e.g., O'Neil, 1981) grew directly out of the nonsexist men's movement. "The feminist movement of the 1970s was the primary stimulus for the men's liberation movement that ultimately evolved into men's studies and the psychology of men" (O'Neil, 2015, p. 6). The goal was to be part of the feminist dialogues regarding restrictive gender roles and ultimately to develop a theory and a research program that explained how sexism and gender roles interacted to produce oppression for both sexes. The broader assumptions about men that drove scholarship during this time period therefore led to GRC being used to support the ideological conclusions regarding masculinity that had been made by the nonsexist men's movement. Said another way, the questions being asked, important though they may have been, arose from specific epistemological perspectives (e.g., O'Neil, 2015):

> Why were men so unhappy and seeking liberation in the men's movements? Why did men have so many problems with women in intimate and work relationships? Why did men communicate differently than women and not express many feelings? Why did men work so much and die earlier than women? Why did men avoid domestic work and fathering roles? Why were men violent? Why did men molest children, fear homosexuals, and become addicted or sexually dysfunctional? Why did men harass, rape, and batter women? How could we get men to change? (p. 17)

As these questions imply, the goal of researchers focusing on men and masculinity during this period was to reaffirm the ideals of feminism by challenging the sociocultural forces that constrained men's choices in ways similar to how they constrained women's choices (e.g., Brooks & Elder, 2016; Levant & Richmond, 2016). The core assumption was that society's culturally embedded gender roles were restrictive in that they prevented individuals from charting their own path as well as selecting activities, behaviors, and values congruent with their sense of themselves (O'Neil, 2015). Said another way, there existed a masculinity ideology independent from femininity that consisted of the "internalization of cultural belief systems about masculinity and male gender, rooted in the structural relationships between the sexes" (Pleck, 1995, p. 19). That relationship, as we have noted elsewhere (e.g., Wester, Heesacker, & Snowden, 2016), was characterized as a trait or group of interrelated traits, assumed to have transtemporal as well as transsituational stability, while being operationalized by the behavioral differences between men and women that, socialized as they were within a patriarchal society, acted to oppress women, maintain patriarchy, and harm men themselves.

Men are expected, for example, to be stoic and unemotional to be defined as masculine. They were taught as boys that real men strive for individual success, are focused in their career, and put power and competition ahead of their family. Violations of those ideologies are punished, both as one grows into adulthood and during that adulthood. Certainly, many men are able to cope with these expectations; others have become too rigid, possibly distorted by the ideologically driven messages so common in today's society regarding how men should and should not behave, such that they are unable to conceive of other behavioral options. The distortion occurs because of perceived or actual pressure to meet stereotypical notions of masculinity, resulting in fears and anxieties about not measuring up to traditional gender role expectations (Vandello & Bosson, 2013). The idea that men should strive for power and financial success solely through competitive means would be an example; behaviors that are functional in one setting became maladaptive when overused or misapplied.

Four empirically derived patterns of GRC (O'Neil, 2015; O'Neil, Good, & Holmes, 1995), measured by the Gender Role Conflict Scale (GRCS; O'Neil et al., 1986), have been linked to many types of men's psychological distress (see Wester & Vogel, 2012, for a review). Each pattern gives voice to those specific aspects of the socialized traditional male role deemed problematic for some men in certain situations. Success, Power, and Competition (SPC), the first GRC pattern, refers to personal attitudes toward success as pursued through power and competition. The second pattern, Restricted Emotionality (RE), is defined as having restrictions and fears about expressing one's feelings. The third pattern, Restricted Affectionate Behavior Between Men (RABBM), represents restrictions in expressing one's tender feelings and thoughts with other men. Finally, the fourth pattern, Conflict Between Work and Family Relationships (CBWFR), discusses restrictions in balancing work, school, and family relations resulting in health problems, over work, stress, and a lack of leisure and relaxation.

The psychological domains of GRC imply problems that occur at four overlapping and complex levels—cognitive, emotional (affective), behavioral, and unconscious—and are caused by restrictive gender roles learned in sexist and patriarchal societies. The cognitive aspect of GRC pertains to thoughts and questions about gender roles, the understanding of which varies based on the developmental level of the boy or man. Dualistic thinkers experience gender roles differently from men with more cognitive complexity. Thinking that one does not meet expected masculine norms or cannot compete can cause GRC because there are no further options. The affective domain is how men feel about their gender roles, including the degree of comfort or conflict they have living out their gender role identities. Negative emotions can lead to dysfunction and GRC. Behavioral aspects of GRC include ways men respond to and interact with others and themselves that produce negative intrapersonal and interpersonal outcomes. Discrimination against men and women based on sexist assumptions are examples of how GRC can be expressed behaviorally. Finally, unconscious GRC encompasses thoughts, feelings, and behaviors related to conflicts with gender roles that are beyond men's awareness.

GRC has also been conceptualized as occurring in four general contexts (or experiences) that give the construct a form. These contexts were defined as GRC within the man (intrapersonal); GRC expressed toward others (interpersonal); GRC experienced from others (also interpersonal); and GRC during gender role transitions. GRC in an intrapersonal context is a man's experience of negative emotions and thoughts about his masculinity that cause personal gender role devaluations, restrictions, and violations. In the interpersonal context, GRC expressed toward others occurs when the man's gender role problems cause him to devalue, restrict, or violate someone else by, for example, telling sexist jokes or committing sexual harassment or violence against women. GRC from others occurs when someone devalues, restricts, or violates another person who deviates from or conforms to masculinity or femininity ideology and norms.

Three personal experiences of GRC are defined as gender role (a) devaluations, (b) restrictions, and (c) violations. Gender role devaluations are negative critiques of self or others when conforming to, deviating from, or violating stereotypical gender role norms of masculinity ideology. An example of this might be when a man is shamed for showing tender emotions in public. He then learns to devalue that part of himself. The second gender-related experience is gender role restrictions, which imply that GRC confines oneself or others to stereotypical and restrictive norms of masculinity ideology and expected gender roles. Gender role restrictions also result in attempts to control people's behavior, limit their own or other's potential, and decrease human freedom. Gender role violations represent the most severe kind of GRC. They occur when men harm themselves, harm others, or are harmed by others because of the more extreme aspects of the socialized male gender role.

Another central concept in the GRC research program is the Gender Role Journey, a framework that can be used to help people examine how gender role socialization, GRC, and sexism have affected their lives. The journey has three empirically derived phases: (a) accepting traditional gender roles; (b) gender role ambivalence, fear, anger, and confusion; and (c) personal and professional activism (O'Neil & Egan, 1992, 1993; O'Neil, Egan, Owen, & Murry, 1993). The journey involves a retrospective analysis of early family experiences with gender roles, making an assessment of one's present situation with sexism, and making decisions about how to act in the future using the three phases. It includes resolving gender role transitions defined as events in a person's gender role development that produces changes in his or her gender role identity, self-assumptions, and gender role schemas. Gender role schemas are ways of thinking about maleness and femaleness based on sex and gender roles that guide attitudes and behaviors. Examples of schemas are power, control, emotionality, success, intimacy, and competition, to name a few. Gender role schemas are related to a person's self-concept and are used to evaluate one's personal adequacy as male or female. The gender role journey phases provide a way to understand the situational aspects of GRC within these schemas.

The purpose of this chapter is to present GRC in a different epistemological context, one that will allow researchers to begin studying gender roles as problem-solving methodologies. We think the science needs to move from treating masculinity as an ideological hegemony under which men and women operate to treating masculinity as a method through which men quickly and without too much forethought solve situational problems, an approach initially called for by Addis, Mansfield, and Syzdek (2010). Research questions would therefore move toward defining how individual men construct both their masculinity and their goals in specific situations. We would investigate the manners in which they might use their masculinity to solve problems, how they evaluate the outcomes, and how they develop as a result of experience. As such, it is not the goal of this chapter to provide a point-by-point review of the extant GRC literature, which is available elsewhere (O'Neil, 2008, 2015; O'Neil & Denke, 2016). This chapter instead briefly summarizes the more recent empirical work. Next, it offers a theoretical framework within which GRC theory can evolve. This is followed by a discussion of how current thinking on social and cultural evolution sheds new light on the gender role experience, as well as how that light can inform GRC theory, clinical practice, and future scholarship.

## GENDER ROLE CONFLICT EXTANT LITERATURE

More than 400 separate studies have used the GRCS, and 208 (52%) of these studies have been published in the psychological literature in 50 journals. Two-hundred and forty doctoral dissertations have used the GRCS, and more than 180 GRC studies were presented at the annual American Psychological Association Annual Convention from 1982 through 2015. When looking outside the United States, 74 studies have been completed outside the United States at 53 institutions in 33 countries, including 10 in Australia; nine in South Korea; seven in Canada; five each in Germany,

Great Britain, and Ireland; two each in Indonesia, Japan, Philippines, Scotland, Hong Kong (China); and single studies in Iran, Iraq, Egypt, China, Hungary, Columbia, Portugal, Taiwan, Poland, Spain, Lithuania, Russia, Tasmania, Costa Rica, Sweden, South Africa, Ghana, Croatia, Turkey, Singapore, Thailand, and Malta. The GRCS has been translated into 20 languages and has been adapted to a shorter form (Wester, Vogel, O'Neil, & Danforth, 2012) as well as a form appropriate for use with adolescent boys (Blazina, Pisecco, & O'Neil, 2005).

The research indicates that GRC significantly relates to men's psychological problems, with 211 studies documenting these relationships (see O'Neil, 2015). In the intrapersonal realm, the psychological domains of GRC (cognitive, affective, and behavioral) have considerable empirical support. Strong empirical data also connect GRC to men's cognitive and affective processes, including significant correlations with men's anxiety, depression, homonegativity, negative identity, anger, and low self-esteem. The cognitive aspects of GRC are evident in the significant correlations with traditional attitudes toward women, stereotyping, antigay attitudes, homophobia, and low sex-role egalitarianism. In the behavioral domain, significant correlations exist between GRC and hostile behavior, spousal criticism, sexually aggressive behaviors toward women, and health risk behaviors.

The GRC patterns of SPC, RE, RABBM, and CBWFR significantly predict symptoms of depression, anxiety, anger, alexithymia, low self-esteem, stress, shame, marital dissatisfaction, homonegativity, homophobia, and restrictive and negative attitudes toward women, gays, and, in one study, racial minorities. Even more striking and disturbing is that GRC has been significantly correlated with positive attitudes toward sexual harassment, rape myths, hostile sexism, and self-reported sexual and dating violence toward women. There is also positive evidence for men's personal experiences of GRC as gender role devaluations, restrictions, and violations (O'Neil, 2015). Sixty specific psychological symptoms of devaluations, restrictions, and violations have been empirically correlated with SPC, RE, RABBM, and CBWFR. Forty-seven of the psychological problems relate to men's possible self-devaluations, restrictions, and violations. Another 19 problem areas relate to men's devaluation and violation of others. Nine important psychological symptoms related to self-devaluations include depression, shame, low self-esteem, internalized forms of oppression related to racism, homonegativity, heterosexism, and negative attitudes about being gay. Twenty-three psychological symptoms related to self-restrictions include stress, anxiety, coping problems, hopelessness, loneliness, and various stigma associated with seeking help to name a few. Eleven self-violating symptoms including substance use and abuse, high-risk behavior, eating disorder symptoms, self-objectification, self-destructiveness, and indices related to suicide.

The research also indicates that GRC relates to men's potential to restrict, devalue, or violate others. The devaluation of others has been empirically linked to seven discriminatory attitudes, including stereotyping of women, homophobic and antigay attitudes, racial bias, sex-role egalitarianism, and spousal criticism. Likewise, GRC relationship with violating others includes violence against women, positive attitudes toward sexual harassment, sexually aggressive behavior, likelihood of forced sex, hostility toward women, dating violence, hostile sexism, rape myths, abusive behavior, and coercion. Furthermore, there is evidence that the patterns of GRC relate to gender role devaluations, restrictions, and violations and significant psychological and interpersonal problems for racially and ethnically mixed groups of males and gay men. In 26 studies, 19 psychological symptoms were correlated with gender role devaluations, restrictions, and violations.

Over the past 10 years, 31 studies have been completed on adult men over 30 years of age, 26 studies on African American men, 10 studies on Mexican American men, nine studies on Asian American men, and 28 studies on gay men. There have been 17 studies assessing age differences in GRC from boyhood to retirement. Twelve studies have been completed on adolescent boys using the GRCS–A (Blazina et al., 2005), and three studies have been completed on retired men's GRC. More than 20 multicultural, diversity, demographic, and moderator variables have been correlated with GRC. The most common demographic variables include race, class, ethnicity, age, stage of life, sexual orientation, sex (women and transgendered people), socioeconomic status (SES), educational level, marital status, work roles, and nationality. Other multicultural indices related to GRC include degrees of acculturation and assimilation, racial and ethnic identity, machismo ideology, cultural values, societal discrimination, and states of vulnerability.

## Current Research on GRC

Although O'Neil's recently published (2015; O'Neil & Denke, 2016) major reviews of the GRC database outline in detail the extant literature surrounding the construct of male GRC, there has been additional research published since those works were in press. In 2015, for example, GRC theory was applied to the experiences of Latino men (Davis & Liang, 2015), Irish boys and adolescents (e.g., O'Beaglaoich, Conway, & Morrison, 2015; O'Beaglaoich, Morrison, Nielsen, & Ryan, 2015), Chinese heterosexual and gay men (Zhang et al., 2015), and Chinese adolescents (e.g., Lu et al., 2015). Also, GRC has been used to explore men's experiences in female-dominated workplaces (Sobiraj, Rigotti, Weseler, & Mohr, 2015) and the experiences of male counselors treating male clients (e.g., Whetstine-Richel, 2015).

## Criticisms of the GRC Paradigm

It is important to note that despite its impact on the extant literature, the GRC paradigm is not without its critics. Many argue, for example, that the research program has failed to assess GRC longitudinally by identifying development tasks and contextual demands that interface with men's socialization (Smiler, 2004). Still others assert that despite its being used to understand the experiences had by men of marginalized groups (e.g., Wester, 2008), the development of the original theory from a primarily Caucasian perspective limits its applicability for men of color and men of different sexual orientations. Still others offer the criticism that both the psychology of men and the GRC construct have become—regardless of the original intent of the scholars—trait based and of limited utility in assessing the situational dynamics of men's gendered behavior. As a result, it has been argued that the current state of GRC does not take into account situational and real-life contingencies that affect men's lives (Addis et al., 2010; Jones & Heesacker, 2012; Smiler, 2004). Addis et al. (2010) proposed a contextual and contingent-based, cue-oriented agenda for studying how gender-relevant cues elicit male behavior. Jones and Heesacker (2012) called for the study of the microcontexts of men's issues—that is, sets of cues, norms, and outcome expectations associated with a temporally limited environment. To be fair, however, seven studies have found that situational dynamics relate to men's GRC (see http://web.uconn.edu/joneil). Overall, the original GRC model did not address the causal questions of how, why, and when a man becomes conflicted with their gender roles.

Largely in response to these criticisms, O'Neil (2015; see also O'Neil & Denke, 2016) presented a social information processing model (e.g., Crick & Dodge, 1994) of GRC that potentially accounted for the impact of contextual cues on men's behaviors. This model includes six cognitive steps that individuals go through to respond to the demands of any given situation: (a) encoding of cues, (b) interpretation of cues, (c) clarification of goals, (d) response access or construction, (e) response decision, and (f) behavioral enactment. During the encoding and interpreting of cues, for example, some men might selectively attend to stimuli based on his long-term mental memory of past events and their relationship to GRC. In essence, he might notice only those cues that, as a man, he was taught to notice—situational primes for competition, for example, or for potential sexual conquests rather than the broader (i.e., non–gender-based) environmental demands. After all this processing, a clarified goal or desired outcome is mentally selected, many times on the basis of an arousal state that is connected to the desired outcome. In the response decision step, the man evaluates the possible responses and selects the most positive one on the basis of masculine outcome expectations, its self-efficacy, and the appropriateness of the response. For men, restricted gender roles can narrow the behavioral options and possibilities. Certainly, O'Neil's (2015) ideas require both a stronger theoretical linkage to the psychology of men literature as well as empirical exploration, but the narrative itself is evidence of GRC's ongoing evolution.

**Conclusion**

Growing, as it did, out of a feminist approach to deconstructing gender roles (e.g., Brooks & Elder, 2016; O'Neil, 2015, Chapter 2), GRC was one of the first theories developed exploring the negative interpersonal and intrapersonal consequences of enacting the male role for men, for women, and for society as a whole. More than 200 published manuscript and 240 dissertations clearly demonstrate that the experience of GRC leads to myriad psychological consequences, as well as broader sociological consequences for those involved in men's lives. This line of research has been of great value to the field of psychology in its identification of consequences associated with masculinity and subsequent development of potential ways mental health professionals can work with men and those around them to develop better lives.

At the same time, however, one of the issues that has not been addressed in the GRC database has been the *functionality* of traditional gender roles, or the degree to which behaviors society has traditionally labeled masculine allow men specifically, but potentially also society in general, to successfully meet situational goals (e.g., Addis et al., 2010). This functionality can explain why traditional gender roles exist and are still endorsed by many men, despite evidence suggesting the behavior can be dysfunctional in some situations. O'Neil's information processing model (O'Neil, 2015; O'Neil & Denke, 2016) has promise here, but it lacks any theoretical specifications regarding the mechanism through which men solve problems. Research has demonstrated that the suppression of any verbal expression of emotions, for example, has been linked to a slowing of the onset and progression of cancer (e.g., Consedine, Magai, & Bonanno, 2002) as well as the regulation of grief (e.g., Bonanno, 2001), even though it is predictive of interpersonal distress. What mechanism allows for this outcome?

## GRC THEORY: THE NEXT GENERATION

Perhaps functionality has not been addressed much to this point within the psychology of men because the nonsexist approach minimized the focus on functional or beneficial aspects of traditional masculinity (see Kiselica, Benton-Wright, & Englar-Carlson, 2016, for a recent exception). This minimization is understandable; the idea that both male and female gender roles served at least some social purposes has been hotly debated, seemingly because of the distinction between intent versus impact of an action (e.g., Korn, 1995; Swim, Hyers, Cohen, & Ferguson, 2001). Intent involves what someone wants or expects to accomplish when engaging in an action. However, when that action produces unexpected or unintended results, whether in addition to or instead of the intended result, intent differs from impact. Although grounded in scholarship and well-intentioned, functional discussions of gender role may have been avoided because of the potential of a functional approach to be misused to justify harmful behaviors and attitudes. Bio-evolutionary perspectives on gender, for example, have often taken a functional approach (see reviews by Geary, Winegard, & Winegard, 2016; Lippa, 2016) and have been misused to justify and excuse sexist or oppressive behaviors, regardless of the scholars' original intent.

To be clear, we do not embrace the "is–ought" fallacy (also known as Hume's guillotine) that lies at the heart of much of the misuse of functional and evolutionary justifications of dysfunctional behavior of men. The is–ought fallacy holds that what *is* also is what *ought* to be. As an example of this fallacy, if men are demonstrably physically aggressive, they *should* be that way, the proof of which *is* that they are that way. We also do not mention functionality as a way to imply that the use of oppressive gender roles is appropriate, nor do we seek to discuss functionality to justify the sexist, patriarchal oppression of women by men across the ages. Instead, some have asserted that it is time to develop a contextual, constructive understanding of masculinity (e.g., Addis et al., 2010). If so, because we already possess a theoretical understanding of the forces that shaped masculinity (and its role in the problematic behaviors of men), then a method through which the men themselves might be determining functionality needs to be articulated.

**Heuristics**

From the perspective of functionality, the construct of masculinity might be better understood as a label individuals (and society) give to the heuristic category that they activate to understand a situation they are in, to evaluate that situation, and to decide on and implement a behavior (e.g., Addis et al., 2010) designed to meet a specific outcome. Heuristics represent a practical approach to problem solving that is not designed to be perfect but instead is considered sufficient for one's immediate goals. Although the concept of heuristics may reflect essentialism, we believe that the heuristics themselves are not essentialist (e.g., Wester & Vogel, 2012). Instead, we believe that heuristics are a construal, affecting how individuals perceive, comprehend, and interpret the world around them, especially in situations in which they are required to infer additional details of content, context, or meaning in specific situations. Indeed, the word *heuristic* comes from "the same root as the word eureka" (Kahneman, 2011, p. 98); heuristics speed up the process of producing a satisfactory solution. They are mental shortcuts that reduce the cognitive load and increase the speed of decision making. Two of the most familiar examples are the *representativeness heuristic* and the *availability heuristic*. The representativeness heuristic involves the judgments made not on a critical examination of the available information but on how similar the prospects are to the prototypes the person holds in his or her mind. Similarly, the availability heuristic occurs when people make judgments about the probability of events by the ease with which examples come to mind. Overuse of these heuristics results in significant errors in cognitive processing, including such well-known examples as confirmation bias—the tendency to search for, interpret, focus on, and remember information in a way that only confirms one's preconceptions—and the base-rate fallacy—the tendency to ignore generic, general information and focus on information pertaining only to a certain case. Indeed, Lee Ross's (1987) concept of naive realism is especially important in the context of construal. It is the conviction all individuals have that they are the ones who are perceiving reality accurately. Essentially, people acknowledge the fact that others make cognitive errors based on their construal but personally think that they form their own thoughts without being affected by such biased processing. Being blinded by this process often leads individuals to commit the fundamental attribution error, also known as the correspondence bias or attribution effect, which is the tendency for people to place an undue emphasis on internal characteristics (i.e., traits) to explain someone else's behavior in a given situation rather than considering the situation's external factors (i.e., states).

When people use heuristics, the ones they use (e.g., male gender role) depend on both the cues they perceive in the situation and on the habit strength of activating that heuristic versus other heuristics. The more frequently an individual uses a heuristic, the more likely it is to be activated. Because gendered thinking is nearly incessant throughout life, and because gendered thinking saturates most cultures and subcultures, and certainly saturates U.S. culture, we believe that for most men, gendered thinking has high habit strength and is cued by lots of environmental features. Furthermore, because GRC involves several interlocking heuristics (e.g., the display of rules regarding emotions, the role of competition in any situation, protecting one's family), when it is activated, there is quite likely to be variability in how it is activated. Indeed, there is likely to be confusion about what heuristic applies best or perhaps whether two or more can appropriately guide behavior in a particular situation. Because of this, one can think of GRC as the outcome of competing and conflicting heuristics activated to guide a men's behavior in a given context. Here is an example: "Do I adhere to the display rules regarding emotion, or do I respond to the emotional needs of my partner? I do not know, and I am therefore conflicted." The point is, at their most fundamental level, heuristics, such as those associated with masculinity, are problem-solving mechanisms that speed up responding in a complex world by minimizing cognitive load.

## Cognition

Kahneman's (2011) book *Thinking, Fast and Slow* is a treasure trove of principles that can guide research and thinking about heuristics, masculinity, and GRC. Here are three examples. Chapter 11 is devoted to anchoring effects. *Anchoring* refers to the fact that people often overly react to the first or a very early piece of information to guide their judgments. They do so often without awareness and even when they express confidence that the information did not affect their judgments. An example of anchoring is when a charitable organization suggests a range of monetary gifts that one could give. Higher suggestions, such as $1,000 (vs. $100), bring higher contributions. How might anchoring be a useful concept in understanding GRC? When men regularly see other men depicted as fearless killers, for example, in the video game *Call of Duty Black Ops III* (a series of individual video games for a variety of gaming consoles that had sold more than 175 million copies since April 2015; source: http://www.wikipedia.org/wiki/Call_of_Duty), it very well could serve as an anchor for concluding how much aggression is appropriate for men and thereby contribute to men's violence and their acceptance or at least tolerance of violent behavior in other men and in boys.

A second example of the usefulness of Kahneman's (2011) book comes from Chapter 7 and the explanation of a heuristic called WYSIATI ("what you see is all there is"). This heuristic leads people to jump to conclusions based only on the limited evidence immediately available. In essence, they overuse a heuristic in part because the is–ought fallacy supercharges the process; because this is how men must behave, and the evidence for the same is all around me, than I also ought to behave this way. Although we explore the mechanism through which this occurs (i.e., system thinking) later in this chapter, suffice it to say that WYSIATI is likely to lead men not to consider factors and information if it is not right in front of them, and it leads to behaviors that appear to the average observer directly in line with the stereotypical understanding of men. Given how gendered society is and how pervasive images and messages of traditional masculinity are, men are quite likely to consider only these obvious and salient traditional gender role characteristics when making behavioral choices.

A third example from Kahneman (2011, Chapter 38) involves the concepts of duration neglect and the focusing illusion. Evidence suggests that people do not systematically and representatively evaluate how positive or negative an experience or a period of life was, nor do they average across all the moments of those situations to conclusively evaluate the event. They instead rely too heavily on the first experiences within a situation. This focusing illusion sets an anchor point for evaluation, and other evaluations are made by adjusting away from that anchor. They compound this error by heuristically evaluating their happiness or unhappiness with a given experience based on two factors: the peak, or when the experience was the most negative, and how quickly the negativity diminishes. This is known as *duration neglect*; if the negativity of an experience diminishes more quickly, the experience is judged to be more painful. In other words, they engage in *focal neglect* by focusing only on one small aspect of the overall experience or just a few selected parts, such as the beginning, the peak, and the end of an experience. They neglect the happiness levels in between. Duration neglect and the focusing illusion may provide the insight needed to understand one of the most curious findings in the GRC literature—namely, if gender role–specific behaviors produce so many adverse effects for men and the people around them, why do they still engage in such behavior? From the duration-neglect perspective, men are mostly processing their experiences heuristically, meaning they are not paying much, if any, attention to the average moment-to-moment consequences of masculinity. Men who engage in focal neglect, only focusing on one particular moment (e.g., the peak moment or the beginning or end of an experience), can preserve the illusion that adhering to GRC beliefs and behaviors produces mostly positive experiences. This focal-neglect effect may be heightened by powerful expectations that traditional gender roles will pay off for men, which may lead to selective attention to only the most positive experiences emanating from gender role beliefs and behaviors.

### Superorganism

Perhaps the most promising explanation for this functionality of the traditional male gender role is the concept of *superorganism* (e.g., Kesebir, 2011). A superorganism is a group of individual organisms of the same species who act in concert and thereby produce an evolutionary advantage over species whose members operate alone, in pairs, or in smaller social groups. Scholars believe that superorganisms evolved to confer an advantage of one species over others by coordinating individual efforts to be more effective in avoiding predators, subduing prey, and engaging in other species-enhancing actions. Indeed, social learning is one of the primary tools of coordinated effort that produces a superorganism; masculinity as a set of behavioral responses passed on via social learning processes, no matter how noxious current society finds the result, would certainly qualify.

The concept of superorganisms as it applies to men requires readers to understand that evolution has two components. The first and better known evolutionary component is biological evolution. Charles Darwin and his colleagues championed the cause of biological evolution, with the result that it is a widely accepted perspective for understanding speciation across time. At the same time that Darwin was developing and articulating notions related to biological evolution, however, Herbert Spencer was developing ideas around the second component of evolution, sociocultural. Sociocultural evolution operates similarly to biological evolution, except that sociocultural evolution occurs rapidly, whereas biological evolution occurs more slowly. Both increase the survivability of the species and improve the functioning of the organism, and they affect each other to confer survivability advantages. This interplay of components reflects a perspective about nature and nurture that we find helpful in understanding GRC.

Haidt (2012) made the case for the application of superorganism concepts to humans, given our tendency toward coordinated efforts and its confirmation of an evolutionary advantage to humans. Socioculturally, for example, behavioral scientists have known for decades that humans subordinate self as members of groups (e.g., combat units, corporations, religious faiths). In the case of the male gender role, the shared beliefs, expectations, customs, and traditions could be considered a group that would result in men acting in concert. It could be argued, therefore, that because humans dominate other species, men dominate women and girls as a consequence of behaving as a superorganism. So traditional masculinity may have developed and been sustained because it resulted in dominance over other species and, within the human species, over children, women, and even men who operated outside of the superorganism (e.g., men of different sexual orientations, men of color). In essence, it increased the odds of survival. But domination has had its costs, for men, for women, and for society, as both feminism and the hundreds of studies on GRC reliably document.

On the biological side, superorganism behavior is supported by emerging neurobiological research. Indeed, evidence suggests that humans are also neurologically predisposed to behave under specific conditions as part of a larger group, subjugating their individualism to the group (e.g., Hölldobler & Wilson, 2009), with marked survival advantages over less socially coordinated species. For example, oxytocin is a neurotransmitter that has been documented to trigger greater trust and generosity toward in-group members, while increasing apprehension about and distrust of out-group members (e.g., Baumgartner, Heinrichs, Vonlanthen, Fischbacher, & Fehr, 2008). This sharpening of in- and out-group boundaries is an essential component of superorganism behavior, of which, we suggest, hegemonic masculinity (e.g., Connell & Messerschmidt, 2005) is an example, built from and sustained by adherence to traditional masculinity. How this propensity is related to men and GRC is that "men" or large groups of men can be understood to be one of those superorganisms, in which members often subordinate self-interest in service of group membership, motivated by a sense of belonging. As objectionable as aspects of the male group might be to other groups, and to society at large, there is little doubt that adopting superorganism status through the development of hegemonic masculinity has facilitated the social dominance of men, but with the tremendous costs documented in many GRC studies.

Obviously not all organisms have both biological and sociocultural evolution. Only organisms capable of complex social behavior, such as humans, benefit from the sociocultural evolutionary processes. This is because the development of both social behavior and culture is necessary for both types of evolution to occur. It can be argued, for example, that the primary benefit of social behavior in humans and other higher animals was the ability to have both sociocultural and biological evolution operating to improve outcomes for the species. Biological evolution influences cultural evolution, but it is also important to note that sociocultural evolution also influences biological evolution. For example, biological evolution produced the social brain, with the development and enlargement of the cortex and particularly the prefrontal cortex, which is centrally involved in social behavior. Without the development of the cortex, complex sociocultural behavior is impossible, and this avenue of superorganism development and maintenance is not possible. Less developed organisms, such as honeybees and schooling fish do sometimes behave as superorganisms, but that behavior is driven by biologically evolved mechanisms, which are slower to develop and modify than behavior changes caused by sociocultural evolution. This notion that sociocultural evolution influences biology refutes the notion that biology exclusively determines men's behavior (e.g., Joel et al., 2015). The traditional idea behind sex-based difference in brain structures is that once a fetus develops testicles, he secretes testosterone, which masculinizes the brain. Joel and her colleagues (2015) used 1,400 individual brain scans to test this theory, focusing on areas traditionally identified as evidenced sex-based differences, including the hippocampus and the inferior frontal gyrus. They found that few people had all of the brain features they might be expected to have based on their sex; averaged across many people sex differences in brain structure do exist, but an individual brain is likely to be just that: individual, with a mix of features. The greater causes of men's behavior therefore include a complex interplay of sociocultural forces, biological forces, and their interplay.

GRC theory can therefore be viewed from this perspective as the harbinger (or a reflection) of sociocultural change. This is because GRC research documents the costs of traditional masculinity, that is, the degree to which traditionally masculine behaviors do, or do not, fit the functionality demands of any current situation. In a world where superorganism status resulted mostly in survival benefits, GRC would occur less, because few conflicts would arise between socialized behaviors and what would be required of boys and men to meet goals in specific situations. However, in today's world, certainly during the past century, society has changed to the extent that the traditional gender model no longer applies; men and women are expected, indeed required, to be functional in domains far outside of what their ancestors would have been required to do. This change requires behaviors beyond the traditionally socialized gender roles. Just as important, the socialized male gender role has produced a host of adverse outcomes of which GRC is a significant component. These adverse outcomes call into question the utility of men's superorganism status as well as the traditional gender role that appears to drive that status. Said another way, the survival benefits are no longer significant enough to justify the oppressive and sexist costs.

For the study of GRC, therefore, it is useful to think about men and their traditional gender roles as resulting from a process that conferred evolutionary benefit through the development of a superorganism. However, as the benefits—to society, to men, and even to women—conferred by superorganism status declined, the social costs increased or emerged, which drew the attention of gender role scholars. The costs of the traditional male gender role have been well documented by the first author and many other scholars. The perspective we take in this chapter is that the traditional male gender role is likely to have developed for reasons that were beneficial to the species in some ways, but it has become costly in many others. As time has passed, the benefits of men acting as a superorganism appear to have diminished, and the costs, through traditional masculinity and the GRC that results, appear to have increased. Indeed, this shift from male hegemony to GRC may be thought of as another example of sociocultural evolution. In modern times and in developed nations, men do far less hunting and gathering. They spend much less time actively defending their territory, their family members, and their property. They spend much more time in sociocultural pursuits, which do not require and do not particularly reward traditional male gender role components. Indeed, we wonder whether the primary reason scholars began unmasking the male gender role when they did was because, by then, gender roles were becoming untenable; the benefits of superorganism status are now significantly outweighed by the societal costs of adhering to the traditional masculinity that has been required to achieve and maintain superorganism status.

## System 1 and 2 Thinking

Male gender roles are socially constructed, and therefore are largely, although not completely, shared among groups of men. This is a critical observation for linking superorganism status to the decision-making methods men use; these social constructions of gender reside, it would seem, as a complex interconnected set of heuristics that activate automatically in response to situational demands. That is, male gender role schemas (O'Neil, 2015) organize a repository of interconnected, relatively simple guideline for behavior that, like all heuristics, take the place of more careful, effortful, and therefore complex analyses that humans are generally reluctant to undertake because we are, in fact, cognitive misers (e.g., Fiske & Taylor, 1984). This perspective therefore suggests that these traditional male gender role components that drive superorganism status are largely automatic. They reflect what Kahneman (2011), among others, has called *System 1 thinking.*

System 1 thinking is automatic and unconscious, emotional and intuitive. It reacts quickly to the environment and quickly produces responses in reaction to the incoming stimuli. This is the critical component linking superorganism status to the problem-solving methodology; System 1 guides responses to the environment as quickly as possible. Through automatic application, a relevant heuristic guides behavior based on decision rules that are simple and largely unexamined. This short reaction time increases the likelihood of survival in situations, which probably confers some evolutionary advantage. Applied to the male gender role, for example, "immediately observable contextual cues [microcontexts; Jones & Heesacker, 2012] . . . activate corresponding stereotypes and belief systems" (Deaux & Major, 1987, p. 374). The presence of a female, for example, might activate specific behavioral patterns in men—whether those behavioral patterns be the display rules regarding emotional expression or the simple act of straightening one's posture to present a more "manly" physique. These belief systems are the heuristics discussed earlier; they contain information about the nature of gender role–appropriate behaviors, data regarding the match between any given situation and one's gender role, and knowledge "about how men and women should behave in various types of situations" (Eagly, 1987, pp. 25–26).

In contrast, *System 2 thinking* is effortful, rational, and intentional. System 2 is the slower, more reflective thinking system. It allows humans to deliberate and consider options carefully. This is the system humans use when they rely on well-articulated reasons and more fully developed evidence. It is reasoning based on what we have learned through careful analysis, evaluation, explanation, and self-correction. This is the system that comes into play when humans are called on to think carefully and solve complex or novel problems. It also is responsible for the review and revision of our behaviors in light of relevant guidelines, rules of procedure, or goal-meeting outcomes. From a superorganism perspective, System 2 is a luxury; it takes time to sort through the numerous potential choices an individual might face in any given moment. Indeed, System 2 decisions are directly influenced by the correct or incorrect application of heuristic maneuvers, correct or incorrect being defined exclusively as the meeting (or not meeting) of situational goals rather than any externally imposed, ideologically based definition. Said another way, it is the meeting (or not meeting) of those goals that is at stake with regard to any evolutionary advantage regardless of how society might evaluate the good or bad of resultant behavior.

People typically rely on System 1 and heuristics, but not always. Context heavily determines System 1 versus System 2 use (although so do individual factors), but the default condition is System 1. However, when people have sufficient motivation to think effortfully (e.g., when they perceive the cost of behavioral errors to be high) and have the available capacity (e.g., not stressed, not anxious, not using available capacity on something else, not multitasking, not fatigued, not intoxicated, not distracted), they will rely on System 2. The point is that a lot of pieces have to fall in place for System 2 thinking to override System 1. Scholars, such as those of us who study men and masculinity (the authors of this chapter included), have tended to overestimate the power of System 2 in everyday lives because we tend to live in our own heads more than most people. For an example of how scholars may not mirror people generally, consider what you are doing now. Readers are reading text that we wrote, both activities that reflect (we hope) deliberate, effortful, and systematic thinking—lots of System 2.

Ironically, even the assumption that there is more System 2 thinking going on than System 1 reflects System 1 thinking. In their classic *Science* article "Judgment Under Uncertainty: Heuristics and Biases," Tversky and Kahneman (1974) blamed the availability heuristic, in which people estimate the likelihood of an event or group of events (e.g., the probability that someone will engage in System 2 thinking) by relying on how many instances of that event readily come to find. Academics probably can readily think of more cases of System 2 thinking—because they do so much of it in their work—than other people, and thus they would overestimate System 2 thinking likelihood and underestimate System 1 thinking.

There are many examples of these dual processing models in psychology, starting with Craik and Lockhart's (1972) analysis of dual processing as an alternative to long-term versus short-term memory; Craik and Tulving's (1975/2004) deep versus shallow memory processing accounting for systematic differences in recall; continuing through research on attitude change and persuasion, such as Petty and Cacioppo's (1985) elaboration likelihood model and the more recent associative-propositional evaluation model (Gawronski

& Bodenhausen, 2006a) in which the interactions between the two types of evaluative mechanisms more holistically explain the attitude change process. However, much of the scholarship on the psychology of men has been, understandably, focused on understanding the consequences of System 1 thinking using samples of what Gawronski and Bodenhausen (2006b) labeled *explicit attitudes* (e.g., p. 745). Evolving beyond a study of those consequences, in effect working toward a comprehension of why men do things through the meaning they assign the concept of masculinity as well as the contexts in which said masculinity is enacted, would require the study of specific System 1 content, as well as an acknowledgment of the role played by System 2 in maintaining System 1.

From this, therefore, male gender role socialization would produce psychological distress only under specific conditions; men being unable to adapt their socialization to current life situations or interpersonal or family demands, for example, might reflect struggles in shifting from System 1 to System 2. Indeed, reconceptualizing GRC as largely the result of System 1 thinking may prove helpful in understanding and addressing the dysfunctions associated with the traditional male gender role. Put simply, we believe that increasing men's System 2 thinking and decreasing men's System 1 thinking will reduce the adverse impact of traditional masculinity on men's behaviors, allowing them to adapt more effectively to the situations they experience, instead of simply and automatically relying on the traditional male gender role.

Linking this work to our earlier discussions of heuristics and superorganisms, we believe that traditional male gender role components drive superorganism status in men and are activated automatically. That is, they are activated quickly and without conscious decision making. They efficiently guide behavior in reaction to the situation. They reflect System 1 thinking. From this perspective, hegemonic masculinity can be viewed as the natural consequence of the traditional male gender producing superiority over other species and over women and girls. The so-called battle of the sexes reflects this competition, as does the feminist movement, which may be viewed as the development of women's superorganism in response to male domination. Indeed, there remain parts of this world where hegemonic masculinity still holds sway; one potential explanation for this could be that the biological and environmental presses experienced in those locations still confer the significant benefits associated with superorganism status. Consider a war-torn nation or a country that is struggling to recover from a long-term environmental disaster. On a smaller level, consider the behavioral patterns evidenced by individuals as well as larger groups of men. Environments where men are much more likely to face real threats of predation while also experience the real need to be effective predators may still confer survival benefits to those affiliated with superorganism status. We raise these examples only to provide anecdotal evidence for the rise of traditional masculinity being part of the sociocultural evolutionary process that was effective in responding to biological and environmental presses in antiquity but that are less beneficial (and more costly) now.

## IMPLICATIONS

The approach presented in this chapter is based on the long history of dual processing models in cognitive and social psychology as well as in the broader psychology of judgment and decision making. From these perspectives, male gender roles organize and activate a set of heuristics that guide behavior in situations that don't facilitate or allow for careful and effortful, System 2 thinking. The particular nature of the situation determines (a) whether heuristics will be used; (b) if so, whether gender heuristics will be used; and (c) if gender heuristics will be used, which ones will be used to guide behavior. In essence, men react to the microcontextual cues present in any given situation and via System 1 instantly determine whether heuristics in general, or gender heuristics specifically, will be used as well as which ones and to what end.

However, one wrinkle in the story of System 1 and System 2 thinking is that according to Haidt (2006), System 2 is sometimes activated to defend System 1–derived conclusions. This fact may explain why men can sometimes logically and somewhat rationally defend an aspect of the male gender role that is clearly dysfunctional, such as avoiding health care when they are sick or attempting to dominate and control those they love. One can embrace and apply a heuristic through System 1 (e.g., men are tough, men should take control), which then commandeers System 2 to justify the action (e.g., men have to be tough or they will not be able to survive, protect their loved ones, or defend the nation in times of war; men should take control because they are the most competent). We suspect that this process is responsible for a phenomenon so many of us who work with men in therapy or who study the psychology of men have encountered; men arguing the value and functionality of their own gender role despite the amount of counter evidence present in their lives.

### Psychotherapy

In general, our perspective involves shifting men in psychotherapy from System 1 to System 2 thinking, akin to but more specific than the approach put forth in Rabinowitz and Cochran's (2002) *Deepening Psychotherapy With Men*. Briefly, Rabinowitz and Cochran asserted that there are four primary "zones" (pp. 9–32) of conflict that men experience in their lives; a discomfort with "being" and a socialized preference for "doing" would be primary examples. Therapists who wish to go deeper in their work with such men need to develop a sense of empathy for such issues and an understanding of the focal conflict underlying those zones and the wounds that precipitated their need for therapy. In the context of the working alliance, therefore, these wounds could be more deeply explored via the specific narratives around each individual life experience—what Rabinowitz and Cochran labeled *portals*.

Our approach would build on Rabinowitz and Cochran's (2002) work by paying attention to the needed shift from System 1 to System 2 thinking, as well as recognizing how System 1 and System 2 interact. The logic for this is that traditional conceptualizations of gender role are instantly and automatically assessed by a staggering array of situations and contexts. Gender is a massively reinforced set of behaviors for most people, and yet the resultant identity often goes unexamined. Indeed, it is an examination through the portal that Rabinowitz and Cochran advocated for, within of course the context of an empathic, supportive therapeutic alliance. However, therapists should be aware of the fact that (a) this is a situation primed for System 2 thinking and (b) System 2 thinking can be used to justify System 1 conclusions. System 2 is the slower, more deliberative thinking system. It is reasoning based on what we have learned through careful analysis, evaluation, explanation, and self-correction—all of which are characteristics of successful psychotherapy. Yet, at the same time, therapists should guard against the defensive stance seemingly exhibited by many clients as they argue the value and functionality of their own gender role.

Norbert Schwarz and colleagues (Schwarz, Strack, Kommer, & Wagner, 1987) documented an ingenious use of System 1 to influence behavior, which has therapeutic implications. The essence of the approach is that if an individual struggles too hard to list examples of something, that individual will infer that said something is rare. Conversely, when individuals are able to easily come up with examples, they conclude that the something is quite common. What makes this a classic example of System 1 is that this effect is related to the amount of cognition required to complete the task. For example, therapists could ask clients to list a dozen examples of when the traditional male gender role benefitted them. When clients struggle to complete this long list, which is quite likely, their System 1 thinking will conclude that the traditional male gender role hasn't really benefitted them all that much. Likewise, asking men to list only one or two examples of when operating independently of male gender roles was beneficial is quite likely to produce requested examples and the System 1 conclusion will be that there are plenty of benefits of operating independently of traditional male gender roles. These approaches work because in System 1 thinking, ease of retrieval is often substituted for frequency—a process readers should recognize from our earlier discussion of scholars' likely overestimation of System 2 thinking via the availability heuristic (Tversky & Kahneman, 1974). If people can recall examples easily, they conclude that there must be lots of examples, but if examples are difficult to recall, there must not be many of them. Changing list length changes ease of retrieval and therefore the conclusions about frequency, with the hapless System 1–thinking client none the wiser.

We think men will benefit from relying more on System 2 than System 1. System 2 allows men to evaluate their gendered beliefs and behavior thoughtfully and carefully, but in most situations System 1 is the default mode. Thus, therapy should focus not only on men shifting to System 2 while in therapy but also on how to shift to System 2 outside of therapy whenever situations and circumstances invite a gendered response (which for most men is very often). Rabinowitz and Cochran's (2002) approach is an example of one method therapists might use to stimulate the shift; developing an empathic awareness of the client's conflict zones as well as identifying a portal through which their narrative can be accessed and explored would provide the client with the luxury of exploring those options, evaluating the source as well as the functionality of those options, and ultimately being challenged by the therapist to consider newer, more adaptive options.

It is also important to provide men with psychoeducation aimed at developing an awareness of situations that make System 2 thinking difficult (e.g., fatigue, substance use, very stimulating situations). One option is to suggest that men develop coping skills to attenuate such System 2–diminishing elements. The reevaluation and integrating process involves the deconstruction of masculine stereotypes and restricted gender roles detailed in O'Neil's (2015) Gender Role Journey is relevant here; when men redefine and integrate new definitions of masculinity (change their gender role schemas), they have concluded that the old notions of masculinity (the stereotypes) no longer work for them. Under these conditions, System 1 thinking can be replaced with System 2 thinking, understanding of course that the defensive use of System 2 needs to be dealt with in the context of psychotherapy.

**Future Research**

O'Neil's (2015) text contains several chapters on new directions for GRC research, including multiple context-based and information processing approaches that can be used to generate new empirical questions. Building on these, the ideas presented in this chapter need to be theoretically fleshed out and empirically validated. Indeed, one of our first recommendations would be for the psychology of men to develop measures of implicit masculine self-concepts and attitudes which reflect System 1 thinking so that the concepts raised in this chapter could be evaluated empirically. This would represent a significant shift, given that the psychology of men has, for the most part, relied on self-report measures of explicit attitudes from which the field has drawn fairly sweeping conclusions about men and their characteristics (for specific discussions, see Shields, 2013; Wester et al., 2016; Wester & Vogel, 2012). By unifying (e.g., Greenwald et al., 2002) the study of implicit and explicit attitudes with research on cognitive processes and behavioral observations, the psychology of men could begin to reconcile seemingly contradictory findings, on topics such as men and emotion, while also understanding men and masculinity more holistically. The interaction of associative and propositional evaluation processes might facilitate explicit as well as implicit attitude change, which would in turn could help men switch between System 1 and System 2 (e.g., Gawronski & Bodenhausen, 2006a). More recently, Kahneman (2011) detailed several experiments in which he and his team were able to stimulate System 1 and System 2 thinking, and their research team proposed several conditions under which individuals use (and shift between) these systems. Scholars might consider adopting those approaches in their research and practice of the psychology of men.

Further, System 1 and System 2 thinking needs to be studied to document both the positive and negative consequences of male gender role socialization and GRC. If the superorganism approach has merit, then GRC is most likely to be experienced when traditional notions of masculinity no longer function in ways that allow men to meet their life goals. Also, System 1 thinking rather than System 2 thinking is more likely to result in GRC, internalized oppression, psychological and interpersonal problems, and violence, so descriptive contexts can be identified from men's gender role socialization that help explain how the functionality of gender roles operate and promote both systems. Finally, the role played by situational, biological, unconscious, familial, multicultural, religious, racial, and ethnic contingencies—essentially additional classifications of superorganisms—in system thinking needs exploration.

## Advocacy

It is well known that some of the reasoning behind O'Neil's (2015) text arose from his recognition of the need for a call to action. In his mind, the psychology of men was not moving fast enough to understand the broader impact of male gender role socialization on men, women, and society overall. Admittedly, the specialization had contributed much to documenting the degree to which this construct society has labeled *masculinity* was in part to blame for many of society's ills while also being linked to the psychological distress experienced by men themselves. Indeed, privilege had a cost, as the

GRC database clearly demonstrates. Yet at the same time, key questions regarding the "why" underneath men's behaviors were not being addressed, and complex questions regarding men's construction of their own masculine identity were only just beginning to be asked. The specialization had no answers when critics pointed out that men's gender roles were changing as the world moved into the 21st century, and it was unclear why so many men did not experience gender role–related problems when so many obviously struggled to adjust their behaviors.

Perhaps progress on these issues has come slowly because it is time to develop a more complex understanding of men's lives based on the functionality of their behavioral choices in particular contexts and to develop, test, and validate a theory that focuses not only on what is learned, but also on how it is employed, in what contexts it is employed, and with what results. For the psychology of men, it is time to ask what is next and to focus on the goals met and unmet by men's gendered behaviors, so that the men affected adversely, and those affected adversely by, their behaviors, may benefit from this new work by having realistic and relevant guidance on what they might do differently to optimize their gender-influenced decisions. O'Neil's (2015) concept of gender role transitions (see pp. 97–99, 108–112) is illustrative here; moving from System 1 to System 2 thinking could be considered akin to a gender role transformation process (see pp. 113–116). The process includes (a) changes with defenses, (b) facing and resolving false gender role assumptions, (c) increased internal dialogue, (d) psychological warfare, and (e) symbol manipulation. As Steve Jobs (1955–2011), who famously had success, power, and competition issues, once said:

> Your time is limited, so don't waste it living someone else's life. Don't be trapped by dogma—which is living the result of other people's thinking. Don't let the noise of other's opinions drown out your own inner voice. And most important, have the courage to follow your heart and intuition. (see http://www.quotationspage.com/quote/38353.html)

It would seem likely that the psychology of men, just like those we work with, is in the process of moving from one stage to the next.

## CONCLUSION

With this chapter we are not, as some might assert, arguing that the past 35 years of GRC scholarship needs to be relegated to history. Nor are we calling for a wholesale rejection of the nonsexist origins of the specialization or the reassertion of patriarchal oppression via evolutionary justification. Instead, what we are calling for is progress. The field needs to progress away from the treatment of masculinity as a hegemonic norm under which men labor; intended or otherwise, such an approach is more positivistic than warranted and has often been used to reify ideological assumptions about what is bad (or good) about masculinity (e.g., Bederman, 2011; Shields, 2013). The field also needs to progress toward a more complex understanding of how men construct and use their own individual identity as a man; we think the System 1/System 2 model, coupled with the conceptualization of manhood as a superorganism, holds promise in this regard. Finally, the field needs to progress toward the application of our theories to the prediction of men's actual behavior, as well as the role played by both the context (including microcontexts; see Jones & Heesacker, 2012) and the system-level thinking processes. This will allow a clearer understanding of functionality to emerge, and, in turn, more thoughtful conversations can begin regarding ideology, society, and the role of gender in the lives of men and women.

## REFERENCES

Addis, M. E., Mansfield, A. K., & Syzdek, M. R. (2010). Is "masculinity" a problem? Framing the effects of gendered social learning in men. *Psychology of Men & Masculinity, 11*, 77–90. http://dx.doi.org/10.1037/a0018602

Baumgartner, T., Heinrichs, M., Vonlanthen, A., Fischbacher, U., & Fehr, E. (2008). Oxytocin shapes the neural circuitry of trust and trust adaptation in humans. *Neuron, 58*, 639–650. http://dx.doi.org/10.1016/j.neuron.2008.04.009

Bederman, G. (2011). Why study "masculinity," anyway? Perspectives from the old days. *Culture, Society & Masculinities, 3*, 13–25. http://dx.doi.org/10.3149/CSM.0301.13

Blazina, C., Pisecco, S., & O'Neil, J. M. (2005). An adaptation of the Gender Role Conflict Scale for adolescents: Psychometric issues and correlates with psychological distress. *Psychology of Men & Masculinity, 6*, 39–45. http://dx.doi.org/10.1037/1524-9220.6.1.39

Bonanno, G. A. (2001). Introduction: New directions in bereavement research and theory. *American Behavioral Scientist, 44*, 718–725. http://dx.doi.org/10.1177/0002764201044005002

Brooks, G. R., & Elder, W. B. (2016). History and future of the psychology of men and masculinities. In Y. J. Wong & S. R. Wester (Eds.), *APA handbook of men and masculinities* (pp. 3–21). http://dx.doi.org/10.1037/14594-001

Connell, R. W., & Messerschmidt, J. W. (2005). Hegemonic masculinity: Rethinking the concept. *Gender & Society, 19*, 829–859. http://dx.doi.org/10.1177/0891243205278639

Consedine, N. S., Magai, C., & Bonanno, G. A. (2002). Moderators of the emotion inhibition–health relationship: A review and research agenda. *Review of General Psychology, 6*, 204–228.

Craik, F. I. M., & Lockhart, R. S. (1972). Levels of processing: A framework for memory research. *Journal of Verbal Learning & Verbal Behavior, 11*, 671–684. http://dx.doi.org/10.1016/S0022-5371(72)80001-X

Craik, F. I. M., & Tulving, E. (2004). Depth of processing and the retention of words in episodic memory. In D. A. Balota & E. J. Marsh (Eds.), *Cognitive psychology: Key readings* (pp. 296–308). New York, NY: Psychology Press. (Reprinted from *Journal of Experimental Psychology: General,* (1975), *104,* 268–294)

Crick, N. R., & Dodge, K. A. (1994). A review and reformulation of social information-processing mechanisms in children's social adjustment. *Psychological Bulletin, 115,* 74–101. http://dx.doi.org/10.1037/0033-2909.115.1.74

Davis, J. M., & Liang, C. H. (2015). A test of the mediating role of gender role conflict: Latino masculinities and help-seeking attitudes. *Psychology of Men & Masculinity, 16,* 23–32. http://dx.doi.org/10.1037/a0035320

Deaux, K., & Major, B. (1987). Putting gender into context: An interactive model of gender-related behavior. *Psychological Review, 94,* 369–389. http://dx.doi.org/10.1037/0033-295X.94.3.369

Eagly, A. H. (1987). *Sex differences in behavior: A social-role interpretation.* Hillsdale, NJ: Erlbaum.

Fiske, S. T., & Taylor, S. E. (1984). *Social cognition.* Reading, MA: Addison-Wesley.

Gawronski, B., & Bodenhausen, G. V. (2006a). Associative and propositional processes in evaluation: An integrative review of implicit and explicit attitude change. *Psychological Bulletin, 132,* 692–731.

Gawronski, B., & Bodenhausen, G. V. (2006b). Associative and propositional processes in evaluation: Conceptual, empirical, and metatheoretical issues: Reply to Albarracín, Hart, and McCulloch (2006), Kruglanski and Dechesne (2006), and Petty and Brin (2006). *Psychological Bulletin, 132,* 745–750. http://dx.doi.org/10.1037/0033-2909.132.5.745

Geary, D. C., Winegard, B., & Winegard, B. (2016). Evolutionary influences on men's lives. In Y. J. Wong & S. R. Wester (Eds.), *APA handbook of men and masculinities* (pp. 211–229). http://dx.doi.org/10.1037/14594-010

Greenwald, A. G., Banaji, M. R., Rudman, L. A., Farnham, S. D., Nosek, B. A., & Mellott, D. S. (2002). A unified theory of implicit attitudes, stereotypes, self-esteem, and self-concept. *Psychological Review, 109,* 3–25. http://dx.doi.org/10.1037/0033-295X.109.1.3

Haidt, J. (2006). *The happiness hypothesis: Finding modern truth in ancient wisdom.* New York, NY: Basic Books.

Haidt, J. (2012). *The righteous mind: Why good people are divided by politics and religion.* New York, NY: Vintage Books.

Hölldobler, B., & Wilson, E. O. (2009). *The superorganism: The beauty, elegance, and strangeness of insect societies.* New York, NY: Norton.

Joel, D., Berman, Z., Tavor, I., Wexler, N., Gaber, O., Stein, Y., . . . Assaf, Y. (2015). Sex beyond the genitalia: The human brain mosaic. *Proceedings of the National*

*Academy of Sciences of the United States of America, 112,* 15468–15473. Retrieved from http://www.pnas.org/content/early/2015/11/24/1509654112

Jones, K. D., & Heesacker, M. (2012). Addressing the situation: Some evidence for the significance of microcontexts with the gender role conflict construct. *Psychology of Men & Masculinity, 13,* 294–307. http://dx.doi.org/10.1037/a0025797

Kahneman, D. (2011). *Thinking, fast and slow.* New York, NY: Farrar, Straus & Giroux.

Kesebir, S. (2011). The superorganism account of human sociality: How and when human groups are like beehives. *Personality and Social Psychology Review, 6,* 233–261.

Kiselica, M. S., Benton-Wright, S., & Englar-Carlson, M. (2016). Accentuating positive masculinity: A new foundation for the psychology of boys, men, and masculinity. In Y. J. Wong & S. R. Wester (Eds.), APA *handbook of men and masculinities* (pp. 123–143). http://dx.doi.org/10.1037/14594-006

Korn, J. B. (1995). Institutional sexism: Responsibility and intent. *Texas Journal of Women and the Law, 4,* 83–124.

Levant, R. F., & Richmond, K. (2016). The gender role strain paradigm and masculinity ideologies. In Y. J. Wong & S. R. Wester (Eds.), APA *handbook of men and masculinities* (pp. 23–49). http://dx.doi.org/10.1037/14594-002

Lippa, R. A. (2016). Biological influences on masculinity. In Y. J. Wong & S. R. Wester (Eds.), APA *handbook of men and masculinities* (pp. 187–209). http://dx.doi.org/10.1037/14594-009

Lu, Q., Kang, X., Li, X., Zheng, H., Liu, X., & Shao, C. (2015). Revision of the Gender Role Conflict Scale—Adolescent for Chinese adolescents. *Chinese Journal of Clinical Psychology, 23,* 17–21.

O'Beaglaoich, C., Conway, R., & Morrison, T. G. (2015). Psychometric properties of the Gender Role Conflict Scale for Adolescents among Irish boys. *Psychology of Men & Masculinity, 16,* 33–41. http://dx.doi.org/10.1037/a0036018

O'Beaglaoich, C., Morrison, T. G., Nielsen, E., & Ryan, T. A. (2015). Experiences of gender role conflict as described by Irish boys. *Psychology of Men & Masculinity, 16,* 312–325. http://dx.doi.org/10.1037/a0037962

O'Neil, J. M. (1981). Male sex-role conflict, sexism, and masculinity: Implications for men, women, and the counseling psychologist. *The Counseling Psychologist, 9,* 61–80. http://dx.doi.org/10.1177/001100008100900213

O'Neil, J. M. (2008). Summarizing 25 years of research on men's gender role conflict using the Gender Role Conflict Scale: New research paradigms and clinical implications. *The Counseling Psychologist, 36,* 358–445. http://dx.doi.org/10.1177/0011000008317057

O'Neil, J. M. (2012). The psychology of men. In E. Altmaier & J. Hansen (Eds.), *Oxford handbook of counseling psychology* (pp. 95–127). New York, NY: Oxford University Press.

O'Neil, J. M. (2015). *Men's gender role conflict: Psychological costs, consequences, and an agenda for change.* http://dx.doi.org/10.1037/14501-000

O'Neil, J. M., & Denke, R. (2016). An empirical review of gender role conflict research: New conceptual models and research paradigms. In Y. J. Wong & S. R. Wester (Eds.), *APA handbook of men and masculinities* (pp. 51–79). http://dx.doi.org/10.1037/14594-003

O'Neil, J. M., & Egan, J. (1992). Men and women's gender role journeys: Metaphors for healing, transition, and transformation. In B. Wainrib (Ed.), *Gender issues across the lifecycle* (pp. 107–123). New York, NY: Springer.

O'Neil, J. M., & Egan, J. (1993). Abuses of power against women: Sexism, gender role conflict, and psychological violence. In E. P. Cook (Ed.), *Women, relationships, and power: Implications for counseling* (pp. 49–78). Alexandria, VA: ACA Press.

O'Neil, J. M., Egan, J., Owen, S. V., & Murry, V. (1993). The Gender Role Journey Measure (GRJM): Scale development and psychometric evaluations. *Sex Roles, 28,* 167–185. http://dx.doi.org/10.1007/BF00299279

O'Neil, J. M., Good, G. E., & Holmes, S. (1995). Fifteen years of theory and research on men's gender role conflict. In R. F. Levant & W. S. Pollack (Eds.), *The new psychology of men* (pp. 164–206). New York, NY: Basic Books.

O'Neil, J. M., Helms, B., Gable, R., David, L., & Wrightsman, L. (1986). Gender role conflict scale: College men's fear of femininity. *Sex Roles, 14,* 335–350. http://dx.doi.org/10.1007/BF00287583

Petty, R. E., & Cacioppo, J. T. (1985). The elaboration likelihood model of persuasion. *Advances in Experimental Social Psychology, 19,* 123–162.

Pleck, J. H. (1995). The gender role strain paradigm: An update. In R. F. Levant & W. S. Pollack (Eds.), *The new psychology of men* (pp. 11–32). New York, NY: Basic Books.

Rabinowitz, F. E., & Cochran, S. V. (2002). *Deepening psychotherapy with men.* http://dx.doi.org/10.1037/10418-000

Ross, L. (1987). The problem of construal in social inference and social psychology. In N. Grunberg, R. E. Nisbett, & J. Singer (Eds.), *A distinctive approach to psychological research: The influence of Stanley Schacter* (pp. 118–150). Hillsdale, NJ: Erlbaum.

Schwarz, N., Strack, F., Kommer, D., & Wagner, D. (1987). Soccer, rooms, and the quality of your life: Mood effects on judgments of satisfaction with life in general and with specific domains. *European Journal of Social Psychology, 17,* 69–79.

Shields, S. A. (2013). Gender and emotion: What we think we know, what we need to know, and why it matters. *Psychology of Women Quarterly, 37,* 423–435. http://dx.doi.org/10.1177/0361684313502312

Smiler, A. (2004). Thirty years after the discovery of gender: Psychological concepts and measures of masculinity. *Sex Roles, 50,* 15–26. http://dx.doi.org/10.1023/B:SERS.0000011069.02279.4c

Sobiraj, S., Rigotti, T., Weseler, D., & Mohr, G. (2015). Masculinity ideology and psychological strain: Considering men's social stressors in female-dominated occupations. *Psychology of Men & Masculinity, 16,* 54–66. http://dx.doi.org/10.1037/a0035706

Swim, J. K., Hyers, L. L., Cohen, L. L., & Ferguson, M. J. (2001). Everyday sexism: Evidence for its incidence, nature, and psychological impact from three daily diary studies. *Journal of Social Issues, 57,* 31–53. http://dx.doi.org/10.1111/0022-4537.00200

Tversky, A., & Kahneman, D. (1974). Judgment under uncertainty: Heuristics and biases. *Science, 185,* 1124–1131. http://dx.doi.org/10.1126/science.185.4157.1124

Vandello, J. A., & Bosson, J. L. (2013). Hard won and easily lost: A review and synthesis of theory and research on precarious manhood. *Psychology of Men & Masculinity, 14,* 101–113. http://dx.doi.org/10.1037/a0029826

Wester, S. R. (2008). Male gender role conflict and multiculturalism: Implications for counseling psychology. *The Counseling Psychologist, 36,* 294–324. http://dx.doi.org/10.1177/0011000006286341

Wester, S. R., Heesacker, M., & Snowden, S. J. (2016). An elephant in the room: Men's emotion from sex differences to social neuroscience. In Y. J. Wong & S. R. Wester (Eds.), *APA handbook of men and masculinities* (pp. 457–482). http://dx.doi.org/10.1037/14594-021

Wester, S. R., & Vogel, D. L. (2012). The psychology of men: Historical developments, current research, and future directions. In N. A. Fouad (Series Ed.), J. A. Carter & L. M. Subich (Eds.), *APA handbook of counseling psychology: Vol. 1. Theories, Research, and Methods* (pp. 371–396). http://dx.doi.org/10.1037/13754-014

Wester, S. R., Vogel, D. L., O'Neil, J. M., & Danforth, L. (2012). Development and evaluation of the Gender Role Conflict Scale Short Form (GRCS–SF). *Psychology of Men & Masculinity, 13,* 199–210. http://dx.doi.org/10.1037/a0025550

Whetstine-Richel, T. W. (2015). The relationship between gender role conflict and self and other awareness in male counselors treating men. *Dissertation Abstracts International: Section B. The Sciences and Engineering, 75,* 11(E). (UMI No. 3628896)

Zhang, C., Blashill, A. J., Wester, S. R., O'Neil, J. M., Vogel, D. L., Wei, J., & Zhang, J. (2015). Factor structure of the Gender Role Conflict Scale—Short Form in Chinese heterosexual and gay samples. *Psychology of Men & Masculinity, 16,* 229–233. http://dx.doi.org/10.1037/a0036154

# 4

# A CRITICAL DISCURSIVE APPROACH TO STUDYING MASCULINITIES

SARAH SEYMOUR-SMITH

Many investigations of men and masculinity based on the notion of roles sit uneasily between essentialist and performance-based notions of gender. In this chapter, the aim is to outline a *critical discursive psychological* (Edley, 2001; Wetherell & Edley, 1999) approach to studying masculinities that is clearly performance based in that it treats masculinity as a situated, fluid, and nego-tiated set of contingent actions and responses (Edley & Wetherell, 1995). There is a move away from treating masculinity as an internal trait that can be measured, to viewing masculinity as something people "do" or perform in talk such that we would expect different presentations of masculinity over a course of interaction. Just as the way one theorizes gender and masculinity typically determines the methods used in research, so, in turn, does it have an impact on the way that data are collected and the analytic tools used. For the performative stance on masculinity illustrated in this chapter, qualitative research is the best means of inquiry.

http://dx.doi.org/10.1037/0000023-005
*The Psychology of Men and Masculinities*, R. F. Levant and Y. J. Wong (Editors)
Copyright © 2017 by the American Psychological Association. All rights reserved.

Qualitative research aims to prioritize people's experiences and meaning making. However, qualitative research can be broadly glossed into two camps: experiential research, which aims to document people's experiences, views, and practices, and critical research, which aims to interrogate dominant meanings and deconstruct these (Clarke, Ellis, Peel, & Riggs, 2010). Critical discursive psychology is firmly located within the latter "turn to language," taking a social constructionist stance. The turn to language approach challenged the way that we acquire knowledge of the world, creating a shift in epistemology provided through critiques of essentialist understandings of knowledge construction. Traditional approaches to research worked on the assumption that it was possible to pin down an objective and fixed representation of reality. However, the social constructionist movement moved away from the notion of language as a transparent medium used to convey preexisting knowledge to a view of language as the site where we actually constitute knowledge. Thus, language is viewed as being intricately linked to our processes of thinking and reasoning (Potter & Wetherell, 1987), such that texts are never neutral but always constitute a particular version of reality. For example, if students fail an assessment, they may explain their failure differently depending on whether they were talking to parents/carers or to peers. To parents, they might claim that the lecturer was a poor communicator and the guidelines were unclear; to peers, their account might be that they were too busy partying and rushed the work. Discursive psychologists are not concerned with the "truth" of either of these versions; rather, they are interested in the "action" accomplished with the version of reality that is presented; blame and justification for a low grade are evident in both examples presented here but are worked up in different ways, which have an impact on the participant's identity. Social constructionist inquiry is "concerned with explicating the processes by which people come to describe, explain, or otherwise account for the world (including themselves) in which they live" (Gergen, 1985, p. 266), the argument being that individual and collective interests play a part in our descriptions of the world. Taken-for-granted assumptions, such as the binary categories of man and women, are challenged following investigations of how different cultures understand gender (Kessler & McKenna, 1978). Furthermore, social constructionists acknowledge the way that phenomena are historically situated with meanings shifting as a consequence of social processes such as communication, rhetoric, and negotiation across time (Gergen, 1985). Social constructionist research aims to identify the various culturally available ways of constructing social reality and explores their use to highlight the implications for human experience and social practice (Willig, 2005). Thus, the study of masculinities from this perspective takes into consideration the various ways that men's accounts are organized and attend to wider discourses.

In this chapter, the distinct approach of critical discursive psychology is unpacked to highlight how it differs from other forms of qualitative research and thus enable readers to gain some insight into the advantages of the position. Initially, some key influences of a discursive approach to masculinities are discussed, notably the concept of hegemonic masculinity developed from the work of Carrigan, Connell, and Lee (1985) and from later revisions suggested by Connell and Messerschmidt (2005). Next, the section on the "turn to language" discusses the main underpinnings of the theoretical stance used. Following this, a discursive framework for the study of masculinities, as documented by the body of work from Wetherell and Edley, is outlined via key analytic resources. Illustrations of this discursive approach are then provided before suggesting how to conduct and evaluate discursive research. Finally, a critical evaluation of discursive research is offered, and future research is discussed.

## THE INFLUENCE AND DEVELOPMENT OF CONNELL'S WORK ON HEGEMONIC MASCULINITY

Research on men and masculinities owes a significant debt to early feminist research and social constructionist theory. In the 1970s and 1980s, feminists developed the term *patriarchy* to refer to the notion of male power. Patriarchy was understood as a "set of social relations between men, which have a material base, and which though hierarchical, establish or create interdependence and solidarity among men that enable them to dominate women" (Hartmann, 1981, pp. 14–15). Kate Millett (1970) argued that patriarchal power is ubiquitous and that ideological indoctrination is the cause of women's oppression. She believed that women's oppression did not stem from biology but from the social constriction of femininity. In *Sexual Politics*, she demonstrated how patriarchal power created a sexist society. Society is constructed with dominant and subordinate roles. Male gender roles are typically valued more highly than women's gender roles. Celia Kitzinger's (1987) groundbreaking book *The Social Construction of Lesbianism* is a further illustration of how a social constructionist stance is able to effectively critique gay affirmative research for marginalizing the lesbian experience in a similar fashion to mainstream psychology's focus on heterosexual men (Clarke & Peel, 2004).

Building on feminist research, some pro-feminist men started to critically investigate the notion of masculinity (Edley, 2001). What this body of work attempted to do was to further explore how masculinity is linked to power relations in society. In *Gender and Power*, Connell (1987) carefully worked through an analysis of how broad patterns evident in society influence the formation of masculinity. Connell combined this with an account of the complexity of the material circumstances that influence the organization of men's relationships with women, suggesting that men benefit from women's input in both public and private life. Carrigan et al. (1985) viewed masculinity as a set of social processes and argued that change occurred through struggle and negotiation between men and women but also, importantly, between different groups of men.

Critical discursive masculinity research draws heavily on the concept of Connell and her colleagues' work on *hegemonic masculinity*, which recognized that there exists a plurality of masculinities. Hegemonic masculinity refers to the cultural and social power that a dominant form of masculinity holds in exerting ways of being male over other subordinated styles of masculinity (Connell & Messerschmidt, 2005). Hegemonic masculinity represents the ideological construction of masculinity and is argued to serve the interests of dominant men. However, it is not simply the diversity of masculinities that is important but the relations between different kinds of masculinity (Connell, 1995). Connell argued that most men do not really fit the image of the dominant form of masculinity; rather, there is a hierarchy between men. Connell (1987) argued that the "interplay between different forms of masculinity is an important part of how a patriarchal social order works" (p. 183). Hegemonic masculinity does not explicitly refer to physical force, although it could be supported by force; the power it wields is achieved through culture, ascendancy, and persuasion (Connell & Messerschmidt, 2005, pp. 832, 840). An example of this is present in the responses that Laura Bates received during "The Everyday Sexism Project," which she set up to document instances of sexism received by women (and men). During the course of the project, Bates was sent numerous posts from men threatening, in detail, the ways that they would rape her in response to her quiet revolution (Bates, 2014). Thus, hegemonic domination is not a simple matter of enforcement through physical force, but the cultural sanctioning of hierarchy may invoke this explicitly or implicitly. Even though many men may not be able to live up to the ideal of masculinity, they are, in various ways, complicit in sustaining hegemonic masculinity as they gain access to male privilege, however indirectly, from women and other groups of men. As such, it can produce dilemmas for men about whether they are sufficiently masculine. Despite these benefits hegemonic masculinity does not mean total control but that it is a dialogical process that may be disrupted, contested, or resisted at any point (Connell 1987, 1995). Carrigan et al. (1985) argued that our investigations must explore how certain groups of men manage to legitimate and reproduce this position of power. This dialogical theorizing of masculinity is helpful because it can account for changing practices of masculinity (Connell & Messerschmidt, 2005).

Connell's thesis is in accordance with many social constructionist accounts of identity in that she viewed masculinities as plural and relational—constructed in relation to women and to other men. However, Wetherell and Edley (1998) pointed out that Connell's explanation of hegemonic masculinity overlooked the detail of how masculinities emerged in practice. As a result, discursive researchers combined Connell's insights with other theoretical approaches to outline some steps necessary to the analysis of gender practices (Wetherell & Edley, 1998). In later reformulations of the concept, Connell and Messerschmidt (2005) highlighted discursive psychology as beneficial in exemplifying how different constructions of masculinity were deployed tactically at the local level. Before outlining the specific foundations of Wetherell and Edley's approach, it is important to locate their position within the wider "turn to language."

## CRITICAL DISCURSIVE PSYCHOLOGY AND THE "TURN TO LANGUAGE"[1]

As indicated in the introduction to this chapter, critical discursive psychology is heavily influenced by the "turn to language." In light of this, discursive psychology radically differs from other forms of qualitative research in that it places language center stage (Wetherell & Edley, 2014). This has a profound impact on the types of research questions that are addressed and the form of analyses that are undertaken, departing from those traditionally associated with qualitative work. Discursive psychology moves away from the notion of language as a transparent medium used to convey preexisting knowledge that most experiential approaches adhere to, instead viewing language as the site where we actively constitute knowledge. Discursive approaches treat language as action with the primary focus considering how phenomena are constructed, oriented to, and displayed in social interactions. In a sense, then, language "does" things; it performs particular functions. And this focus on action orientation has social, psychological and political implications (Potter & Wetherell, 1987). For example, the phrase "I call my mom every night" could be treated as conveying a piece of information, but the action of calling so frequently functions as a display of "doing being a good daughter/son."

In their pioneering book *Discourse and Social Psychology: Beyond Attitudes and Behaviour*, Potter and Wetherell (1987) set out an approach to discourse that builds on insights from philosophy, sociology, and literary theory. One of the influences that they cite is Austin's (1962) speech act theory. Austin

---

[1]Portions of this section adapted from "Applying Discursive Approaches to Health Psychology," by S. Seymour-Smith, 2015, *Health Psychology, 34*, pp. 371–380. Copyright 2015 by the American Psychological Association.

argued that many of the way we say things can be seen as "speech acts"; such acts not only convey information but also transform reality. Put briefly, a performative speech act, for example, refers to utterances that actually perform what they say. Speech act theory also illustrates the importance of context in interpreting ambiguous utterances. Knowledge of cultural contexts helps us to infer meaning more precisely. Austin's notion of illocutionary force usefully pointed out how this happens. The same statement, such as "shut that door," can be read as an order, a request, or a question, and which it is depends on the context (Wetherell & Potter 1988). The fictional character of Sheldon from the popular culture show *The Big Bang Theory* provides numerous humorous displays of Austin's ideas. Sheldon is a senior theoretical physicist at Caltech and shares an apartment with Leonard. Sheldon struggles with social interaction and often takes questions literally, as displayed in the following example:

Leonard: You'll never guess what just happened.

Sheldon: You went out in the hallway, stumbled into an interdimensional portal, which brought you 5,000 years into the future, where you took advantage of the advanced technology to build a time machine, and now you're back, to bring us all with you to the year 7010, where we are transported to work at the think-a-torium by telepathically controlled flying dolphins?

Leonard: No. Penny kissed me.

Sheldon: Who would ever guess that?

Although obviously played up for the humor, this example demonstrates how Sheldon takes literally Leonard's question and proposes a (ridiculous) candidate answer. Sheldon similarly displays a lack of understanding about the rules of social interaction in that he disrupts the implicit rules of conversation. Notably, Leonard's question is a ruse (or story preface) to encourage Sheldon to ask him to reveal what happened; in effect Leonard's question was requesting permission to tell his news. This focus on action and attention to the sequential aspects of talk leads us to consider a further influence of discursive psychology: conversation analysis.

Sacks (1992) developed *conversation analysis*, an innovative approach to the study of talk in interaction. Sacks developed his ideas from working on detailed transcriptions of tape-recorded talk that allowed him to focus on members' routine accomplishment of sense making in situ. On the basis of early observations of phone calls to the Suicide Prevention Center, Sacks argued that talk was organized and designed in a detailed way. Sacks came to prioritize the organization of talk-in-interaction "in its own right, as a 'machinery' independent of individual speakers, which provides the resources drawn upon by speakers in constructing their participation in any given interaction" (Hutchby & Wooffitt, 1998, p. 35). A central argument for conversation analysis is that patterns in interaction are recursive and participants consistently use the same techniques in different circumstances, but these resources are also context sensitive (Hutchby & Wooffitt, 1998). A main concern of conversation analysis is the organization and orderly accomplishment of turn-taking in interaction or the "sequential order of talk" and the various kinds of interaction work achieved as a consequence (Hutchby & Wooffitt, 1998). A focus on the sequential unfolding of talk establishes that "participants themselves actively analyze the ongoing production of talk to negotiate their own, situated participation in it" (Hutchby & Wooffitt, 1998, p. 38). For example, the following data are taken from a study in which robots were used to help engage children with intellectual and learning disabilities. The task here is for the child to identify the animal card that the robot asks them to find.

*Robot:* Can you show me the pig?

*Child:* Pig?

*Teacher:* Yes.

*Child:* [points to pig card]

Before this extract, the robot had not been clear in its command, and thus the child incorrectly identified the animal. As a consequence, in the second turn (utterance), we see the child orient to the task, but he also seeks clarification that he heard "pig" correctly. Once the teacher has confirmed that his understanding is correct (with her "yes"), the child picks the right card. Through second turns, speakers reveal that they have understood the content and intended action of the prior turn. This is referred to as *participants' orientation*, a key resource for discursive psychology in examining how talk and associated actions are treated as accountable and "consequential." Studying masculinity from this perspective places emphasis on grounding analytic observations about gender on the meanings and understandings of the participants themselves (Edley & Wetherell, 2008). Rather than imposing an analytic gloss that gender is analytically important, we are able to demonstrate that it is important to the participants themselves by the way that they refer to gender in talk.

In addition to the importance of examining the sequential details of talk-in-interaction, Wetherell (1998) argued for an inclusion of the broader, historical "argumentative texture" that infiltrate our discursive worlds (Laclau, 1993; Laclau & Mouffe, 1987). Therefore, a further influence for critical discursive psychology has been the work of the French social theorist Michel Foucault. Whereas a conversation analytic approach can be termed a *bottom-up* approach in that it focuses on how talk accomplishes actions and is closely tied to the data, approaches that draw on Foucault have in contrast been described as *top-down* (Edley & Wetherell, 1997). Top-down positions place more emphasis on issues of power and ideology and the broader pattern of social relations in which talk and texts are embedded.

In his work, Foucault's goal was not to "find truths" but to investigate the constitution of truth through discourse. Foucault examined what was required, in particular historical periods, to create the social spaces for knowledge to be constituted (Dreyfus & Rabinow, 1982). He used the term *episteme*, for instance, to refer to the sets of relations and discursive regularities that can be discovered in a particular period of time. A further key concept for Foucault was that of *discursive formation*. Here it is argued that some modes of thought are allowed, while others are stifled or made invisible (Storey, 1993). Foucault (1972) argued that these discursive formations regularly transformed into new discursive formations. In doing so, he rejected the idea that truths are universal and timeless; rather, discursive formations sustain a "regime of truth" that changes throughout historical periods (Storey, 1993). Foucault placed the body at the center of the struggles between different formations of power and was interested in how the body was regulated by different discursive formations. He believed that the body was produced through discourse, and he was critical of the traditional notion of the subject who was constructed as a fully conscious, stable, and independent being. In contrast to this, Foucault viewed the subject as being produced through discourse and then positioned by discourse. In this way, the subject operated within the limits of the episteme, the discursive formation, and the regime of truth at any particular period and culture. Subjects are produced by discourse, and discourse also makes a place for the subject. The subject cannot stand outside of the regulating power of these, and Foucault's contribution to the notion of the subject was to consider how the subject is produced in different historical periods (Hall, 2001). For example, Foucault's work considered how gay men are presented differently across historical periods. Therefore, in addition to a focus on the sequential production of masculinity grounded in participant's understandings, Edley and Wetherell (2008) were keen to go beyond this to situate their analysis of masculinity within broader culturally available discourses. Critical discursive psychology held on to the importance of history and culture and developed the concept of positioning, as we see in the next section.

## A CRITICAL DISCURSIVE APPROACH TO MASCULINITY: KEY ANALYTIC RESOURCES

In their critical discursive approach to the study of masculinities, Wetherell and Edley aimed to capture the paradoxical relationship that exists between discourse and identity I have described here (Edley, 2001; Edley & Wetherell, 2008; Wetherell & Edley, 2014). Building on Connells's notion that people are constrained by social structure, their aim was to see what this "constraint" looked like in practice. However, attempting to articulate a mode of analysis that captures how identity is contextually produced for particular occasions yet permeated and mediated by historical and cultural discourses is no mean feat. To negotiate the analytic process of both these traditions, one must be able to combine the broad interpretative identification of power, ideology, and inequality that is not necessarily grounded in the interaction at hand with the bottom-up analysis of the turn-by-turn display of gender identification as a participants' concern. Wetherell and Edley's discursive psychology approach to masculinity thus focuses on the ideological construction of masculinities as they unfold on the ground (Wetherell & Edley, 1998). Over the course of a number of studies, Wetherell and Edley considered the practical accomplishment of how masculinities emerged in practice. A key focus was on accountability, which they argued depends on the coproduction of all parties in social interaction such that "people are accountable to each other in interaction and thus departures from 'what everybody knows to be appropriate' require explanation and create 'trouble' in interaction which will need repair" (Wetherell & Edley, 1998, p. 161). For example, somebody may meet a friend who has had a baby and comment on how pretty the baby is. Babies can be hard to identify as male or female, and if this comment was made about a male baby, the parent may correct their friend as "pretty" is not typically a favorable compliment for a baby boy; this creates some "trouble" in the interaction, which the friend will need to address. Masculinity from this perspective is viewed as the way that meanings of masculinity flow across texts and contexts and how individual men establish and then reflect and often rework these meanings in relation to ideological dilemmas (Billig, 2001) that they encounter in their talk.

For a discursive approach, then, the theorization of subjectivity is crucial. In their account of subjectivity, Wetherell and Edley (1998) combined the notion that individuals are positioned by discourses in the Foucauldian sense yet actively re-create positions for themselves, especially in response to "trouble." How men position themselves in relation to hegemonic masculinity is "regulated by shared forms of sense making which are consensual although contested, which maintain male privilege, which are largely taken for granted, and which are highly invested" (Wetherell & Edley, 1999 p. 351).

Wetherell and Edley (1998) argued that an adequate discourse analysis of gender practice should move to "large" data sets where one can identify discursive patterns across a variety of settings. To explicate the dual nature of gender practice as both constituted and constitutive, Wetherell and Edley developed three key analytic concepts—*interpretative repertoires*, *ideological dilemmas*, and *subject positions*—that form the basis of a critical discursive analytic approach.

## Interpretative Repertoires

The notion of *interpretative repertoire* was first developed by Gilbert and Mulkay (1984) and later by Potter and Wetherell (1987) to describe a broad unit that makes sense of social life. An interpretative repertoire is a recognizable routine of arguments, descriptions, and evaluations found in people's talk often distinguished by familiar clichés, anecdotes, and tropes and often marked by vivid metaphors. Interpretative repertoires are the commonplaces (Billig, 2001) of everyday conversation and the building blocks through which people develop accounts and versions of significant events and through which they perform social life. Interpretative repertoires are "what everyone knows." Indeed, the collectively shared social consensus behind an interpretative repertoire is often so established and familiar that only a fragment of the argumentative chain needs to be formulated in talk to form an adequate basis for the participants to jointly recognize the version of the world that is developing. Interpretative repertoires represent relatively coherent ways of talking about things and are part of our shared social understanding. After time spent coding the data for interpretative repertoires, a sense of recognition of various patterns develops, and there is a feeling that the majority of ways that a topic is talked about have been noted (Edley, 2001). Once it has been possible to check through these interpretative repertoires, it is often possible to see that they are drawn on in different ways.

A good example of interpretative repertoires is illustrated in Edley and Wetherell's (2001) exploration of men's constructions of feminism and feminists. Two competing interpretative repertoires were prevalent in their data. The first was a liberal feminist repertoire of women simply wanting equality, presented in a rational and neutral manner. However, this was contrasted with a more elaborate and embodied account of feminism that evaluated feminists in terms of their (unappealing) physical appearance, sexual orientation, and (negative) attitude toward men. Edley and Wetherell (2001) noted that participants in their study moved between these two interpretative repertoires as they made sense of ideological and interactional consequences.

## Ideological Dilemmas

Another analytic concept that discursive researchers use to link discourse with wider concerns than the surrounding text is the concept of ideological dilemmas. When individuals speak, they draw on terms that are culturally, historically, and ideologically available (Billig, 2001). *Ideology* is defined here as the common sense of society, which appears natural, inevitable, and unquestioned. Billig et al. (1988) argued against the Marxist notion that ideologies were coherent and integrated sets of ideas that served the interests of the ruling class. Instead, they suggested that theorists of ideology have missed a critical feature, the notion of the *thinking individual*. Their point is that individuals are not merely passive receivers of knowledge. Billig et al. referred to the notion of *lived ideologies*, which are said to be the beliefs, values, and practices of particular societies or cultures. However, it is important to realize that these lived ideologies are not all coherent or integrated (Edley, 2001). Indeed, Billig et al. noted that much everyday discourse is organized around dilemmas and involves arguing and puzzling over these. Ideology, they argued, comprises contrary themes, and without these "individuals could neither puzzle over their social worlds nor experience dilemmas" (p. 2). Through these contrary themes, we develop our rhetorical skills as we think through socially shared beliefs and argue their merits. Billig (2001) claimed that in discussions one can hear individuals "jostling" with the contrary themes of common sense. A crucial feature of lived ideologies is their usefulness as rich and flexible resources for social interaction (Edley, 2001). They represent different arguments and ways of viewing the world, and often we move between contradictory themes depending on the flow of talk. From this perspective of ideology, the interest is in examining the "social preconditions for dilemmas in order to show how ordinary life, which seems far removed from the dramas of wolves and precipices, is shaped by dilemmatic qualities" (Billig et al., 1988, p. 9).

To illustrate the concept of ideological dilemmas, a study about men's imagined futures opened up discussions of fatherhood (Wetherell & Edley, 1999). When the issue of how men would combine work and child care arose, the men resisted the idea of paying others to look after their children. Stemming from this discussion one participant, Aaron, is caught in an ideological dilemma as he attempts to negotiate between being a good, hands-on father yet balancing this with his desire to have a career. Contradictory positions are encountered between his construction of an egalitarian relationship and his wish for his partner to be the main caregiver. The analysis centers on the way that the men attempt to justify their positions in the ideological field through various strategies and how this has implications on their identity as men.

## Subject Positions

The idea that there are various competing interpretative repertoires that people draw on in their talk means that individuals have access to a whole range of rhetorical opportunities and thus indicates the possibility of human agency (Edley, 2001). *Subject positions* refer to the various ways that the self is positioned through interpretative repertoires or the ways that the self is invoked or negotiated in interaction. Common to discursive and social constructionist research (Gergen, 1999) is the claim that identity (personhood) is constituted and reconstituted through discourse and is thus flexible, contextual, relational, situated, and inflected by power relations. Davies and Harre (1990) argued that identity is always an open question with a shifting answer depending on the positions made available through talk, in interaction and conversations. The story lines of everyday conversations provide us with a position to speak from, and they allow the positioning of others as characters with roles and rights. Subject positions also open up possibilities for shifting resistances. From the perspective of critical discursive psychology, subject positions are important for a number of reasons. First, they accomplish certain things in interactional contexts. Second, the subject positions evident in discourse around men tell us something about the range of ways that men can construct themselves in particular cultural contexts. This also tells us something about the broader ideological context (Edley, 2001). The identity positions that come into play in conversation can at various points be either welcome or unwelcome. More important, analytically, we can go consider how subject positions come to be "troubled" and "untroubled" (Wetherell, 1998). We can effectively track "the emergence of different and often contradictory or inconsistent versions of people, their characters, motives, states of mind and events in the world—and [ask] why this (different) formulation at this point in the strip of talk?" (Wetherell, 1998, p. 395).

By considering all the positions in play in a stretch of talk, including those that might be relevant but are absent, we become aware of what is invoked by certain positions. Often we realize that we present ourselves as having inconsistent subject positions, and "troubled" subject positions need careful attention. Subject positions in Wetherell's (1998) argument are not already constituted or determined by discourses but are actively constituted in response to emergent conversational activities. Analysis should take into account the "argumentative threads displayed in participants' orientations" (Wetherell, 1998, p. 404).

Such argumentative threads are evident in Edley and Wetherell's (1997) study about the construction of masculine identities. The analysis focuses on how members of a subordinated group of male students negotiated their place in the school hierarchy. By invoking the cultural resource of the "new man," the participants were able to distinguish themselves from the dominant male identity of the rugby players (a group they did not belong to). Moreover, a further interesting strategy was to accept a discredited identity of "wimp" by redefining "wimps" as incorporating mental strengths that the rugby players did not possess.

Wetherell and Edley laid the groundwork for a critical discursive psychology of masculinities and conducted numerous studies of masculinities that demonstrated their approach. Their work included an analysis of the construction of masculine identities (Edley & Wetherell, 1997), the negotiation of imaginary positions (Wetherell & Edley, 1999), and the construction of feminism and feminists (Edley & Wetherell, 2001). In turn, their approach was taken up by numerous other researchers of masculinity. The following section outlines some research related to men's health issues.

## DISCURSIVE PSYCHOLOGY IN PRACTICE: SOME EMPIRICAL ILLUSTRATIONS

Discussing a critical discursive approach in the abstract does not always convey the scope and type of analysis that is conducted. Therefore, this section showcases some empirical illustrations in the context of men's health to flesh out the approach. Please note that the data excerpts are transcribed with a Jefferson (2004) style transcription notation that captures some of the way that the speech is delivered (see Appendix). Readers new to this mode of data transcription may find the extracts more difficult to follow than usual, but it is necessary for this type of analysis.

### Constructing Male Patients

The first example examines the contradictory discursive framework through which doctors and nurses constructed their male patients (Seymour-Smith, Wetherell, & Phoenix, 2002). Three interpretative repertoires—women are health conscious and responsible, while men are not; men don't talk about emotional issues; and men are the serious users of the health service—evidenced a contradictory discursive framework. The following extract references the first interpretative repertoire.

*Extract 1*[2]

Taken from an interview with a male doctor.

1. Interviewer so:o there are more women using the practice
2. [than men
3. Dr. Crawford [oh yeah
4. yeah I would say so
5. Interviewer (1) mm (.) do you why do you think that is?
6. Dr. Crawford erm two reasons I think firstly (.) women's health
7. is very
8. much in (.) the news

---

[2]Extracts 1–4 from "'My Wife Ordered Me to Come': A Discursive Analysis of Doctors' and Nurses' Accounts of Men's Use of General Practitioners," by S. Seymour-Smith, M. Wetherell, and A. Phoenix, 2002, *Journal of Health Psychology, 7*, pp. 253–267. Copyright 2002 by Sage Publications. Reprinted with permission [analysis amended].

9. Interviewer: yeah
10. Dr. Crawford and women are much more health conscious I
11. would think
12. than men are (.) so they also tend to come to the surgery
13. with children [so they know their way
14. Interviewer [mm
15. Dr. Crawford here and they get to know the doctors and they are
16. comfortable with it
17. Interviewer right
18. Dr. Crawford erm (.) so I think it's a combination of things
19. Interviewer mm
20. Dr. Crawford ermm (1) that's probably a lot to do with it
21. they they
22. come for smears they come for ante-natal care so it isn't
23. a big deal to them to come (.) whereas men tend I think to
24. hide their health problems and pretend everything is all
25. right
26. Interviewer right
27. Dr. Crawford so and they don't come 'til their wife makes
28. them an
29. appointment
30. Interviewer (.) I've heard that so many times ((laughs))
31. Dr. Crawford oh yeah absolutely mm (.) it's it's amazing you
32. know they
33. just do not come you find records remarkably little in
34. [(.) for a lot of men who have got
35. Interviewer [mm
36. Dr. Crawford problems but won't admit it

The interpretative repertoire constructs women as more health conscious and familiar with health issues from the media, their own medical needs, and in their role as caretakers of children's health. Women are thus also deemed as more "comfortable with" coming to the surgery through their engagement in these mundane activities (Line 13). In contrast, men are constructed as more reluctant and hide their health problems (Lines 24 and 36), and this is evidenced by their records (Line 33). Within this repertoire men are positioned as childlike by the doctor as they "don't come 'til their wife makes an appointment." The interviewer receives this construction as something that she is familiar with (as indicated in the section on interpretative repertoires).

A formulaic response was noted across the first two repertoires, and this was often presented as a story and frequently worked up as a joke. Formulaic responses have a canonical flavor, a sense of "what men are like."

*Extract 2*

Taken from an interview with a male doctor.

1. Sarah do many of the men (.) er bring their partners with them to
2. the consultation?
3. Dr. Hall difficult to know whether they bring them or whether
4. their
5. partner says I'm coming ((laughs))
6. Sarah ((laughs))

*Extract 3*

Taken from an interview with a female doctor.

1. Sarah do many of the men bring their partners with them to the
2. consultation?
3. Dr. Frome (1) some
4. Sarah some?
5. Dr. Frome (yes) some do
6. Sarah right
7. Dr. Frome some are <u>dragged</u> by their partners
8. Sarah right ((laughs))
9. Dr. Frome ((laughs))
10. Sarah does that ha happen (1) quite often or
11. Dr. Frome (.) or you'll get the er opening line (.) <u>she sent me</u>
12. Sarah yeah=
13. Dr. Frome =you know
14. Sarah ((laughs)) yeah

*Extract 4*

Taken from an interview with a male doctor.

1. Sarah do many of the men bring their (.) <u>partners</u> with them to
2. the consultation=
3. Dr. Andrews =<u>no:oo</u> ((laughs))
4. Sarah no? ((laughs))
5. Dr. Andrews many of the partners bring their <u>men</u> to the con-
6. sultation
7. [((laughs))
8. Sarah [ ((LAUGHS)) really?
9. Dr. Andrews <u>oh yes</u> (.) <u>or:r</u> the men come in and say my <u>wife</u> has
10. ordered me to come

Responses to the question "Do many men bring their partners with them to the consultation?" typically produced a comic response from the doctors. Without presenting a detailed analysis of these data extracts (for further discussion, see Seymour-Smith, Wetherell, & Phoenix, 2002), a number of points can be made. First, female partners are portrayed as health supervisors to men, effectively positioning men as childlike. Second, the timing and sequencing of the comedy (e.g., extract 4, lines 3–5, with the latched, brief, negative response accompanied by laughter but without any elaboration) signal some conversational expectation is being broken for effect and cues the listener that some kind of revelation is about to be unfolded. The way that the responses are played out orient to some culturally shared knowledge about men—with laughter displaying mutual co-orientation and affiliation (Glenn, 1991). Third, at one level, men are criticized in this discourse, yet the critique does not bite or quite engage. It is worked up in a humorous and tolerant way with the evaluative accent positioning of the male patient as "hapless and helpless."

The discourse of our sample of health care professionals can be seen as a simple reflection and description of doctors' and nurses' everyday experiences of the men in their care, but such descriptions are also deeply implicated in the formation and continuation of the "reality" of the male patient. The interpretative repertoire positions men and women differently such that the discursive environments created through these formulations of the male patient are likely to have some clear practical consequences for the ways in which men negotiate health and illness.

Through a consideration and orientation to the wider cultural environment via interpretative repertoires plus an examination of how men are positioned within these, a discursive analysis demonstrates how hegemonic masculinity was valorized and indulged while simultaneously critiqued. The attention to the sequential aspect of how this plays out adds support to this analysis; there's evidence within the social interaction of how this is treated by the participants. The interviewer is treated as a coparticipant within the analysis—something often missed in other forms of qualitative research where an isolated participant quote may be taken out of the context in which it is produced (Potter & Hepburn, 2005).

## Men's Negotiation of a Troubled Self-Help Group Identity

The second example comes from a set of interviews with men who had testicular cancer and women who had breast cancer (Seymour-Smith, 2008). The set of interviews formed part of a larger study about men's health, but all the participants in this particular study belonged to a self-help group. One of the questions asked to all participants in the wider study was whether they considered attending a self-help group when they were ill. Because members of this particular cohort were recruited via the support groups they attended, the interviewer still asked the question but added that of course she knew they did. What happened in response to this question became the focus of the analysis because it caused "trouble" for the men. Whereas women unproblematically accepted the positioning by the interviewer of belonging to a self-help group, the men resisted the self-help group identity, stating things such as, "It was the last thing I wanted." What became apparent was that the men were resisting the identity and activities associated with belonging to a "stereotypical" support group. Indeed, the men routinely oriented the identity and activities that such stereotypes invoke, as can be seen in the following extract.

*Extract 5*[3]

Taken from an interview with Cal and Paul.

1. Paul    I think they expect to come along and find a load of ill
2. people=
3. Cal     =yeah yeah [((laughs))
4. Paul    [and you know [inaudible due to over talking]
5. Sarah   [yeah
6. Cal     [yeah it's er I think it's erm a bit of a I always use this one
7. but a bit of an alcoholics anonymous thing (2)
8. Sarah   yeah
9. Cal     stand up you know my names Cal Jackson I've had
10. testicular
11. cancer and then burst into tears and all that sort of thing and
12. blokes don't like that sort of [thing
13. Sarah   [they just think I'm not going
14. to do that
15. Cal     I don't want anybody to cry in front of me or anything
16. like
17. that=
18. Sarah   =no
19. Cal     so they don't want to come along

Immediately before this extract, Cal and Paul had been discussing the problem of getting men to attend the self-help group to which they both belong. Paul claims that men might expect to find "a load of ill people." Cal sets up a familiar image of self-help group, Alcoholics Anonymous, and dramatizes the activities of this type of group as bursting into tears. Of

[3]Extracts 5–7 from "'Blokes Don't Like That Sort of Thing': Men's Negotiation of a 'Troubled' Self-Help Group Identity," by S. Seymour-Smith, 2008, *Journal of Health Psychology, 13*, pp. 798–803. Copyright 2008 by Sage Publications. Reprinted with permission [analysis amended].

interest to an analysis of hegemonic masculinity, Cal states, "Blokes don't like that sort of thing." Later, he changes footing (*footing* refers to how the mode and frame of conversation is determined; the stance taken by speakers indicates their alignment to the topic under discussion; Goffman, 1983) and says, "I don't want anybody to cry in front of me or anything like that." Another self-help group member, Matt, also built up a comical portrayal of support groups as being "like a mother's meeting" and being "touchy feely." It appeared that the existence of stereotypical notions of self-help groups was troubling for men because of the potential for being likened to an—arguably gendered—stereotypical self-help group member. In some sense, then, the way the interviewer positioned the men as members of a self-help group effectively challenged their masculine identity, and this "trouble" was evident in their responses. How, then, did the men explain their presence at self-help groups? How did they manage this troubled identity? In the extract that follows, Matt narrates his eventual involvement in a support group.

*Extract 6*

Taken from an interview with Matt.

1. Matt    but it (1) one of the guys I work with (.) <u>he</u> went down
2. with
3. it about 18 months after I had it
4. Sarah    mm
5. Matt    and er he went along (1) 'cos he was probably <u>more</u>
6. <u>that</u> sort
7. of person that=
8. Sarah    =right =
9. Matt    =would do that sort of thing you know
10. Sarah    yeah
11. Matt    I suppose I am now because I went along but (1) I
12. (.) I it
13. (.) when I first saw it I thought (.) no it's not for me it
14. was ((unclear))
15. Sarah    yeah
16. Matt    [then he sort of like
17. Sarah    [so did he tell you about it?
18. Matt    yeah he he rung me up 'cos we weren't working
19. together he'd
20. left and moved to another company by this point (.) and he
21. rung up and he said do you want to come along he says 'cos
22. it's really good

23. Sarah    mm
24. Matt    and erm I sort of had a thought about it (1) I won't go
25. and then I thought yeah I will so I just went along to one
26. meeting not expecting a <u>lot</u> erm

Matt accounts for his change of decision to attend the group through a narrative about how a guy from work became involved in the group because it was "really good." Matt formulates his friend as "probably <u>more that</u> sort of person that . . . would do that sort of thing you know," leaving open the full explanation of what that type of person might be. However, whatever that person might be occasions Matt to reflexively add that he is perhaps that type of person now. In doing so, Matt is caught in an ideological dilemma. He has previously positioned himself as not being the type of person who would attend a self-help group. What follows is a construction of this initial awareness of the group as being "not for me" (Line 10), and even deciding "I won't go" (Line 20). However, he presents a change of heart with "then I thought yeah I will so I just went along to <u>one</u> meeting <u>not</u> <u>expecting a lot</u>" (Lines 21–22, emphasis added).

The added value of a discursive approach in contrast to some other forms of qualitative analysis is that it is capable of attending to the contradictions of the presentation of identity, mapping the dilemma and the way the participant positions himself.

This construction of self-help groups as not being beneficial (not expecting a lot, or not wanting an emotional outlet) was a familiar pattern in the men's accounts. The way that the men negotiated their involvement was by constructing their group as proactive, as we can see in Nick's excerpt.

*Extract 7*

Taken from an interview with Nick.

1. Sarah    so what's it like when you've <u>been</u> to the meetings
2. then=
3. Nick    =it suits me 'cos there's not a lot of people <u>there</u>
4. Sarah    yeah
5. Nick    erm (.) you know 'cos <u>I'm not one for</u> (.) you know er
6. maybe the
7. stereotypical [erm you know view of self-help groups we all
8. get
9. Sarah    [ ((laughs)) yeah
10. Nick    round in a circle and start crying and feel sorry for
11. yourself
12. Sarah    mm right=

13. Nick     = I mean I'm not into that=
14. Sarah    =no=

[Lines omitted]

15. Nick     erm (.) I probably didn't consider too much somebody
16. coming at
17. to the meeting after I started and talking to them and <u>how</u>
18. <u>useful I would be</u> but just getting involved and perhaps
19. <u>sharing</u> in some of the
20. Sarah    mm
21. Nick     good things that Cal and the others are doing
22. Sarah    mm mm
23. Nick     erm so you know and and feeling that you know <u>I ought</u>
24. <u>to put</u>
25. something back in =
26. Sarah    =right

[Lines omitted]

27. Nick     =YES <u>that's right</u> for me it's about <u>saving lives</u>
28. Sarah    yeah
29. Nick     it's about stopping people dying of cancer
30. Sarah    mm
31. Nick     for me
32. Sarah    mm yeah
33. Nick     ultimately 'cos (.) that's why you talk about it=
34. Sarah    =yeah

Common to the other men, Nick makes relevant the activities associated with stereotypical self-help groups and distances himself from the problematic activity of crying and feeling sorry for yourself. The turning point for Nick is constructed as a realization that he could be potentially useful to newcomers attending the group (Lines 15–21). In doing this, Nick, as with the other men, built up his and their membership in the group around giving something to the group rather than being in receipt of something from the group. This proactive version of what constitutes a self-help group member wards off other potentially problematic identities (e.g., being in receipt of support, crying), producing a more "legitimate" male identity.

One could conclude that these were men who were perhaps rejecting hegemonic masculine ideals through attending a self-help group, as men participate in self-help groups to a lesser extent than women (Thiel de Bocanegra, 1992). However, the careful management of identity that was involved in the men's accounts meant that they are in some ways complicit because they do not necessarily challenge gendered power relations. Men's identities were constructed in relation to who they were not (Wetherell & Edley, 2014). Specifically, they were not men who cried or belonged to stereotypical support groups. By formulating a proactive group membership, the men constructed their identity in a way that conformed to the dominant characteristics of strength and not weakness (see also Wetherell & Edley, 1999, for a similar pattern in the men that they interviewed). This also echoes the point that Connell (1995) made about the subordination of identities that are not viewed as legitimate (see also Edley & Wetherell, 1997, on a discussion of the wimp). The analysis demonstrates how men resist, negotiate, and refashion or reappropriate hegemonic masculinity (Wetherell & Edley, 2014).

The discursive climate in which this group of men exist places restrictions on potential performances of masculinity. By employing the methods of discursive psychology, it is possible to unpack the complexity of this performativity through a consideration of how men are positioned in the interaction and how they attend to this and rework their own position as a consequence. However, in this instance, the resistance to being positioned as a man who attends a support group had a material consequence for the members of the self-help group: They changed the name of their group from "testicular cancer self-help group" to a new name that omitted the troubling "self-help" concept. This highlights the value of a discursive approach because it has implications for the way that men's health is promoted. First, the name of self-help groups should be carefully considered, especially if men are to be attracted. Second, perhaps health education campaigns need to consider targeting men in ways that appeal, or even conform, to what we could describe as hegemonic masculine ideals (e.g., bravado, humor, discretion).

### African Caribbean Men and the Digital Rectal Exam

Focusing on men's discursive practice in situations where they are doing identity work illustrates any ideological consequences that may, or may not, lead to the maintenance of power inequalities (Wetherell & Edley, 2014). In addition, a discursive approach is able to consider the shifting dynamics of the broader social context as it plays out in social interaction. Furthermore, men are not just men; masculinity intersects with social class and ethnicity, in addition to other variables (Wetherell & Edley, 2014). The last empirical illustration comes from a study that examined the poor prognostic outcomes of African Caribbean men in the United Kingdom with prostate cancer (Seymour-Smith et al., in press). Interviews were conducted with African Caribbean men with and without prostate cancer. The data excerpt that follows comes from part of an interview in which barriers to help seeking were being discussed.

*Extract 8*

Taken from an interview with Derek, a man without prostate cancer.

1. Derek hmm I don't <u>really</u> want a doctor to be examining my
2. (.) you
3. know my[back bottom
4. Sarah    [yeah yeah yeah
5. Derek you know it's (.) [it's you know
6. Sarah [it's just one of those things isn't it
7. Derek there's no other way you can say it
8. Sarah I know
9. Derek but it's that we (.) have got
10. Sarah that <u>fear</u> of that=
11. Derek =a lot of Jamaican men kind of have got that here and
12. there
13. Sarah WHY↑ (.) so <u>why</u> do you think it (.) because I think
14. <u>white</u> men (.) have that fear as well but why↑ why do you
15. think it's <u>more</u> (.) Jamaican (.) sort of issue?
16. Derek well hmm okay heh heh
17. Sarah heh heh heh 'cos it (.)it's useful for me know that (.)
18. to know
19. how to overcome it
20. Derek erm it's (0.2) I think it's an (.)it's it's (0.1) it's <u>not</u> as
21. prevalent as <u>back</u> in the (.) erm (.)how can I say back in
22. the (.) the the past generations [if you like
23. Sarah [yeah yeah
24. Derek it's not as erm it's it's kind of erm:m it's getting(0.1)
25. we're we're becoming more er:::m erm:mmm(0.2) <u>less</u> homo-
26. phobic
27. Sarah okay (.)that's good (£)
28. Derek I think that's the word
29. Sarah so do think that's what it is [all about tha:at
30. Derek [yeah <u>yes</u>(.) yes
31. Ja Jamaica unfortunately
32. Sarah has got that <u>stig</u>[ma:a that of
33. Derek [has got the homophobia is it's a <u>thing</u>
34. Sarah <u>yeah</u>
35. Derek (.) <u>men</u> <u>do not</u>
36. Sarah    do that
37. Derek you don't play [with another man
38. Sarah [yeah yeah=
39. Derek =you know what I'm saying

40. Sarah yeah no (.) [no I get that
41. Derek [so even (.)even a <u>doctor</u>
42. Sarah it's stil[l
43. Derek [even though [it's a <u>doctor</u>
44. Sarah [seen as (.) yeah yeah
45. Derek we have in the <u>past</u> (.) not really been erm (.) erm
46. <u>willing</u>
47. Sarah yeah=
48. Derek =to allow a <u>doctor</u> [to examine certain parts of your
49. Sarah [ok yeah
50. Derek your body
51. Sarah yeah no I understand that
52. Derek and (.)and that is it (.)it's kind of <u>taboo</u>
53. Sarah yeah(.)
54. Derek I think a man does not you know erm [do that to
55. <u>another</u> man

The majority of men in the study constructed the digital rectal exam (DRE) as a barrier. In Extract 8, Derek explains that he doesn't want a doctor to examine his "back bottom." The interviewer claims that White men have a similar fear of DRE and asks why it is more of a Jamaican issue. Derek makes links to homophobia, with Jamaican men viewing contact "in certain parts of your body" as "taboo." Derek positions Jamaican men as not "playing" with another man, and this it seems extends to a physical examination by a doctor (Lines 35–41). However, what is interesting in the account is the various shifts in footing (Goffman, 1983) that Derek makes throughout his explanation—initially he locates himself within this discourse (Line1), then this is broadened out to "a lot of Jamaican men" (Line 11), then to "the past generations" (Line 22), to "Jamaica" (Line 31), "men" (Line 55), "you" (line 33), "we" (Line 45), "your" (Line 50), and "a man" (Line 54). In doing so, he variously positions himself as falling prey, or rising above, this legacy of homophobic thinking. A critical discursive approach thus focuses on the performance of identity, noting the shifts that arise from the actions being accomplished at various points in the interaction.

Although DRE was routinely constructed as problematic, a progressive narrative was also identified, as illustrated in the following extract.

*Extract 9*

Taken from an interview with Joel, a man with prostate cancer.

1. Sarah    so moving away from your particular experience what
2. do you

3. think might be the reasons why other <u>men</u> in your situation
4. might dela:ay looking (.)you know se (.)er doing something
5. about <u>symptoms</u> of prostate cancer
6. Joel I think some men just embarrassed
7. Sarah yeah
8. Joel but then you know but you know they're touching your bum
9. Sarah right
10. Joel and [things like some men embarrassed
11. Sarah [a lot of people have said that
12. Joel a lot of black men like that
13. Sarah I know the people have said that it's
14. Jack yeah they do=
15. Sarah = white men don't [like it either but people have
16. Joel [yeah yeah I don't know about white men
17. but a lot of black men like that
18. Sarah yeah
19. Joel you know what I mean (.) it just like that you know but it's
20. not <u>big deal?</u>
21. Sarah no if you have to do it don't you?=
22. Joel =but I mean my doctor said to me when I had one he
23. just like
24. that (course Joel) no problem but we embarrassed just like that
25. if he (.)if he didn't do that to me I wouldn't have been around
26. today
27. Sarah exactly it's worth it isn't it

As with Derek in Extract 8, Joel constructs DRE as problematic for "Black men" due to embarrassment about "touching your bum." The interviewer again raises the issue that White men do not like DRE, possibly to prompt further explanation of why this is such a troubled identity for the African Caribbean community. Joel invokes active voicing of his doctor, which effectively removes some of the difficulty associated with "owning up" to digressing from the cultural associations with DRE. His "take-home" message is that without DRE, he would not be alive.

Having a DRE troubles African Caribbean men's hegemonic masculine identity with the stigmatization (as they typically construct it) of being associated with gay sexual acts. However, by paying attention to how men discursively manage this ideological dilemma of seeking help demonstrates that a hegemonic identity can be managed via a pragmatic approach. Furthermore, progressive narratives about homophobia are also possible to track through the microanalysis of footing shifts.

# CONDUCTING AND EVALUATING CRITICAL DISCURSIVE WORK ON MASCULINITIES

The preceding discussion has situated a critical discursive psychological approach to masculinity within the turn to language, overviewed the key analytic resources, and illustrated these via empirical research. But how does one make the move to actually conducting a discursive study?

First of all, the study needs to fit within the remit of the field. Those used to conducting qualitative research will need to shift their focus of study from treating language as a transparent medium used to access participants' "inner workings" and move to a consideration of how language constitutes the social world. The focus switches to the study of language in use and research questions aim to consider construction and function (Potter & Wetherell, 1987; Taylor, 2001).

Critical discursive analysis is a fairly labor-intensive approach; thus, the amount of data one can work on can be relatively small. Enough data are needed to map out interpretative repertoires and other patterns across texts or interviews but not so much that the project at hand becomes unworkable. Ten interviews lasting between 45 and 90 minutes would probably be sufficient, but work in this area will vary dramatically depending on the specific research question. At some point, the researcher will note that he or she has reached a point of saturation where the same patterns keep reappearing and nothing more is gained from further data collection.

For researchers conducting interviews, it is important to think carefully about designing questions that stimulate interpretative contexts in the interview. For example, the same issue could be addressed more than once in an interview, as in Potter and Wetherell's work on racism where they questioned participants about equality across different topics. This allowed them to analyze the general features of equal rights from a variety of responses (Potter & Wetherell, 1987, p. 164). In contrast to much other qualitative research, the questions become just as much of a topic of analysis as the interviewee's responses (Potter & Wetherell, 1987). This can clearly be seen in the earlier section on support group identity where we saw that one question became the starting point for the subsequent analysis. When interviewing from a critical discursive perspective, the interviewer is treated as a coparticipant in the interaction and is subject to the same scrutiny as the participant. Thus, in some senses, the framework allows a more interactive style of interviewing because the interviewer is not treated as a neutral person. However, it is still important to ask the same questions to all participants to systematically cover the issues under study.

A good transcript that indicates a sense of how the talk was delivered is crucial to undertaking critical discursive research. Although it is tempting to pay a professional transcriber to do the job, a major advantage of transcribing one's own data is that the material becomes very familiar, providing a good level of immersion in the data even before coding. If time constraints are an issue, such that a professional transcriber is employed to do the job, it is important to at least listen to the data to monitor the "accuracy" of the work. In contrast to other forms of qualitative research, transcription requires more than simply writing down what was said during the interaction. If one takes seriously the focus on the sequential production of talk, then a more detailed and nuanced reflection of what happened is needed. A Jefferson style transcription used for conversation analysis is useful if it is a simplified version (see the Appendix for description of the transcription symbols). Interview data should include the interviewer's contributions, as indicated earlier.

When coding the data, the goal is to look at patterns across the data set that stem from analytic noticings or are guided by the research question. Coding makes the data manageable but should be done as inclusively as possible (Potter & Wetherell, 1987; Willig, 2005). It is important to note that coding is typically conducted with the specific research question in mind, but this means that there may be other aspects of discourse that are not analyzed in the current project that could be revisited at a later date (Willig, 2005). It is useful to produce a data file for each pattern (note that one data extract may appear across one or more data files where relevant) because this helps in the analytic stage. When doing this, it is important to note where each data extract came from so that, during the analysis stage, you can easily locate the data extract to consider the context surrounding its production.

The skills required in analyzing data from a critical discursive psychological study are developed over time as one attempts to make analytic sense of the coding. There is no straightforward recipe of steps that can be simply described; it is more of an organic process of immersion and of returning time and again to your findings to present the patterns in a way that is both systematic and thorough. The patterns one initially finds may need revising if they do not adequately account for the phenomena or leave too many exceptions to the rule (Potter & Wetherell, 1987). A systematic analysis of the interactional context in which accounts are produced, attention to variability across accounts, and a consideration of the construction of discourse need to be examined. A useful start might be to map out the interpretative repertoires and then consider the more intricate work of outlining the subject positions these open up. Ideological dilemmas can be tracked within the accounting work that participants undertake in attending to contradictive repertoires and subject positions. A focus on action orientation of accounts requires a consideration of the context in which the interaction is produced and a thorough exposition of the consequences for participants in the interaction (Willig, 2005). Analysis is not about tidying up the data to present an overarching, simplistic summary;

rather, it is about interrogating our own assumptions and making sense of the often contradictory accounts (Potter & Wetherell, 1987).

Writing up the analysis is slightly different from other qualitative approaches. The layout is similar with a few exceptions. First, the way that data extracts are presented should not isolate the context of the participants' words. Interview data should include the interviewer's contributions, or at least provide some summary of the context in which the account was produced. The analysis section provides a demonstration of how the researcher reached his or her claims, almost akin to a mathematician including the notation of workings out rather than merely presenting the final calculation. The analysis should be built up in a coherent manner, developed over the course of each analytic section. Detailed interpretation needs to be grounded in the data extracts that are presented so that the reader can assess their validity. Sneaking in claims that are not "evidenced" with analysis of data extracts is considered poor form. A few data extracts from a data file should suffice to convey the pattern under investigation. As a consequence, the analysis section is often longer than other qualitative reports.

The evaluation of critical discursive research lies partly in the adherence to the preceding guidance. Reviewers will assess the coherence of the analytic claims and decide whether the analysis falls short of satisfactorily addressing the research question. Readers are able to assess the validity of the analysis through the availability of the data that is presented. A further validity check is to consider whether the analysts' claims are oriented to by the participants. For example, when analyzing ideological dilemmas, the analysis needs to be grounded in the way that participants display this. For example, referring back to Extract 6, in Line 9, Matt displayed that he has produced a contradiction about his ideology toward support groups with the phrase "I suppose I am now." Above all, the analysis should be fruitful; it should make sense of the discourse and generate novel findings (Potter & Wetherell, 1987).

# APPRAISAL

In this chapter a critical discursive psychological framework for studying men and masculinities has been proposed, with key analytic resources identified and illustrated. A critical discursive perspective allows the researcher to consider the variation of identities displayed in men's accounts. The way men talk about themselves allows us to investigate the complex, dynamic way that masculinities are created, negotiated, and deployed, demonstrating that identity fluctuates within each participant (Wetherell & Edley, 2014). Critical discursive psychology offers a sophisticated means of tracking men's identities as they emerge in practice for particular rhetorical purposes. Attention to the broader cultural environment in which masculinities are located is combined with a microfocus on the conversational context in which these emerge and are played out. It also considers what ideology looks like in practice and how men may resist or negotiate their position within discourses of masculinity on a moment-by-moment basis. Edley and Wetherell's critical discursive approach has been taken up by numerous other researchers (Gough, 2009; Seymour-Smith, 2008; Seymour-Smith et al., 2002; Willott & Griffin, 1997).

Of course, critical discursive psychology is does not exist without critique. The field of discursive psychology is not a unitary project. The approach discussed here differs from the form of discursive psychology that is more heavily influenced by insights from conversation analysis (CA; Edwards & Potter, 1992; Hepburn & Wiggins, 2007; Potter, 1996; Potter & Wiggins, 2007). This CA-aligned approach rejects the concept of hegemonic masculinity deployed by Wetherell and Edley. Instead, the preference is to explore whether participants themselves orient to hegemonic masculinity and argue that invoking hegemonic forms of masculinity are intrinsically linked to any discursive work that is being accomplished at that point (Speer, 2001; Stokoe, 2012). Furthermore, the concept of interpretative repertoires is deemed over-interpretative because it is more of an analyst's frame of reference and stipulates a microform of analysis grounded in the participants' talk.

Finally, CA-aligned discursive psychologists favor the study of "naturally occurring" data to examine the way that gender is made relevant by the participants themselves rather than beginning with preconceived research questions about masculinity (Potter & Hepburn, 2005; Stokoe & Smithson, 2001). Readers may peruse these and other debates in more detail (Billig, 1999a, 1999b; Edley & Wetherell, 2008; Potter & Hepburn, 2005; Schegloff, 1997, 1998, 1999a, 1999b; Seymour-Smith, 2015; Speer, 2001; Stokoe, 2012; Stokoe & Smithson, 2001; Wetherell, 1998; Wooffitt, 2005).

## FUTURE RESEARCH

One could undertake numerous possible research projects using a critical discursive research perspective. Thus far, we have seen how critical discursive psychology can be applied to areas such as men's health, fatherhood, male constructions of feminism, and school hierarchies. Suggestions for new areas of research might include a focus on "problem" male identities. For example, some researchers have already studied the identities of men who are on probation (Willott & Griffin, 1999) and male sex offenders (Lea & Auburn, 2001; Winder, Gough, & Seymour-Smith, 2015), but these could be updated or expanded to include a focus on male perpetrators of violence or male prisoner identities. New discursive research on masculinities could also focus on recent phenomena such as the prevalent "lad culture" in UK universities. Lad culture is broadly depicted as homosocial bonding centered on "banter" (often misogynistic); it emerges across social media sites such as "Uni Lad" and "True Lad," and within UK university social cultures, it is typically centered on sport and drinking (Bates, 2014; Phipps & Young, 2015).

Taking lad culture as an example, there are a number of routes one could pursue to explore the phenomenon. An interview-based study could be conducted with male students to identify their sense-making practices around issues such as banter, drinking culture, and the objectification of women. Another route could be to explore how these issues are negotiated by male students in a focus group setting. Here one could track how hegemonic forms of masculinities are negotiated and potentially resisted. Finally, interactions between male and female students in naturalistic settings could explore how lad culture operates and is negotiated and resisted. This approach would be able to also consider whether female students are complicit with lad culture. One could video record "predrinking" (or "preloading") sessions that occur before social events within residence halls. Such research would be ground-breaking in that it would be able to examine lad culture in situ.

I hope that a critical discursive approach to the study of masculinities will engage some readers of this chapter. The approach, like any position, does not offer the answer to all questions concerning masculinity. It lends itself to particular types of research questions and is not suited to others; however, this book offers numerous other means of theorizing and analyzing masculinity. It is merely hoped that this chapter provides some grounds for developing new insights.

## APPENDIX: TRANSCRIPTION NOTATION[4]

| | |
|---|---|
| [ ] | Square brackets mark the start and end of overlapping speech. Position them in alignment where the overlap occurs. |
| ? | Rising intonation. |
| ↑↓ | Vertical arrows precede marked pitch movement, over and above normal rhythms of speech. They are for marked, hearably significant shifts; and even then, the other symbols (full stops, commas, question marks) mop up most of that. Like with all these symbols, the aim is to capture interactionally significant features, hearable as such to an ordinary listener—especially deviations from a commonsense notion of "neutral" which admittedly has not been well defined. |
| Underlining | Signals vocal emphasis; the extent of underlining within individual words locates emphasis, but also indicates how heavy it is. |
| CAPITALS | Mark speech that is obviously louder than surrounding speech (often occurs when speakers are hearably competing for the floor, raised volume rather than doing contrastive emphasis). |
| (0.4) | Numbers in parentheses measure pauses in seconds (in this case, four tenths of a second). Place on new line if not assigned to a speaker. |
| (.) | A micropause, hearable but too short to measure. |
| (guess) | Text in single brackets represents transcriber's "best guess." |
| ((text)) | Additional comments from the transcriber (e.g., context or intonation). |
| she wa::nted | Colons show degrees of elongation of the prior sound; the more colons, the more elongation. I use one per syllable length. |
| heh heh | Voiced laughter. Can have other symbols added, such as underlining, pitch movement, or extra aspiration. |
| £ | Smiley voice. |
| .hhh | Inspiration (in-breaths); proportionally as for colons. |

## REFERENCES

Austin, J. L. (1962). *How to do things with words*. London, England: Oxford University Press.

Bates, L. (2014). *Everyday sexism*. London, England: Simon & Schuster.

---

[4]From "Glossary of Transcript Symbols With an Introduction," by G. Jefferson, in G. H. Lerner (Ed.), *Conversation Analysis: Studies From the First Generation* (pp. 13–31), 2004, Amsterdam, the Netherlands: John Benjamins. Copyright 2004 by John Benjamins. Adapted with permission.

Billig, M. (1999a). Conversation analysis and the claims of naivety. *Discourse & Society, 10*, 572–576. http://dx.doi.org/10.1177/0957926599010004007

Billig, M. (1999b). Whose terms? Whose ordinariness? Rhetoric and ideology in conversation analysis. *Discourse & Society, 10*, 543–558. http://dx.doi.org/10.1177/0957926599010004005

Billig, M. (2001). Discourse, rhetorical and ideological messages. In M. Wetherell, S. Taylor, & S. Y. Yates (Eds.), *Discourse theory and practice: A reader* (pp. 210–221). London, England: Sage.

Billig, M., Condor, S., Edwards, D., Gane, M., Middleton, D., & Radley, A. (1988). *Ideological dilemmas: A social psychology of everyday thinking.* London, England: Sage.

Carrigan, T., Connell, R., & Lee, J. (1985). Hard and heavy: Toward a new sociology of masculinity. In M. Kaufman (Ed.), *Beyond patriarchy* (pp. 139–192). New York, NY: Oxford University Press.

Clarke, V., Ellis, S. J., Peel, E., & Riggs, D. (2010). *Lesbian, gay, bisexual, trans and queer psychology: An introduction.* http://dx.doi.org/10.1017/CBO9780511810121

Clarke, V., & Peel, E. (2004). The social constructionism of lesbian: A reappraisal. *Feminism & Psychology, 14*, 485–490. http://dx.doi.org/10.1177/0959353504046861

Connell, R. W. (1987). *Gender and power.* Cambridge, England: Polity Press.

Connell, R. W. (1995). *Masculinities.* Cambridge, England: Polity Press.

Connell, R. W., & Messerschmidt, J. W. (2005). Hegemonic masculinity: Rethinking the concept. *Gender & Society, 19*, 829–859. http://dx.doi.org/10.1177/0891243205278639

Davies, B., & Harre, R. (1990). Positioning: The discursive production of selves. *Journal for the Theory of Social Behaviour, 20*, 43–63. http://dx.doi.org/10.1111/j.1468-5914.1990.tb00174.x

Dreyfus, H. L., & Rabinow, P. (1982). *Michel Foucault: Beyond structuralism and hermeneutics.* Brighton, England: Harvester Press.

Edley, N. (2001). Analysing masculinity: Interpretative repertoires, ideological dilemmas and subject positions. In M. Wetherell, S. Taylor, & S. J. Yates (Eds.), *Discourse as data: A guide for analysis* (pp. 189–228). London, England: Sage.

Edley, N., & Wetherell, M. (1995). *Putting men in perspective.* Hemel Hemstead, England: Harvester Wheatsheaf.

Edley, N., & Wetherell, M. (1997). Jockeying for position: The construction of masculine identities. *Discourse & Society, 8*, 203–217. http://dx.doi.org/10.1177/0957926597008002004

Edley, N., & Wetherell, M. (2001). Jekyll and Hyde: Men's constructions of feminism and feminists. *Feminism & Psychology, 11*, 439–457. http://dx.doi.org/10.1177/0959353501011004002

Edley, N., & Wetherell, M. (2008). Discursive psychology and the study of gender: A contested space. In K. Harrington, L. Litosseliti, H. Sauntson, J. Sunderland (Eds.), *Gender and language research methodologies* (pp. 161–173). Basingstoke, England: Palgrave Macmillan.

Edwards, D., & Potter, J. (1992). *Discursive psychology*. London, England: Sage.

Foucault, M. (1972). *The archaeology of knowledge* (A. M. S. Smith, Trans.). New York, NY: Harper.

Gergen, K. J. (1985). The social constructionist movement in modern psychology. *American Psychologist, 40*, 266–275. http://dx.doi.org/10.1037/0003-066X.40.3.266

Gergen, K. J. (1999). *An invitation to social constructionism*. London, England: Sage.

Gilbert, G. N., & Mulkay, M. (1984). *Opening Pandora's box: A sociological analysis of scientists' discourse*. Cambridge, England: Cambridge University Press.

Glenn, P. J. (1991). Current speaker initiation of two-party shared laughter. *Research on Language and Social Interaction, 25*, 139–162. http://dx.doi.org/10.1080/08351819109389360

Goffman, E. (1983). The interaction order. *American Sociological Review, 48*, 1–17. http://dx.doi.org/10.2307/2095141

Gough, B. (2009). A psycho-discursive approach to analysing qualitative interview data, with reference to a father–son relationship. *Qualitative Research, 9*, 527–545. http://dx.doi.org/10.1177/1468794109343624

Hall, S. (2001). Foucault: Power, knowledge and discourse. In M. Wetherell, S. Taylor, & S. J. Yates (Eds.), *Discourse theory and practice: A reader* (pp. 72–81). London, England: Sage.

Hartmann, H. (1981). The unhappy marriage of Marxism and feminism: Towards a more progressive union. In L. Sargent (Ed.), *Women and revolution* (pp. 172–189). London, England: Pluto.

Hepburn, A., & Wiggins, S. (2007). Discursive research: Themes and debates. In A. Hepburn & S. Willig (Eds.), *Discursive research in practice: New approaches to psychology and interaction* (pp. 1–28). http://dx.doi.org/10.1017/CBO9780511611216.001

Hutchby, I., & Wooffitt, R. (1998). *Conversation analysis*. Cambridge, England: Polity Press.

Jefferson, G. (2004). Glossary of transcript symbols with an introduction. In G. H. Lerner (Ed.), *Conversation analysis: Studies from the first generation* (pp. 13–31). Amsterdam, the Netherlands: John Benjamins.

Kessler, S., & McKenna, W. (1978). *Gender: An ethnomethodological approach*. New York, NY: Wiley.

Kitzinger, C. (1987). *The social construction of lesbianism*. London, England: SAGE.

Laclau, E. (1993). Politics and the limits of modernity. In T. Docherty (Ed.), *Postmodernism: A reader* (pp. 329–343). London, England: Harvester Wheatsheaf.

Laclau, E., & Mouffe, C. (1987). Post Marxism without apologies. *New Left Review, 166*, 79–106.

Lea, S., & Auburn, T. (2001). The social construction of rape in the talk of a convicted rapist. *Feminism & Psychology, 11*, 11–33. http://dx.doi.org/10.1177/0959353501011001002

Millett, K. (1970). *Sexual politics*. Garden City, NY: Doubleday.

Phipps, A., & Young, I. (2015). "Lad culture" in higher education. Agency in the sexualisation debates. *Sexualities, 18*, 459–479. http://dx.doi.org/10.1177/1363460714550909

Potter, J. (1996). *Representing reality: Discourse, rhetoric and social construction*. http://dx.doi.org/10.4135/9781446222119

Potter, J., & Hepburn, A. (2005). Qualitative interviews in psychology: Problems and possibilities. *Qualitative Research in Psychology, 2*, 281–307. http://dx.doi.org/10.1191/1478088705qp045oa

Potter, J., & Wetherell, M. (1987). *Discourse and social psychology: Beyond attitude and behaviours*. London, England: Sage.

Potter, J., & Wiggins, S. (2007). Discursive psychology. In N. K. Denzin & Y. S. Lincoln (Eds.), *The Sage handbook of qualitative research* (pp. 73–90). http://dx.doi.org/10.4135/9781412956253.n153

Sacks, H. (1992). *Lectures on conversation* (Vols. 1 & 2). Oxford, England: Blackwell.

Schegloff, E. A. (1997). Whose text? Whose context? *Discourse & Society, 8*, 165–187. http://dx.doi.org/10.1177/0957926597008002002

Schegloff, E. A. (1998). Reply to Wetherell. *Discourse & Society, 9*, 413–416. http://dx.doi.org/10.1177/0957926598009003006

Schegloff, E. A. (1999a). Naivete vs. sophistication or discipline vs. self-indulgence: A rejoinder to Billig. *Discourse & Society, 10*, 577–582. http://dx.doi.org/10.1177/0957926599010004008

Schegloff, E. A. (1999b). Schegloff's texts as "Billig's data": A critical reply. *Discourse & Society, 10*, 558–572. http://dx.doi.org/10.1177/0957926599010004006

Seymour-Smith, S. (2008). "Blokes don't like that sort of thing": Men's negotiation of a "troubled" self-help group identity. *Journal of Health Psychology, 13*, 785–797. http://dx.doi.org/10.1177/1359105308093862

Seymour-Smith, S. (2015). Applying discursive approaches to health psychology. *Health Psychology, 34*, 371–380. http://dx.doi.org/10.1037/hea0000165

Seymour-Smith, S., Brown, D., Cosma, G., Shopland, N., Battersby, S. & Burton, A. (in press). "I really don't want a doctor to be examining, you know, my back bottom": The digital rectal examination as a barrier to prostate cancer diagnosis in African-Caribbean men. *Psycho-Oncology*. http://dx.doi.org/10.1002/pon.4219

Seymour-Smith, S., Wetherell, M., & Phoenix, A. (2002). "My wife ordered me to come!": A discursive analysis of doctors' and nurses' accounts of men's use of general practitioners. *Journal of Health Psychology, 7*, 253–267. http://dx.doi.org/10.1177/1359105302007003220

Speer, S. A. (2001). Reconsidering the concept of hegemonic masculinity: Discursive psychology, conversation analysis and participants orientations. *Feminism & Psychology, 11*, 107–135. http://dx.doi.org/10.1177/0959353501011001006

Stokoe, E. H. (2012). Categorical systematics. *Discourse Studies, 14*, 345–354. http://dx.doi.org/10.1177/1461445612441543

Stokoe, E. H., & Smithson, J. (2001). Making gender relevant: Conversation analysis and gender categories in interaction. *Discourse & Society, 12*, 217–244. http://dx.doi.org/10.1177/0957926501012002005

Storey, J. (1993). *Introductory guide to cultural theory and popular culture.* New York, NY: Harvester Wheatsheaf.

Taylor, S. (2001). Locating and conducting discourse analytic research. In M. Wetherell, S. Taylor, & S. J. Yates (Eds.), *Discourse as data: A guide for analysis* (pp. 5–48). London, England: Sage.

Thiel de Bocanegra, H. (1992). Cancer patients' interest in group support programs. *Cancer Nursing, 15*, 347–352.

Wetherell, M. (1998). Positioning and interpretative repertoires: Conversation analysis and post-structuralism in dialogue. *Discourse & Society, 9*, 387–412. http://dx.doi.org/10.1177/0957926598009003005

Wetherell, M., & Edley, N. (1998). Gender practices: Steps in the analysis of men and masculinities. In K. Henwood, C. Griffin, & A. Phoenix (Eds.), *Standpoints and differences: Essays in the practice of feminist psychology* (pp. 161–173). London, England: Sage.

Wetherell, M., & Edley, N. (1999). Negotiating hegemonic masculinity: Imaginary positions and psycho-discursive practices. *Feminism & Psychology, 9*, 335–356. http://dx.doi.org/10.1177/0959353599009003012

Wetherell, M., & Edley, N. (2014). A discursive psychological framework for analysing men and masculinities. *Psychology of Men & Masculinity, 15*, 355–364. http://dx.doi.org/10.1037/a0037148

Wetherell, M., & Potter, J. (1988). Discourse analysis and the identification of interpretative repertoires. In C. Antaki (Ed.), *Analysing everyday explanation: A casebook of methods* (pp. 168–183). London, England: Sage.

Willott, S., & Griffin, C. (1997). "Wham, bam' am I a man?" Unemployed men talk about masculinities. *Feminism & Psychology, 7*, 107–128. http://dx.doi.org/10.1177/0959353597071012

Willott, S., & Griffin, C. (1999). Building your own lifeboat: Working-class male offenders talk about economic crime. *British Journal of Social Psychology, 38*, 445–460. http://dx.doi.org/10.1348/014466699164266

Winder, B., Gough, B., & Seymour-Smith, S. (2015). Stumbling into sexual crime: The passive perpetrator in accounts by male Internet sex offenders. *Archives of Sexual Behaviour, 44*, 167–180.

Willig, C. (2005). *Introducing qualitative research in psychology: Adventures in theory and method.* Maiden Head, England: Open University Press.

Wooffitt, R. (2005). *Conversation analysis and discourse analysis: A comparative and critical introduction.* http://dx.doi.org/10.4135/9781849208765

# 5

# A REVIEW OF SELECTED THEORETICAL PERSPECTIVES AND RESEARCH IN THE PSYCHOLOGY OF MEN AND MASCULINITIES

ANTHONY J. ISACCO AND JAY C. WADE

The field of psychology of men and masculinities has benefited from the development of theoretical perspectives over the past 30 years. In addition to the major theoretical perspectives described in Chapters 1 through 4, we present six theoretical perspectives in this chapter: masculine gender role stress (MGRS), male reference group identity dependence, conformity to masculine norms, precarious manhood, positive psychology–positive masculinity (PPPM), and masculinity contingency. The concepts of MGRS, male reference group identity dependence, and conformity to masculine norms were published between 1987 and 2003 and are comparatively more established with more research literature. The emergent concepts of precarious manhood, PPPM, and masculinity contingency were published between 2008 and 2015 and show promise for new avenues of research. In this chapter, we describe each theoretical perspective, review psychometric evidence and empirical findings, and provide an analytic critique of the literature.

http://dx.doi.org/10.1037/0000023-006
*The Psychology of Men and Masculinities*, R. F. Levant and Y. J. Wong (Editors)

MGRS is a theoretical construct that was developed by Eisler and Skidmore (1987). MGRS integrates stress and coping literature with theories and research pertaining to masculine gender role socialization. Men may feel intense demands to uphold male gender roles and learn to adopt increasingly rigid gender roles as a way to avoid social punishment and gain social rewards for being masculine. MGRS is one possible outcome of male gender role rigidity (McCreary et al., 1996). It is defined as "the cognitive appraisal of specific situations as stressful for men" (Eisler & Skidmore, 1987, p. 125). Men experience stress in situations that they appraise as a challenge to their masculine role or situations that elicit fears that they are not meeting societal expectations for masculinity. The theoretical perspective posits that men with higher levels of MGRS would be at greater risk for negative physical and psychological health outcomes, such as cardiovascular illness, anxiety, and anger (Eisler & Skidmore, 1987). MGRS predicts that the negative relationship between high levels of MGRS and negative health outcomes is more salient for men than for women because of the male gender socialization process (McCreary et al., 1996). Eisler (1995) explained that a central assumption of MGRS is that societal demands on men to rigidly adhere to culturally approved masculine roles and behaviors may have negative health consequences for some men.

## Masculine Gender Role Stress Scale: Description and Psychometric Evidence

The Masculine Gender Role Stress Scale (MGRSS) was developed by Eisler and Skidmore (1987) to measure the degree to which men cognitively appraise how stressful specific situations are to their masculinity. The MGRSS was developed through classical test theory. The initial items were generated with a sample of male and female undergraduate students using an open-ended sentence completion technique. Participants were asked to provide responses about stressful attributes to "being a man." Those responses were given to 50 trained raters; the raters assessed the degree of stress that the response may elicit in men and in women. Two selection criteria were used: (a) items had to be significantly more stressful for men than women and (b) the mean rating on items assessed to be stressful for men had to be in the moderate-to-high range.

The MGRSS consists of 40 items, measured on a Likert scale (0 = *not at all stressful*; 5 = *extremely stressful*). Scores can range from 0 to 200, with higher scores indicating more masculine gender role stress. A total score is calculated by summing the items. Sample items include the following: How stressful would it be "telling someone you feel hurt by what they said?" and "having a female boss?" The items are clustered into five empirically derived factors: (a) *Physical Inadequacy* is defined as the inability of men to meet masculine standards of physical fitness, sexual prowess, and muscular physique; (b) *Emotional Inexpressiveness* assesses situations that require the expression of tender emotions such as love, fear, and hurt; (c) *Subordination to Women* assesses situations that entail men being outperformed by women, such as having a female boss or being with a woman who makes more money; (d) *Intellectual Inferiority* is defined by situations that question men's rational abilities, lack of ambition, indecisiveness, or uncertainty; and (e) *Fear of Performance Failure* is concerned with potential failures in work and sex, which reflect men's perceptions of achievement.

Psychometric evidence for the MGRSS has been collected in various studies that have examined three criteria for construct validity: (a) MGRS will be different for men and women, (b) MGRS is a distinct construct from masculinity, and (c) MGRS is associated with negative health outcomes (e.g., anxiety and anger). The initial scale consisted of 66 items that underwent preliminary validation using factor analysis techniques with a sample of 173 male and female undergraduate students. The preliminary validation and some subsequent studies have found support for construct validity (Eisler, 1995; Eisler & Skidmore, 1987; Eisler, Skidmore, & Ward, 1988). McCreary et al. (1996) did not find gender differences between male and female samples and asserted that MGRS may be measuring similar constructs such as gender role conflict and strain. Two week test–retest reliability of the scale has been reported at $r = .93$, although few studies have reported on such reliability evidence (Skidmore, 1988). The internal consistency for the overall scale has been more widely reported and has ranged between $\alpha = .88$ and .94 (Swartout, Parrott, Cohn, Hagman, & Gallagher, 2015). The internal consistency has been less reported for the five factors. The internal consistency for the five factors has been reported to range between .76 and .84 for Performance Failure, .80 to .83 for Subordination to Women, .68 to .79 for Physical Inadequacy, .64 to .74 for Intellectual Inferiority, and .65 to .70 for Emotional Inexpressiveness (Efthim, Kenny, & Mahalik, 2001; Moore et al., 2008).

An abbreviated MGRSS has been developed using item response theory (Swartout et al., 2015). The new scale development effort aimed to create a psychometrically sound measure of MGRS that was shorter, easier to complete by participants, and accessible in clinical and research settings. The study included more than 2,000 participants who were recruited through a large university and an urban community setting. The analyses yielded a 15-item scale of MGRS with solid psychometric evidence. The authors concluded that the new, abbreviated scale was warranted and promising but in need of replication and further psychometric evidence to support its widespread applicability and use.

## Empirical Support

A search of PsycINFO (as of June 2015) identified approximately 30 articles and book chapters that had examined MGRS. The concept has generated several empirical investigations and is considered an established construct in the psychology of men and masculinity scholarship. Eisler (1995) provided an initial analysis and summary of the first wave of MGRS scholarship and reported overall support for the construct. He reported that men experienced stress in situations that prompt them to feel pressure to conform to masculinity stereotypes and rigid cultural norms of masculinity. As mentioned earlier, results on the validity of the MGRS construct have been mixed. In support of the construct, Eisler did not find a significant association between the MGRSS and scores on the Personal Attributes Questionnaire, which measures sex-typed masculinity. Men with higher scores on the MGRSS demonstrated higher levels of anger, fear, and engagement in high-risk behavior. Current research has continued to report associations between high levels of total MGRS scores and scores from the MGRS subscales and negative health outcomes in various samples of men.

Using a sample of undergraduate men with an experimental design, those scoring higher on MGRS had higher levels of verbal aggression, irritation, anger, jealousy, and physical aggression compared with men with lower scores on the MGRSS (Eisler, Franchina, Moore, Honeycutt, & Rhatigan, 2000). In a similar experimental study by Moore and Stuart (2004), the Eisler et al. (2000) findings were largely replicated and were also consistent with Franchina, Eisler, and Moore's (2001) findings: "High MGRS men reported greater attributions of negative intent to partner behavior in masculine gender-relevant and gender-irrelevant situations compared with low MGRS men" (Moore & Stuart, 2004, p. 139). Higher levels of MGRS have been associated with higher levels of anger, anxiety, and poorer health behaviors in undergraduate samples (Eisler, Skidmore, & Ward, 1988). High levels of MGRS among men have also been associated with less emotional expression and increased fears of emotional expression (e.g., Robertson, Lin, Woodford, Danos, & Hurst, 2001). When men feel a threat to their masculinity and become stressed, they experience negative health outcomes.

Most studies used the MGRSS total score in data analysis, but some studies have used the subscales to report more complex findings. In a nuanced analysis with a clinical sample of violent men, Moore and colleagues (2008) reported that Performance Failure was linked to psychological aggression, Physical Inadequacy to sexual coercion, and Intellectual Inferiority to injury (psychological aggression, sexual coercion, and injury represent three subscales on a measure of intimate partner violence). Efthim, Kenny, and Mahalik (2001) investigated MGRSS subscales in relation to shame, guilt, and externalization in a sample of undergraduate students; those scholars reported that Emotional Inexpressiveness and Subordination to Women was associated with externalization and inexpressiveness of guilt; Physical Inadequacy and Fear of Performance Failure was associated with guilt, a tendency to blame other, and to experience shame; four of the five factors (all except Subordination of Women) were associated with shame. Continued examination of the subscales in future research may help to identify trends of associations with positive and negative outcomes.

**Analytic Critique**

Men, particularly those with a rigid and high level of adherence to traditional masculinity, continue to experience stress in situations that are contrary to that sense of masculinity. Thus, MGRS is still a lived experience by men and a viable theoretical construct for continued empirical efforts. However, some groups of men may experience situational stress for reasons in addition to their masculine gender role. Jakupcak, Osborne, Michael, Cook, and McFall (2006) examined MGRS in a sample of male military veterans with posttraumatic stress disorder symptoms. Military situations and culture often prompt men to exhibit traditional masculine norms, which is integrated into their military role and identity. The demands and culture of the military represent an obvious overlap with societal experiences of traditional masculinity. MGRS focuses solely on stress from gender socialization, whereas other factors of stress, such as combat situations, may also be interplaying in men's experiences. MGRS is perhaps limited by not taking into account different environmental triggers to stress. Researchers have begun to examine MGRS at the subscale level, which fits with the direction of current scholarship in the psychology of men and masculinity to avoid analyzing a "global" masculinity ideology. Eisler (1995) asserted that not all aspects of traditional masculinity are detrimental to men's health or cause stress, which is congruent with current studies at the subscale level as well as with recent theories that downplay the generalizing of negative aspects of traditional masculinity. The use of subscales is important to better pinpoint what specific aspects of male gender roles are stressful and detrimental to men's health.

Going deeper beyond subscales, the more sophisticated use of item-level analysis has accounted for changes to male gender socialization. Swartout and colleagues (2015) suggested that some gender roles may be changing and thus, influencing MGRS in new ways. The implication is that societal expectations for men are changing, and some items to measure MGRS may need to change accordingly. Men may have more flexible perceptions of workplace and family gender roles and, as a result, experience less stress when romantically involved with more successful women. The utility and relevance of items such as "being married to someone who makes more money than you" and "being with a women who is more successful than you" need to be reevaluated in contemporary groups of men. On the other hand, male participants continued to express high levels of stress due to fears of being perceived as gay; the authors suggested that continued stress in that regard among heterosexual men in the United States may be more static. The continued examination of MGRS theory, construct validity, and the scale at deeper levels is a positive sign that MGRS theory remains current, predictive, and explanatory of men's experiences of stress related to masculinity norms.

Eisler (1995) reported inconclusive data on the proposed association between MGRS and cardiovascular risk or disease. Indeed, linking a specific psychological construct to such a severe physical ailment is challenging. A promising area of growth for MGRS theory and research is to further develop and integrate the biological aspects of stress into the theory. Stress research has exploded during the past 10 to 15 years in regard to how stress is connected to biological and physiological health. Biomarkers of stress (e.g., cortical, insulin, testosterone) have become important and insightful variables in research studies of health and well-being. Moore and Stuart (2004) conducted one study of MGRS that also included physiological variables (skin conductance levels and heart rates). Continued integration of biopsychosocial factors may produce a more comprehensive picture of how MGRS affects cardiovascular risk and disease as well as other psychological and physical ailments.

## MALE REFERENCE GROUP IDENTITY DEPENDENCE

Male reference group identity dependence is a theory of male identity developed by Wade (1998) to provide a psychological explanation for differences among men in their masculinity ideology and other gender-related phenomena. The theory is based on two theories: ego identity development theory (Erikson, 1968) and reference group theory (Sherif, 1962). Ego identity development refers to the work of the ego in the developmental process of formulating an identity. A reference group is a group to which an individual psychologically orients himself or herself, regardless of actual membership, and it serves as the source of the individual's norms, attitudes, and values. Male identity statuses describe how ego identity and male reference groups interact to form a male's gender role self-concept. The gender role self-concept is one's self-concept with regard to gender roles and includes one's gender-related attributes, attitudes, and behaviors (McCreary, 1990).

Male reference group identity dependence is defined as the extent to which a male is dependent on a male reference group for his gender role self-concept (Wade, 1998). Four postulates form the theoretical foundation for the theory. Postulate 1 asserts that *males identify with other males to the extent that they feel psychological relatedness to a particular group of males or to all males.* Psychological relatedness is a feeling or sense of connectedness, belonging, similarity, or commonality, in particular with regard to reference groups. A lack of psychological relatedness is experienced as a feeling or sense of isolation, alienation, and anomie. As such, this postulate describes three possible levels of psychological relatedness: (a) a lack of psychological relatedness to other males, (b) psychological relatedness to a particular group of males, and (c) psychological relatedness to all males. Postulate 2 asserts that *three levels of ego identity are associated with three levels of psychological relatedness to other males.* An undifferentiated or unintegrated ego identity is associated with a lack of psychological relatedness to other males. In an undifferentiated ego, the self-concept is largely undefined, and in an unintegrated ego, the self-concept is fragmented. A conformist ego identity is associated with psychological relatedness to a particular group (or image) of males. In a conformist ego, the self-concept is externally defined. An integrated ego identity is associated with psychological relatedness to all males. In an integrated ego, the self-concept is internally defined. Postulate 3 asserts that *three levels of psychological relatedness to other males are associated with how males use reference groups for their gender role self-concept.* When there is a lack of psychological relatedness, there is no male reference group for one's gender role self-concept. When there is psychological relatedness to a particular group of males, the gender role self-concept conforms to, or is dependent on, a particular male reference group. When there is psychological relatedness to all males, there is no prepotent male reference group and one's gender role self-concept is self-defined. Postulate 4 asserts that *how males use reference groups for their gender role self-concept is related to their gender-related attitudes and the quality of their gender role experiences.* When there is no reference group for one's gender role self-concept, there will be confusion with regard to gender-related attitudes, and the quality of one's gender role experiences will be marked by feelings of anxiety, insecurity, alienation, and anomie. When the gender role self-concept is dependent on a male reference group, there will be rigid adherence to stereotyped attitudes about gender roles, and the quality of one's gender role experiences will be limited, restricted, and stereotyped. When there is no prepotent male reference group for one's gender role self-concept, one's gender-related attitudes will tend to be flexible, autonomous, and pluralistic, and the quality of one's gender role experiences will be relatively unlimited based on a personally chosen value system. On the basis of these four postulates, three male identity statuses are posited: no reference group, reference group dependent, and reference group nondependent.

According to Wade (1998), the *no reference group* status is characterized by a lack of psychological relatedness to other males, an unintegrated or undifferentiated ego identity, an undefined or fragmented gender role self-concept, and confusion, anxiety, alienation, and insecurity associated with gender role experiences. The *reference group dependent* status is characterized by feelings of psychological relatedness to some males and not others, a conformist ego identity, dependence on a male reference group for one's gender role self-concept, and thereby rigid adherence to gender roles, stereotyped attitudes, and limited or restricted gender role experiences and behaviors. The *reference group nondependent* status is characterized by feelings of psychological relatedness to all males, an integrated ego identity, and an internally defined gender role self-concept that is not dependent on a male reference group. This status is associated with relatively flexible, autonomous, and pluralistic gender-related attitudes, attributes, and behaviors.

## Reference Group Identity Dependence Scale: Description and Psychometric Evidence

Wade and Gelso (1998) operationalized the male reference group identity dependence construct in the form of a self-report instrument, the Reference Group Identity Dependence Scale (RGIDS), that assesses feelings of psychological relatedness to other males. The RGIDS was developed using a sample of 344 male undergraduate students. Using a pool of 47 items, exploratory factor analysis resulted in a four-factor structure of 30 items corresponding to the three hypothesized male identity statuses. The No Reference Group Subscale measures feelings of disconnectedness from other men or a lack of psychological relatedness to other men. The Reference Group Dependent Subscale measures feelings of connectedness or psychological relatedness to some males and not others. The reference group nondependent status items formed two subscales that were labeled *Reference Group Nondependent Similarity*, which measures feelings of connectedness or psychological relatedness with all males, and Reference Group Nondependent Diversity, which measures appreciation of differences in males. Respondents are asked to report the degree to which they agree or disagree with statements representing feelings and beliefs about oneself as male, other males, and their relationships with other males.

On the basis of nine published studies, the internal consistency reliability Cronbach alphas for the subscales have ranged as follows: No Reference Group, .73–.82; Reference Group Dependent, .53–.72; Reference Group Nondependent Similarity, .70–.82; and Reference Group Nondependent Diversity, .56–.80. Wade and Gelso (1998) reported test–retest reliability over a 4-week period: No Reference Group = .67, Reference Group Dependent = .30, Reference Group Nondependent Diversity = .68, and Reference Group Nondependent Similarity = .60. Wade developed an adult version of the

RGIDS (RGIDS–A; Wade, 2001) for use with noncollege populations of adult men. The RGIDS–A consists of 28 items with the same four factors. On the basis of three published studies, the Cronbach alphas were as follows: No Reference Group, .77, .79, .83; Reference Group Dependent, .57, .67, .77; Reference Group Nondependent Similarity, .77, .83, .95; Reference Group Nondependent Diversity, .69, .76, .91.

## Empirical Support

In the initial validation study of the RGIDS, Wade and Gelso (1998) hypothesized male identity statuses to be differentially related to ego identity status, gender role conflict, and psychological functioning (i.e., anxiety/depression symptomatology, social anxiety, self-esteem). As predicted, the no reference group status related positively to identity diffusion and poor psychological functioning, reference group dependent related positively to identity foreclosure and gender role conflict, and reference group non-dependent related positively to identity achievement (Similarity subscale) and no gender role conflict (Diversity subscale). A contrary finding was reference group dependent also related positively to identity achievement. Overall, the initial study demonstrated some support for the theory.

Wade and Brittan-Powell (2000) examined how RGIDS statuses related to identity aspects (personal, social, and collective), belongingness, and a universal-diverse orientation (appreciating similarities and differences among people). Consistent with theory, the no reference group status was associated with not viewing collective aspects of identity as important to one's sense of self, and with a sense of disconnectedness between self and others. Reference group dependent was associated with viewing the social aspects of one's identity as important and feeling a sense of connectedness. The diversity aspect of reference group nondependent was related to viewing the personal aspects of one's identity as important, feeling a sense of connectedness, and a universal-diverse orientation, whereas Similarity related to collective identity.

Moradi, Velez, and Parent (2013) examined the identity statuses as they relate to traditional masculinity ideology and two dimensions of men's gender-based collective identity: affirmative evaluation of collective identity and importance of collective identity. Consistent with theory, the no reference group status related to not having an affirmative evaluation of collective identity, reference group dependent related to the importance of collective identity, and the nondependent status related to an affirmative evaluation of collective identity. In addition, the similarity dimension of the nondependent status related to traditional masculinity ideology, which was contrary to theory.

Wade and colleagues investigated male identity statuses as predictors of romantic relationship quality (Wade & Coughlin, 2012; Wade & Donis, 2007).

In a mixed sample of heterosexual and gay men, consistent with theory the no reference group status was associated with poor relationship quality in both groups. However, for the heterosexual men, reference group dependent related positively to relationship quality, whereas the diversity dimension of the nondependent status related negatively. This finding is contrary to theory. In a sample of adult men, Wade and Coughlin (2012) investigated masculinity ideology as a mediator in the relationship between male identity status and relationship satisfaction. Results were generally consistent with theory. No reference group was associated with traditional masculinity, which accounted for dissatisfaction in one's relationship. Reference group dependent was associated with traditional masculinity, which accounted for low relationship satisfaction. Reference group nondependent (Diversity) was associated with nontraditional masculinity, which accounted for high relationship satisfaction.

Male identity statuses were examined for their relationship to men's attitudes about race and gender equity in an undergraduate sample and a sample of professional White men (Wade, 2001; Wade & Brittan-Powell, 2001). In the undergraduate sample, reference group dependent was associated with negative attitudes about racial diversity and women's equality, and attitudes conducive to the sexual harassment of women. The diversity aspect of the nondependent status related to positive attitudes about racial diversity and not having sexual harassment proclivities. However, unexpectedly the similarity aspect was associated with having negative attitudes toward gender equality as well as endorsing a traditional masculinity ideology. In the sample of professional men the relationships were generally the same and consistent with theory. However, the similarity aspect did not significantly correlate with the other variables of interest.

Two studies have examined the relationship between male identity status and masculinity in relatively unique samples of men. Saez, Casado, and Wade (2009) examined the relationship between male identity status and hypermasculinity in a sample of Latino men of diverse ethnicities: primarily Dominican, Cuban, and Puerto Rican. As expected, the nondependent status (Diversity) related negatively to hypermasculinity. Contrary to theory, the reference group dependent identity related negatively to hypermasculinity. In a study of male batterers at a treatment facility in Canada (Mendoza & Cummings, 2001), the male identity statuses correlated with traditional masculinity and gender role conflict, consistent with theory. The Similarity subscale did not significantly correlate with masculinity, and, contrary to theory, related negatively to help-seeking.

Wade (2008) examined the relationships between male reference group identity dependence, masculinity ideology, and health-related attitudes and behaviors in a sample of urban African American men. Exploratory factor analysis was conducted using 42 of the original 47 RGIDS items to develop the RGIDS–AA for use with this sample of adult African American men, which consists of 23 items and three factors that correspond to the three male identity statuses. Results from the study were consistent with theory. The reference group nondependent status related positively to personal wellness, whereas the no reference group and reference group dependent statuses were associated with a lifestyle contrary to personal wellness. Furthermore, in a test of mediation, nontraditional masculinity fully mediated the relationship between the nondependent identity status and health promoting behaviors.

### Analytic Critique

Wade (1998) developed a theory of male identity to address the question of why men vary in their masculinity ideology and in their conformity to gender role standards. Male reference group identity dependence (MRGID) theory describes the psychological processes influencing how engaged or disengaged males are with traditional male role norms. The theory does not specify any particular form of masculinity as ideal or problematic; rather, overly rigid adoption or adherence to masculine norms or the lack of behavioral flexibility can be problematic (Smiler, 2004). Wade proposed ego identity development as the basis for male identity statuses (Postulate 2) that underlie conformity and flexibility in this regard. Research supports the relationship to ego identity status, except for the finding that the reference group dependent status related to identity achievement as well as identity foreclosure in college men.

Feelings of psychological relatedness to other males is the basis of male identity in MRGID theory (Postulate 1). Consistent with theory, the identity statuses relate to men's *gender-based* collective identity (Moradi, Velez, & Parent, 2013) and more generally to the importance of personal, social, and collective aspects of identity and feelings of connectedness between self and others (Wade & Brittan-Powell, 2000). Further support for the theory is found in research with a sample of men dissatisfied with their same-sex attraction who had pursued sexual orientation change efforts (Karten & Wade, 2010). Participants' highest endorsement was for the no reference group status, and their lowest was for the similarity aspect of reference group nondependent, whereas in other research samples, no reference group has consistently been found to have the lowest endorsement.

The male identity statuses are associated with how males use reference groups for their gender role self-concept (Postulate 3). Future research should investigate whether a male has a reference group, his psychological relatedness to other males, and, if so, the extent to which he conforms to the gender role norms of the reference group. Nevertheless, this postulate leads to the assertion that male identity statuses will be differentially related to one's gender-related attitudes and experiences (Postulate 4). No reference group has related negatively to trait masculinity (Wade & Brittan-Powell, 2001) and positively with gender role conflict (Mendoza & Cummings, 2001), which is consistent with MRGID theory. However, the research shows more of a consistent and predictable relationship to poor psychosocial functioning than gender-related attitudes. The reference group dependent identity has shown some mixed findings in relation to gender-related attitudes and experiences. In most studies, the findings are consistent with theory, demonstrating a positive relationship to traditional masculinity ideology and gender role conflict, as well as other gender-related experiences (e.g., health behaviors, race and gender equity, relationship quality). In some studies, no relationship was found to masculinity ideology. It is possible that the reliability of the scale has contributed to the lack of finding significant results. The Reference Group Dependent subscale has the lowest reliability of the four scales, with most Cronbach's alpha below .70. Future research could identify males who score high on the Reference Group Dependent Subscale and follow up with qualitative inquiry to identify items that may better represent the feelings and beliefs associated with this identity status.

Central to the reference group nondependent identity are the two dimensions of feelings of similarity to all men and appreciation of diversity in men, as revealed in the development of the RGIDS and RGIDS-A. The similarity dimension has generally not been supported in the research, which has shown that men who feel they are similar to all other men can have traditional attitudes about masculinity. It appears that appreciation of diversity in men better captures this identity status. Male reference group identity dependence theory is a psychodynamic theory that complements the social constructionist view of gender roles. As a theory of male identity, it enriches our understanding of the psychology of men and masculinity and offers another avenue through which researchers and practitioners can conceptualize men's issues.

## CONFORMITY TO MASCULINE NORMS

Conformity to masculine norms is a theoretical model developed by Mahalik (2000) to explain the process involved in men's conformity to gender role norms. The theory is grounded in the social psychology literature on social norms, conformity, and compliance. Conformity to masculine norms is defined as meeting societal expectations for what constitutes masculinity in one's public or private life. Four hypotheses form the theoretical foundation for the model: (a) sociocultural influences, particularly the influence of the most dominant or powerful groups in a society, shape the gender role expectations and standards that constitute gender role norms; (b) gender role norms of the powerful in a society are communicated to individuals through descriptive norms (what is typically done in a social group), injunctive norms (what is approved or disapproved by others), and cohesive norms (what is done by popular people); (c) group and individual factors filter an individual's experience of gender role norms; and (d) these group and individual factors affect the extent to which the individual conforms, or does not conform, to specific gender role norms. Group factors include influences such as socioeconomic status, race, ethnic culture, and religion. Individual factors include influences such as age, personality, and aspects of identity (e.g., male, ethnic, religious, and gay identity). Further, there are benefits and costs to men for both conforming and not conforming to the masculinity norms of the dominant culture in society. For example, conforming aids males in developing their identity as men and provides social and financial rewards. However, research shows the costs can be the psychological and physical health problems that are associated with enacting certain traditional male role norms. Thus, a benefit of nonconformity is avoiding these problems. On the other hand, nonconformity to masculine gender norms may result in being negatively evaluated and rejected by others.

## Conformity to Masculine Norms Inventory: Description and Psychometric Evidence

Mahalik and colleagues (2003) developed the Conformity to Masculine Norms Inventory (CMNI) to assess the extent that an individual male conforms or does not conform to the actions, thoughts, and feelings that reflect masculinity norms in the dominant culture in U.S. society. Items were developed to reflect conformity to masculine norms along a continuum (extreme conformity, moderate conformity, moderate nonconformity, extreme nonconformity) and the affective, behavioral, and cognitive aspects of masculine norms. Behavioral conformity to masculine norms is acting in ways to meet societal expectations for men. Affective conformity is feeling proud or happy when conforming to gender role norms and feeling ashamed if not conforming. Cognitive conformity is believing those things that men and women are expected to believe. The CMNI was developed using a sample of 752, comprising mostly male undergraduate students. Using a pool of 144 items representing 12 distinct masculinity norms, exploratory factor analyses resulted in a 94-item inventory with an 11-factor structure. The 11 factors formed the masculinity norms subscales labeled as follows: Winning, Emotional Control, Risk-Taking, Violence, Power Over Women, Dominance, Playboy, Self-Reliance, Primacy of Work, Disdain for Homosexuals, and Pursuit of Status.

Higher scores on a subscale reflect the more one conforms to the masculine norm. CMNI raw scores can be transformed to $t$ scores for each subscale and total score and interpreted to categorize respondent's degree of conformity or nonconformity (Mahalik, Talmadge, Locke, & Scott, 2005).

Studies using the CMNI have reported subscale reliabilities generally in the range of .63 to .93 and test–retest reliability over a 2- to 3-week period showed correlations ranging from .51 to .90. Dominance and Pursuit of Status subscales most often have had the lowest reliabilities. There are several shorter versions of the CMNI developed through factor analyses or by selecting fewer items for each subscale. Eleven-item, 22-item, 29-item (eight factors), 46-item (nine factors), and 55-item versions of the CMNI exist. The CMNI–11 is based on the highest loading item from each of the 11 CMNI subscales (Mahalik, Burns, & Syzdek, 2007), and the CMNI-22 uses the two highest-loading items (Owen, 2011). Similarly, item selection for the CMNI-55 is based on the five highest item loadings with one additional item added to the Dominance scale because it only has four items in the CMNI-94 (Owen, 2011). The CMNI–46 (Parent & Moradi, 2009) retained only the strongest indicators of each masculine norm and eliminated the Dominance and Pursuit of Status subscales because of their low reliability and weak validity. Hsu and Iwamoto (2014) found the CMNI–46 to be a measure that was more theoretically consistent for White American men than Asian American men. They developed a 29-item version of the CMNI that resulted in the elimination of the Primacy of Work subscale and did not significantly differ across racial groups in terms of the number and types of factors.

**Empirical Support**

A search on PsycINFO identified 81 studies published in academic journals that had used a version of the CMNI as of April 2015. The CMNI has been used in research with various samples of men: college students, gay men, outpatient mental health clients, college football players, adult working men, prisoners, nurses, rodeo cowboys, stay-at-home fathers, men sexually abused in childhood, veterans, men with spinal cord injury, and men with prostate cancer. Additionally, research has been conducted with men of diverse ethnicities and nationalities: Asian American, Black American, Australian, Hong Kong Chinese, Kenyan, and Italian. Consequently, there is considerable research to demonstrate external validity.

In the initial validation study (Mahalik et al., 2003), most of the CMNI subscales differentiated men from women and men who reported high-risk behavior from those who did not. The CMNI related as expected with three other masculinity measures: the Brannon Masculinity Scale, the Gender Role Conflict Scale, and the Masculine Gender Role Stress Scale. Additionally, higher conformity to masculine norms was associated with negative attitudes toward seeking psychological help, the desire to be more muscular, and psychological distress. Several other studies have found similar results with regard to attitudes toward help-seeking for academic help (Wimer & Levant, 2011) and for psychological help (Hammer, Vogel, & Heimerdinger-Edwards, 2013). There has been additional research on body image concerns showing that conformity to masculine norms predicted greater muscle dissatisfaction and muscularity-oriented disordered eating (Griffiths, Murray, & Touyz, 2015). Such concerns have been shown in a range of samples as well. In gay men, conformity to masculine norms was associated with distress if one's body did not resemble his personal physical ideal (Kimmel & Mahalik, 2005). In college football players, the norms of risk taking, emotional control, and primacy of work were positively related to the drive for muscularity (Steinfeldt, Gilchrist, Halterman, Gomory, & Steinfeldt, 2011). Lastly, in young men from the United States, the United Kingdom, Australia, and Sweden, conformity to masculine norms related positively to drive for muscularity, leanness, and fitness in all four countries (Gattario et al., 2015).

Conformity to masculine norms and psychological functioning has been examined in diverse samples as well. For example, in male veterans, conformity was associated with more severe self-reported symptoms of post-traumatic stress (Morrison, 2012) and lower psychological well-being (Alfred, Hammer, & Good, 2014). Conformity to masculine norms related to lower self-esteem and more psychological distress in Black men (Mahalik, Pierre, & Wan, 2006) and depression in Australian men (Rice, Fallon, & Bambling, 2011). In men with a history of sexual abuse during childhood, those whose responses to masculine norms met the criteria for high conformity were 230% more likely to have attempted suicide in the past year than participants who did not meet the criteria for high conformity to masculine norms (Easton, Renner, & O'Leary, 2013). At the subscale level of analysis, conformity to the masculine norm of risk-taking negatively related to psychological distress in those men classified as "risk avoiders," whereas for men classified as "detached risk-takers," the masculine norm of violence negatively related to psychological distress while the masculine norms of playboy, self-reliance, and risk-taking were positively related (Wong, Owen, & Shea, 2012). In Asian American men, the norm of winning was negatively associated with depressive symptoms, while the norm of dominance related positively to depressive symptoms (Iwamoto, Liao, & Liu, 2010).

Research shows a relationship between men conforming to masculine norms and their health behaviors, romantic relationships, and social attitudes. Such men are more likely to engage in behaviors that are not conducive to good health (Hamilton & Mahalik, 2009; Levant, Wimer, & Williams, 2011; Mahalik, Levi-Minzi, & Walker, 2007), be dissatisfied with their romantic relationships (Burn & Ward, 2005), and hold sexist attitudes and unfavorable attitudes toward gay men (Keiller, 2010; Smiler, 2006). At the subscale level of analysis, conformity to the norms of dominance and primacy of work related positively to the health behavior of preventive self-care, whereas the pursuit of status norm related negatively (Levant et al., 2011). Conforming to the playboy norm was associated with low relationship satisfaction (Burn & Ward, 2005) and favorable attitudes toward lesbians (Keiller, 2010). Additionally, studies have revealed predictors of conformity to masculine norms. Men in rural communities endorsed conformity to masculine norms to a stronger degree than men in urban communities (Hammer et al., 2013). Older men and more educated men are less likely to conform to masculine norms (Hammer et al., 2013; Rice et al., 2011). In Black men, using Whites as the racial reference group for one's racial identity was associated with conforming to masculine norms (Mahalik et al., 2006).

## Analytic Critique

Conformity to masculine norms is a theoretical model that explains why men will conform or not conform to gender role standards. Mahalik (2000) has used U.S. society as a point of reference. Accordingly, males learn what standards and expectations are associated with being masculine in U.S. society. In constructing the CMNI, items were developed to represent masculinity norms of the dominant group in U.S. society—White middle- and upper-class heterosexuals. Some research on the 11 masculinity norms raises questions about whether primacy of work and pursuit of status norms are norms that are associated with being masculine (or male) in the United States: Men and women did not differ in their endorsement of primacy of work and pursuit of status norms (Mahalik et al., 2003). However, support for the overall norms being representative of the dominant racial group in U.S. society is reflected in the finding that when Black men use Whites as the racial reference group for their racial identity, they are more likely to conform to masculine norms of the dominant group in society (Mahalik et al., 2006). In other words, Black men who identify with Whites are more likely to conform to the masculinity norms of Whites, and their endorsement of such norms is a validation of the norms being representative of the dominant racial group. Additionally, although Mahalik focused on societal norms in his model, Wong, Horn, Gomory, and Ramos (2013) argued that CMNI items reflect personal norms because the items focus on respondents' personal affect, cognitions, and behaviors rather than their perceptions of other men's behavior or attitudes (i.e., what most men feel, think, believe, and do). Further, Wong et al. noted that conformity to masculine norms may also occur at a more proximal level because the norms of groups that men belong to (e.g., male colleagues, sports teams, or religious groups) may have more of an influence on men's lives than societal norms.

The theory provides an explanation of variability among men with regard to conformity to dominant masculinity norms. There is research supporting variability among men with respect to age, racial identity, community, and education. More research that explicates this variability would advance our understanding of why and which group and individual factors have an influence on conformity. Future research could potentially use $t$ scores with the CMNI, as recommended by Mahalik et al. (2005), for a more nuanced analysis of the costs and benefits of nonconformity, as well as conformity, by examining how the degree of conformity relates to an outcome variable (i.e., extreme conformity, moderate conformity, moderate nonconformity, extreme nonconformity). For example, future research can test whether conformity to masculine norms exhibits a curvilinear relationship with other outcomes, such that extreme conformity and nonconformity (but not moderate conformity) are positively related to deleterious outcomes.

## PRECARIOUS MANHOOD

Precarious manhood is an emergent, interdisciplinary theory in the psychology of men and masculinities. Developed by Vandello and Bosson (2013) and colleagues (Vandello, Bosson, Cohen, Burnaford, & Weaver, 2008), the theory has three main tenets. First, manhood is a precarious social status that is elusive and must be achieved or earned. Second, the status of manhood is tenuous and impermanent. Third, manhood requires public demonstrations to achieve the social status because manhood is primarily confirmed by others. Integrated throughout those three tenets is the assertion that precarious manhood is in contrast to womanhood, the latter of which is viewed as a status that flows more naturally from biological changes and remains secure once achieved (Vandello & Bosson, 2013). The precarious manhood line of scholarship was introduced in 2008 (Vandello et al., 2008). The authors (Vandello & Bosson, 2013) detailed historical influences on precarious manhood, such as early psychoanalytic theories of gender development and contemporary theories of men and masculinity (e.g., gender role stress, gender role strain, gender role conflict). Evolutionary psychology and social role theory represent primary theoretical roots of precarious manhood (Vandello et al., 2008). The belief that manhood is uncertain, a failure-prone process (i.e., not all men achieve the status), and anxiety-provoking represents the common thread among the various psychological theories that have influenced precarious manhood. In addition to psychological theories, precarious manhood has acknowledged overlap with anthropological findings from preindustrial societies that require boys to successfully complete a ritual of strength, bravery, and endurance to transition into manhood (Vandello & Bosson, 2013). In current Western societies, there appear to be fewer institutionalized rituals for men to earn their manhood status, which may exacerbate men's anxieties and uncertainties.

### Empirical Support

Much of the empirical base for precarious manhood has been generated by the primary developers of the theory through a series of experimental studies with primarily White, middle-class undergraduate students in the United States (see Bosson, Vandello, Burnaford, Weaver, & Wasti, 2009; Vandello et al., 2008; Weaver, Vandello, Bosson, & Burnaford, 2010). There is not a precarious manhood self-report measure to date and thus no psychometric evidence to review. The experimental design to test the first tenet (i.e., manhood is elusive and hard-won) included providing participants with a list of fake proverbs and straightforward opinion statements about precarious manhood or precarious womanhood (Vandello et al., 2008). Participants were also asked about their beliefs regarding the essential nature of manhood versus womanhood and were rated on a Likert-type scale (1 = *not at all true*; 7 = *very true*). Both male and female participants attributed the notion and transition to manhood more to social factors than to physical factors. Comparatively, the notion of womanhood was attributed more to physical factors; the transition to womanhood was attributed equally to social and physical factors. The researchers (Vandello et al., 2008) concluded that there is evidence to support Tenet 1, which posits that manhood (more than womanhood) is an elusive and uncertain status that must be earned through social achievement.

The experimental design to test the second tenet (i.e., manhood is tenuous and easily lost) included asking participants to interpret the meaning behind two ambiguous statements: (a) "lost manhood" and (b) "lost womanhood" (Vandello et al., 2008). Participants attributed more social causes than physical reasons to the first statement and the opposite pattern was observed for the second statement. Participants also explained that interpreting statements for lost manhood was easier than ones about lost womanhood. The researchers concluded that there is evidence to support Tenet 2. Weaver et al. (2010) used an experimental design with two parts to assess Tenet 3 (i.e., manhood requires action and public proof). First, the researchers asked male and female participants to complete open-ended statements that began with "A real man . . ." or "A real woman. . . ." The sentences were coded for action verbs, assuming that statements about men would contain more action verbs and statements about women would contain more stable words indicative of enduring, internal qualities. Male participants used more action verbs to describe a real man than they did when describing a real woman. Female participants did not vary in how they completed the two sets of sentences. The researchers concluded that there is support for the part of Tenet 3 regarding manhood requiring action. To test the second part of Tenet 3 (i.e., manhood requires public proof), the researchers (Weaver et al., 2010) asked male and female participants to read a fake police report about a bar fight between two people of the same sex over an opposite-sex romantic interest. The perpetrator was considered the person responsible for initiating the fight with a kick or punch after a public insult by the other person, who was considered the victim. Participants rated the perpetrator's behavior based on situational or dispositional causes (or both). Female participants and those who rated a female victim provided more dispositional causes for the perpetrators violent behavior. Male participants rated the perpetrator's violent behavior using more situational causes. The researchers concluded that there is support for the second part of Tenet 3.

## Analytic Critique

Precarious manhood is a nascent theory that has emerged from a few studies using rigorous experimental design. The experimental designs are a strength of the precarious manhood research agenda, allowing researchers to draw causal inferences. Addis and Schwab (2013) questioned the internal validity of the experimental designs and considered it risky to conflate statistical significance between group differences (men and women). Replication of the studies using more diverse participants will strengthen the external generalizability of the findings. Future research on precarious manhood would benefit from a longitudinal design to test the extent to which precarious manhood changes over time and whether men respond to social factors differently at different developmental stages. Heesacker and Snowden (2013) expressed concern that precarious manhood is another deficit model of masculinity and lacks a more complete conceptualization of manhood. Chrisler (2013) argued that womanhood is also a difficult status to achieve and worried that precarious manhood harkened back to old ideas about gender (i.e., manhood is difficult and womanhood is easy). Bosson and Vandello (2013) responded to those critiques and clarified that (a) comparing groups (men and women) is helpful to understand how people experience gender; (b) precarious manhood is not a deficit model per se but does illustrate some difficulties that men experience; and (c) precarious manhood and data from associated studies does not indicate that women "have it easier" than men in an objective, literal sense. Bosson and Vandello continued to assert that men are at a greater risk of losing their manhood status if men violate socially prescribed gender roles of masculinity than women are of losing their womanhood status if women violate socially prescribed gender roles of femininity. We emphasize the reality that women are at risk and validate some women's perspectives that their womanhood status can be just as precarious, if not more, than men's status. Precarious manhood is a promising emergent theory in the psychology of men and masculinities. Scholars are in continued debate about its assumptions, tenets, findings, and implications. It is unclear how precarious manhood research can be translated to inform psychological interventions that help boys and men to deal with negative social factors and find peace in their own identity as a man.

## POSITIVE PSYCHOLOGY–POSITIVE MASCULINITY

PPPM is an emergent theoretical perspective in the psychology of men and masculinities. PPPM has been developed by Kiselica, Englar-Carlson, and colleagues beginning in the early 2000s (e.g., Englar-Carlson & Kiselica, 2013). Their goal has been to present a complementary perspective to the gender role strain paradigm by identifying the strengths of traditional masculinity in U.S. male populations. Thirty years of research in the psychology of men has led to a deep understanding of the problems that men experience from restricted gender role socialization, but examining strengths and healthy male development was a comparative gap. PPPM has sought to identify and promote socialized male strengths, which can be integrated into clinical practice with male clients. A primary hypothesis is that PPPM may foster positive emotions in male clients by focusing on positive masculinity during counseling (Kiselica, Benton-Wright, & Englar-Carlson, 2016).

**Empirical Support**

PPPM is based on three theoretical and empirical foundations: (a) positive psychology, (b) positive masculinity, and (c) adolescent and young adult fathers. Positive psychology reemerged in the field of psychology in the late 1990s to challenge the status quo deficit model and to promote theories, research, and interventions that promote human well-being and flourishing. PPPM contends that the new psychology of men was too focused on a deficit model of male development and traditional male socialization. In a study investigating connections between traditional masculinity and positive psychology constructs, Hammer and Good (2010) reported that risk-taking, primacy of work, and pursuit of status were positively associated with personal courage, autonomy, endurance, and resilience, whereas winning, emotional control, self-reliance, and pursuit of status were negatively associated with courage, grit, personal control, autonomy, and resilience. The complex associations between masculinity and positive psychology are still equivocal. PPPM has adopted a positive masculinity perspective. Kiselica et al. (2016) defined *positive masculinity* as "prosocial attitudes, beliefs, and behaviors of boys and men that produce positive consequences for self and others" (p. 126). PPPM has identified 11 healthy characteristics of positive masculinity: (a) Male Relational Styles; (b) Male Ways of Caring; (c) Generative Fatherhood; (d) Male Self-Reliance; (e) Worker-Provider Tradition; (f) Men's Respect for Women; (g) Male Courage, Daring, and Risk-Taking; (h) Group Orientation of Boys and Men; (i) Male Forms of Service; (j) Men's Use of Humor; and (k) Male Heroism (Kiselica et al., 2016). These characteristics are considered to emerge from the male gender socialization process but are not considered biological/innate traits exclusive to men, but rather human strengths that can be learned and developed by all people. These strengths are not mutually exclusive, and not all men exhibit all of them.

The scholars who developed PPPM have always had an eye toward applying the paradigm to clinical interventions (Englar-Carlson & Kiselica, 2013). A good portion of PPPM's clinical perspective is based in theory and research related to adolescent and young fathers. Interventions with adolescent and young fathers included some components consistent with a PPPM perspective such as career counseling and job placement services (worker-provider role), outreach efforts in places that men congregate, such as athletic spaces (male ways of relating), and infusing humor into clinical conversations. Summarizing 3 decades of research, Kiselica et al. (2016) asserted that identifying and accentuating masculinity strengths in interventions with adolescent and young fathers had positive benefits, such as improved retention in programs, favorable attitudes toward treatment, improved employment and educational rates, and increased father involvement in their child's life.

Taken together, the theoretical and empirical foundations have contributed to an emergent clinical approach to assisting male clients. Englar-Carlson and Kiselica (2013) suggested that mental health practitioners use the PPPM approach as a helpful tool for theoretical conceptualizations of male clients. Practitioners are urged to actively work with male clients to identify strengths, which can help build rapport and frame the intervention with male clients. Identification of strengths is considered therapeutic in and of itself, while a strength-based approach may help to improve treatment adherence more specifically with male clients. Practitioners may find that using a strength-based perspective with some male clients facilitates appropriate and culturally congruent emotional expression and treatment-seeking behaviors (Englar-Carlson & Kiselica, 2013). The goal of mental health interventions that use a PPPM perspective is to help boys and men develop and enact the 11 male-socialized strengths.

**Analytic Critique**

PPPM has been a welcome addition to the psychology of men and masculinities because men, communities, practitioners, and researchers have been yearning for a positive guide to the healthy development of boys and men. Some critiques of PPPM include a general lack of empirical investigation of the concepts and hypotheses and a lack of a psychometrically sound positive masculinity scale. Ideologically, some scholars (Levant, 2008) have argued that the field would be better served by examining and promoting human strengths rather than highlighting a gendered perspective to strengths. Clinically, PPPM has yet to undergo rigorous clinical trials, using experimental designs, of its effectiveness in various samples of boys and men. Thus, the connection among theory, research, and practice is nascent and in need of additional development.

## MASCULINITY CONTINGENCY

The concept of masculinity contingency was recently developed by Burkley, Wong, and Bell (2016) to explain individual variability in the importance of perceiving oneself as masculine and sensitivity to masculinity threats. Masculinity contingency is based on the concept of contingencies of self-worth (Crocker & Wolfe, 2001), which refers to what people believe they need to be or do to have value and worth as a person, and the consequences of those beliefs. Thus, *masculinity contingency* is defined as the degree to which a man's self-worth is derived from his sense of masculinity. The more a man's self-worth is contingent on his sense of masculinity, the more likely his self-esteem will increase in response to positive feedback about his masculinity and decrease in response to negative feedback about his masculinity. If information or feedback about the self is consistent with his masculine self-concept, it will confirm his sense of self, whereas information or feedback that is inconsistent is potentially threatening to his sense of self. High masculinity contingency would generally be associated with negative personal and social outcomes because self-esteem is less stable and fluctuates more in response to feedback when masculinity is a contingency of self-worth. For example, basing one's self-worth on other's validation of one's masculinity may result in depression when it is not validated or in alcohol abuse to gain validation of one's masculinity. Burkley et al. (2016) correspondingly distinguished between two types of masculinity contingency: *contingency threat* refers to the extent that a man's self-worth is threatened by a lack of his masculinity, whereas *contingency boost* refers to the extent that a man's self-worth is boosted by confirmation of his masculinity. Negative outcomes would be more associated with the threat aspect of masculinity contingency than the boost aspect, because defending oneself against a threat to one's masculinity would have more impact than attempts to confirm one's masculinity.

## Masculinity Contingency Scale:
## Description and Psychometric Evidence

The masculinity contingency construct was operationalized in the form of a self-report instrument, the Masculinity Contingency Scale (MCS; Burkley et al., 2016), that assesses the extent to which a man's self-worth is threatened by a lack of masculinity or boosted by confirmations of masculinity. The MCS is a 10-item scale developed through factor analytic procedures and comprises an overall scale and two related subscales: MCS-Threat and MCS-Boost. Items describe an internal contingency of masculinity (e.g., "When I act manly, I feel good about myself"). Burkley et al. (2016) conducted four studies to assess the reliability and validity of the MCS. Internal consistency reliability Cronbach's alphas for the overall scale and subscales ranged from .91 to .93. Two-week test–retest reliability correlations ranged from .68 to .72. Confirmatory factor analyses supported a hierarchical model with two latent factors loading on a higher order, superordinate factor. The correlation between both factors was .57.

### Empirical Support

Empirical support for the masculinity contingency construct was provided in the initial validation study of the MCS (Burkley et al., 2016). Masculinity contingency, as well as the latent factors of Threat and Boost, was positively associated with traditional gender role attitudes, rape myth acceptance, conformity to masculine norms, gender role conflict, benevolent sexism, hostile sexism, homophobia, and centrality of masculine identity, and negatively associated with pro-feminist attitudes. Overall masculinity contingency and contingency threat were negatively related to trait self-esteem and social desirability. Consistent with theory, in most instances, threat to masculinity was more strongly related to negative outcomes than boost to masculinity. Additionally, overall masculinity contingency predicted benevolent sexism, homophobia, and self-esteem after controlling for the other masculinity-related variables (i.e., gender role conflict, conformity to masculine norms, and centrality of masculine identity). Contingency threat and contingency boost differentially predicted or did not predict these outcomes, and when they were significant predictors, they had greater predictive power than overall masculinity contingency.

### Analytic Critique

Burkley et al. (2016) proposed the concept of masculinity contingency to explain why for some men masculinity will have negative personal and social outcomes. The concept contributes to the psychology of men and masculinity by focusing on the consequences of men staking their self-worth on their sense of his masculinity. Drawing on the theory of contingencies of self-worth, which states that people base their self-worth on certain domains over others, masculinity contingency focuses on the domain of the masculine self-concept. The differentiation of threat and boost to one's masculinity enriches our understanding of how masculinity as a contingency of self-worth operates. Support for the concept is demonstrated with regard to internal contingencies of masculinity, that is, contingencies that reflect intrinsic aspects of the self. Evidence of the impact of external contingencies of masculinity, that is, contingencies that rely on others' opinions, would provide further support for the concept.

What is lacking is a yet deeper understanding of why men would base their self-worth on their sense of masculinity and why this domain would be salient. Contingencies of self-worth theory speculates that people invest more effort in the domains in which their self-esteem is contingent perhaps because they care more about succeeding in these domains or want to validate that they have those qualities or characteristics on which their self-esteem depends (Crocker, Brook, Niiya, & Villacorta, 2006). The concept of masculinity contingency would be enhanced by offering hypotheses that explain what underlies high versus low masculinity contingency. The concept has potential for explaining men's psychosocial functioning in diverse cultural and social groups because the focus is on the link between masculinity (as a social construct) and a man's feelings of self-worth rather than the masculinity ideology of a culture or social group. Additionally, the concept has utility for clinical and program interventions by focusing on the connection between feelings of self-worth and masculine identity.

## SUMMARY

Six psychological theoretical perspectives about men and masculinities were presented in this chapter. Explanations of human cognitions, emotions, and behaviors benefit from empirical examination and validation. To that point, MGRS, male reference group identity dependence, and conformity to masculine norms have undergone years of empirical investigation and are poised to continue to be used in future research and clinical efforts. By comparison, precarious manhood, masculinity contingency, and PPPM are all emergent theoretical perspectives in need of more research to fully elucidate there explanatory and clinical utility. The psychology of men and masculinity has been identified as a field in need of more theoretical diversity. We urge researchers and practitioners to examine, use, and further develop the six perspectives presented in this chapter. Such efforts will contribute to a more diverse psychology of men and masculinities, which will increase our understanding of the lived experiences of men.

## REFERENCES

Addis, M. E., & Schwab, J. R. (2013). Theory and research on gender are always precarious. *Psychology of Men & Masculinity, 14*, 114–116. http://dx.doi.org/10.1037/a0030960

Alfred, G. C., Hammer, J. H., & Good, G. E. (2014). Male student veterans: Hardiness, psychological well-being, and masculine norms. *Psychology of Men & Masculinity, 15*, 95–99. http://dx.doi.org/10.1037/a0031450

Bosson, J. K., & Vandello, J. A. (2013). Manhood, womanhood, and the importance of context: A reply to commentaries. *Psychology of Men & Masculinity, 14*, 125–128. http://dx.doi.org/10.1037/a0032437

Bosson, J. K., Vandello, J. A., Burnaford, R. M., Weaver, J. R., & Wasti, S. A. (2009). Precarious manhood and displays of physical aggression. *Personality and Social Psychology Bulletin, 35*, 623–634. http://dx.doi.org/10.1177/0146167208331161

Burkley, M., Wong, Y. J., & Bell, A. C. (2016). The Masculinity Contingency Scale (MCS): Scale development and psychometric properties. *Psychology of Men & Masculinity, 17*, 113–125.

Burn, S. M., & Ward, A. Z. (2005). Men's conformity to traditional masculinity and relationship satisfaction. *Psychology of Men & Masculinity, 6*, 254–263. http://dx.doi.org/10.1037/1524-9220.6.4.254

Chrisler, J. C. (2013). Womanhood is not as easy as it seems: Femininity requires both achievement and restraint. *Psychology of Men & Masculinity, 14*, 117–120. http://dx.doi.org/10.1037/a0031005

Crocker, J., Brook, A. T., Niiya, Y., & Villacorta, M. (2006). The pursuit of self-esteem: Contingencies of self-worth and self-regulation. *Journal of Personality, 74*, 1749–1771. http://dx.doi.org/10.1111/j.1467-6494.2006.00427.x

Crocker, J., & Wolfe, C. T. (2001). Contingencies of self-worth. *Psychological Review, 108*, 593–623. http://dx.doi.org/10.1037/0033-295X.108.3.593

Easton, S. D., Renner, L. M., & O'Leary, P. (2013). Suicide attempts among men with histories of child sexual abuse: Examining abuse severity, mental health, and masculine norms. *Child Abuse & Neglect, 37*, 380–387. http://dx.doi.org/10.1016/j.chiabu.2012.11.007

Efthim, P. W., Kenny, M. E., & Mahalik, J. R. (2001). Gender role stress in relation to shame, guilt, and externalization. *Journal of Counseling & Development, 79*, 430–438. http://dx.doi.org/10.1002/j.1556-6676.2001.tb01990.x

Eisler, R. M. (1995). The relationship between masculine gender role stress and men's health risk: The validation of a construct. In R. Levant & W. Pollack (Eds.), *A new psychology of men* (pp. 207–225). New York, NY: Basic Books.

Eisler, R. M., Franchina, J. J., Moore, T. M., Honeycutt, H. G., & Rhatigan, D. L. (2000). Masculine gender role stress and intimate abuse: Effects of gender relevance of conflict situations on men's attributions and affective responses. *Psychology of Men & Masculinity, 1*, 30–36. http://dx.doi.org/10.1037/1524-9220.1.1.30

Eisler, R. M., & Skidmore, J. R. (1987). Masculine gender role stress: Scale development and component factors in the appraisal of stressful situations. *Behavior Modification, 11*, 123–136. http://dx.doi.org/10.1177/01454455870112001

Eisler, R. M., Skidmore, J. R., & Ward, C. H. (1988). Masculine gender-role stress: Predictor of anger, anxiety, and health-risk behaviors. *Journal of Personality Assessment, 52*, 133–141. http://dx.doi.org/10.1207/s15327752jpa5201_12

Englar-Carlson, M., & Kiselica, M. S. (2013). Affirming the strengths in men: A positive masculinity approach to assisting male clients. *Journal of Counseling & Development, 91*, 399–409. http://dx.doi.org/10.1002/j.1556-6676.2013.00111.x

Erikson, E. H. (1968). *Identity youth and crisis*. New York, NY: Norton.

Franchina, J. J., Eisler, R. M., & Moore, T. M. (2001). Masculine gender role stress and intimate abuse: Effects of masculine gender relevance of dating situations and female threat on men's attributions and affective responses. *Psychology of Men & Masculinity, 2*, 34–41. http://dx.doi.org/10.1037/1524-9220.2.1.34

Gattario, K. H., Frisén, A., Fuller-Tyszkiewicz, M., Ricciardelli, L. A., Diedrichs, P. C., Yager, Z., . . . Smolak, L. (2015). How is men's conformity to masculine norms related to their body image? Masculinity and muscularity across Western countries. *Psychology of Men & Masculinity, 16*, 337–347. http://dx.doi.org/10.1037/a0038494

Griffiths, S., Murray, S. B., & Touyz, S. (2015). Extending the masculinity hypothesis: An investigation of gender role conformity, body dissatisfaction, and disordered eating in young heterosexual men. *Psychology of Men & Masculinity, 16*, 108–114. http://dx.doi.org/10.1037/a0035958

Hamilton, C. D., & Mahalik, J. R. (2009). Minority stress, masculinity, and social norms predicting gay men's health risk behaviors. *Journal of Counseling Psychology, 56*, 132–141. http://dx.doi.org/10.1037/a0014440

Hammer, J. H., & Good, G. E. (2010). Positive psychology: An empirical examination of beneficial aspects of endorsement of masculine norms. *Psychology of Men & Masculinity, 11*, 303–318. http://dx.doi.org/10.1037/a0019056

Hammer, J. H., Vogel, D. L., & Heimerdinger-Edwards, S. R. (2013). Men's help seeking: Examination of differences across community size, education, and income. *Psychology of Men & Masculinity, 14*, 65–75. http://dx.doi.org/10.1037/a0026813

Heesacker, M., & Snowden, S. J. (2013). Pay no attention to that man behind the curtain: The challenges, causes, and consequences of precarious manhood. *Psychology of Men & Masculinity, 14*, 121–124. http://dx.doi.org/10.1037/a0031369

Hsu, K., & Iwamoto, D. K. (2014). Testing for measurement invariance in the Conformity to Masculine Norms—46 across White and Asian American college men: Development and validity of the CMNI–29. *Psychology of Men & Masculinity, 15*, 397–406. http://dx.doi.org/10.1037/a0034548

Iwamoto, D. K., Liao, L., & Liu, W. M. (2010). Masculine norms, avoidant coping, Asian values and depression among Asian American men. *Psychology of Men & Masculinity, 11*, 15–24. http://dx.doi.org/10.1037/a0017874

Karten, E. Y., & Wade, J. C. (2010). Sexual orientation change efforts in men: A client perspective. *The Journal of Men's Studies, 18*, 84–102. http://dx.doi.org/10.3149/jms.1801.84

Keiller, S. W. (2010). Masculine norms as correlates of heterosexual men's attitudes toward gay men and lesbian women. *Psychology of Men & Masculinity, 11*, 38–52. http://dx.doi.org/10.1037/a0017540

Kimmel, S. B., & Mahalik, J. R. (2005). Body image concerns of gay men: The roles of minority stress and conformity to masculine norms. *Journal of Consulting and Clinical Psychology, 73*, 1185–1190. http://dx.doi.org/10.1037/0022-006X.73.6.1185

Kiselica, M. S., Benton-Wright, S., & Englar-Carlson, M. (2016). Accentuating positive masculinity: A new foundation for the psychology of boys, men, and masculinity. In Y. J. Wong & S. R. Wester (Eds.), *APA handbook of men and masculinities* (pp. 123–143). http://dx.doi.org/10.1037/14594-006

Jakupcak, M., Osborne, T. L., Michael, S., Cook, J. W., & McFall, M. (2006). Implications of masculine gender role stress in male veterans with Posttraumatic stress disorder. *Psychology of Men & Masculinity, 7*, 203–211. http://dx.doi.org/10.1037/1524-9220.7.4.203

Levant, R. F. (2008). How do we understand masculinity? An editorial. *Psychology of Men & Masculinity, 9*, 1–4. http://dx.doi.org/10.1037/1524-9220.9.1.1

Levant, R. F., Wimer, D. J., & Williams, C. M. (2011). An evaluation of the Health Behavior Inventory—20 (HBI–20) and its relationships to masculinity and attitudes towards seeking psychological help among college men. *Psychology of Men & Masculinity, 12*, 26–41. http://dx.doi.org/10.1037/a0021014

Mahalik, J. R. (2000, August). *A model of masculine gender role conformity.* Paper presented at the 108th Annual Convention of the American Psychological Association, Washington, DC.

Mahalik, J. R., Burns, S. M., & Syzdek, M. (2007). Masculinity and perceived normative health behaviors as predictors of men's health behaviors. *Social Science & Medicine, 64*, 2201–2209. http://dx.doi.org/10.1016/j.socscimed.2007.02.035

Mahalik, J. R., Levi-Minzi, M., & Walker, G. (2007). Masculinity and health behaviors in Australian men. *Psychology of Men & Masculinity, 8*, 240–249. http://dx.doi.org/10.1037/1524-9220.8.4.240

Mahalik, J. R., Locke, B. D., Ludlow, L. H., Diemer, M. A., Scott, R. P. J., Gottfried, M., & Freitas, G. (2003). Development of the Conformity to Masculine Norms Inventory. *Psychology of Men & Masculinity, 4*, 3–25. http://dx.doi.org/10.1037/1524-9220.4.1.3

Mahalik, J. R., Pierre, M. R., & Wan, S. S. C. (2006). Examining racial identity and masculinity as correlates of self-esteem and psychological distress in Black men. *Journal of Multicultural Counseling and Development, 34*, 94–104. http://dx.doi.org/10.1002/j.2161-1912.2006.tb00030.x

Mahalik, J. R., Talmadge, W. T., Locke, B. D., & Scott, R. P. J. (2005). Using the conformity to masculine norms inventory to work with men in a clinical setting. *Journal of Clinical Psychology, 61*, 661–674. http://dx.doi.org/10.1002/jclp.20101

McCreary, D. R. (1990). Multidimensionality and the measurement of gender role attributes: A comment on Archer. *British Journal of Social Psychology, 29*, 265–272. http://dx.doi.org/10.1111/j.2044-8309.1990.tb00905.x

McCreary, D. R., Wong, F. Y., Wiener, W., Carpenter, K. M., Engle, A., & Nelson, P. (1996). The relationship between masculine gender role stress and psychological adjustment: A question of construct validity? *Sex Roles, 34*, 507–516. http://dx.doi.org/10.1007/BF01545029

Mendoza, J., & Cummings, A. L. (2001). Help-seeking and male gender-role attitudes in male batterers. *Journal of Interpersonal Violence, 16*, 833–840. http://dx.doi.org/10.1177/088626001016008006

Moore, T. M., & Stuart, G. L. (2004). Effects of masculine gender role stress on men's cognitive, affective, physiological, and aggressive responses to intimate conflict situations. *Psychology of Men & Masculinity, 5*, 132–142. http://dx.doi.org/10.1037/1524-9220.5.2.132

Moore, T. M., Stuart, G. L., McNulty, J. K., Addis, M. E., Cordova, J. V., & Temple, J. R. (2008). Domains of masculine gender role stress and intimate partner violence in a clinical sample of violent men. *Psychology of Men & Masculinity, 9*, 82–89. http://dx.doi.org/10.1037/1524-9220.9.2.82

Moradi, B., Velez, B. L., & Parent, M. C. (2013). The theory of male reference group identity dependence: Roles of social desirability, masculinity ideology, and collective identity. *Sex Roles, 68*, 415–426. http://dx.doi.org/10.1007/s11199-013-0258-3

Morrison, J. A. (2012). Masculinity moderates the relationship between symptoms of PTSD and cardiac-related health behaviors in male veterans. *Psychology of Men & Masculinity, 13*, 158–165. http://dx.doi.org/10.1037/a0024186

Owen, J. (2011). Assessing the factor structures of the 55- and 22-item versions of the Conformity to Masculine Norms Inventory. *American Journal of Men's Health, 5*, 118–128. http://dx.doi.org/10.1177/1557988310363817

Parent, M. C., & Moradi, B. (2009). Confirmatory factor analysis of the Conformity to Masculine Norms Inventory and development of the Conformity to Masculine Norms Inventory—46. *Psychology of Men & Masculinity, 10*, 175–189. http://dx.doi.org/10.1037/a0015481

Rice, S., Fallon, B., & Bambling, M. (2011). Men and depression: The impact of masculine role norms throughout the lifespan. *The Australian Educational and Developmental Psychologist, 28*, 133–144. http://dx.doi.org/10.1375/aedp.28.2.133

Robertson, J. M., Lin, C., Woodford, J., Danos, K. K., & Hurst, M. A. (2001). The (un) emotional male: Physiological, verbal, and written correlates of expressiveness. *The Journal of Men's Studies, 9*, 393–412. http://dx.doi.org/10.3149/jms.0903.393

Saez, P. A., Casado, A., & Wade, J. C. (2009). Factors influencing masculinity ideology among Latino men. *The Journal of Men's Studies, 17*, 116–128. http://dx.doi.org/10.3149/jms.1702.116

Sherif, M. (1962). The self and reference groups: Meeting ground of individual and group approaches. *Annals of the New York Academy of Sciences, 96*, 797–813. http://dx.doi.org/10.1111/j.1749-6632.1962.tb50163.x

Skidmore, J. R. (1988). Cardiovascular reactivity in men as a function of masculine gender role stress, type-A behavior, and hostility. *Dissertation Abstracts International, 49*(4B), 1401. (UMI No. 8804430)

Smiler, A. P. (2004). Thirty years after the discovery of gender: Psychological concepts and measures of masculinity. *Sex Roles, 50*, 15–26. http://dx.doi.org/10.1023/B:SERS.0000011069.02279.4c

Smiler, A. P. (2006). Conforming to masculine norms: Evidence for validity among adult men and women. *Sex Roles, 54*, 767–775. http://dx.doi.org/10.1007/s11199-006-9045-8

Steinfeldt, J. A., Gilchrist, G. A., Halterman, A. W., Gomory, A., & Steinfeldt, M. C. (2011). Drive for muscularity and conformity to masculine norms among college football players. *Psychology of Men & Masculinity, 12*, 324–338. http://dx.doi.org/10.1037/a0024839

Swartout, K. M., Parrott, D. J., Cohn, A. M., Hagman, B. T., & Gallagher, K. E. (2015). Development of the abbreviated masculine gender role stress scale. *Psychological Assessment, 27*, 489–500.

Vandello, J. A., & Bosson, J. K. (2013). Hard won and easily lost: A review and synthesis of theory and research on precarious manhood. *Psychology of Men & Masculinity, 14*, 101–113. http://dx.doi.org/10.1037/a0029826

Vandello, J. A., Bosson, J. K., Cohen, D., Burnaford, R. M., & Weaver, J. R. (2008). Precarious manhood. *Journal of Personality and Social Psychology, 95*, 1325–1339. http://dx.doi.org/10.1037/a0012453

Wade, J. C. (1998). Male reference group identity dependence: A theory of male identity. *The Counseling Psychologist, 26*, 349–383. http://dx.doi.org/10.1177/0011000098263001

Wade, J. C. (2001). Professional men's attitudes toward race and gender equity. *The Journal of Men's Studies, 10*, 73–88. http://dx.doi.org/10.3149/jms.1001.73

Wade, J. C. (2008). Masculinity ideology, male reference group identity dependence, and African American men's health related attitudes and behaviors. *Psychology of Men & Masculinity, 9*, 5–16. http://dx.doi.org/10.1037/1524-9220.9.1.5

Wade, J. C., & Brittan-Powell, C. S. (2000). Male reference group identity dependence: Support for construct validity. *Sex Roles, 43*, 323–340. http://dx.doi.org/10.1023/A:1026695209399

Wade, J. C., & Brittan-Powell, C. S. (2001). Men's attitudes toward race and gender equity: The importance of masculinity ideology, gender-related traits, and reference group identity dependence. *Psychology of Men & Masculinity, 2,* 42–50. http://dx.doi.org/10.1037/1524-9220.2.1.42

Wade, J. C., & Coughlin, P. (2012). Male reference group identity dependence, masculinity ideology, and relationship satisfaction in men's heterosexual romantic relationships. *Psychology of Men & Masculinity, 13,* 325–339. http://dx.doi.org/10.1037/a0026278

Wade, J. C., & Donis, E. (2007). Masculinity ideology, male identity, and romantic relationship quality among heterosexual and gay men. *Sex Roles, 57,* 775–786. http://dx.doi.org/10.1007/s11199-007-9303-4

Wade, J. C., & Gelso, C. J. (1998). Reference Group Identity Dependence Scale: A measure of male identity. *The Counseling Psychologist, 26,* 384–412. http://dx.doi.org/10.1177/0011000098263002

Weaver, J., Vandello, J., Bosson, J., & Burnaford, R. (2010). The proof is in the punch: Gender differences in perceptions of action and aggression as components of manhood. *Sex Roles, 62,* 241–251. http://dx.doi.org/10.1007/s11199-009-9713-6

Wimer, D. J., & Levant, R. F. (2011). The relationship of masculinity and help-seeking style with the academic help-seeking behavior of college men. *The Journal of Men's Studies, 19,* 256–274. http://dx.doi.org/10.3149/jms.1903.256

Wong, Y. J., Horn, A. J., Gomory, A. M. G., & Ramos, E. (2013). Measure of Men's Perceived Inexpressiveness Norms (M2PIN): Scale development and psychometric properties. *Psychology of Men & Masculinity, 14,* 288–299. http://dx.doi.org/10.1037/a0029244

Wong, Y. J., Owen, J., & Shea, M. (2012). A latent class regression analysis of men's conformity to masculine norms and psychological distress. *Journal of Counseling Psychology, 59,* 176–183. http://dx.doi.org/10.1037/a0026206

# II

# MEN'S MENTAL AND PHYSICAL HEALTH

# 6

# MEN'S DEPRESSION AND HELP-SEEKING THROUGH THE LENSES OF GENDER

MICHAEL E. ADDIS AND ETHAN HOFFMAN

The social construction and learning of gender are intimately tied to the way people experience, express, and respond to problems in their lives. This is particularly true in the context of men's mental health. Common masculine social norms such as self-reliance and emotional control can make it difficult for men to seek help when they are suffering, or even to acknowledge their own subjective distress. Moreover, the actions involved in marking oneself as appropriately masculine in particular contexts can produce significant variations in the way men account for emotional distress, depending on who is listening and what is at stake in a particular interaction (Schwab, Addis, Reigeluth, & Berger, 2015). Gender is a ubiquitous aspect of mental health, present in contexts ranging from formal diagnostic criteria to the ways individuals label, communicate, and cope with problems in their lives.

This chapter explores intersections between gender and mental health through a more focused frame of research on depression and help-seeking

http://dx.doi.org/10.1037/0000023-007
*The Psychology of Men and Masculinities*, R. F. Levant and Y. J. Wong (Editors)

in men's lives. We begin by summarizing and critically reviewing the vast literature on sex differences in the epidemiology of major depression. After considering some conceptual and pragmatic limitations of the sex differences research paradigm, we consider theory and research related to masculinity and depression. We address issues related to the diagnosis of depression (e.g., do men tend to be underdiagnosed relative to women, and how might the diagnostic criteria for depression themselves be gendered?) and also coping with depression (e.g., how are masculinities involved in the ways different men respond to depression?). We then turn to a critical review of research on masculinity and help-seeking, particularly in relation to mental health.

Throughout the chapter several themes emerge, including the following:

1. There is ample evidence that the social construction and learning of hegemonic masculine gender norms is associated with negative perceptions (e.g., stigma) of both depression and help-seeking.
2. It is not clear that hegemonic masculine gender norms play a direct causal role in the way men experience, express, and respond to depression, including their decisions regarding help-seeking.
3. It appears that numerous contextual factors influence whether individual men will acknowledge distress, use the label *depression* or other formal terms to describe their experience, consider seeking help from a professional, and so on. These contextual factors may or may not be considered gendered depending on how masculinity is conceptualized and studied. Nonetheless, they often point to potential points of intervention to facilitate personal recognition of emotional distress and adaptive help-seeking (Addis & Mahalik, 2003).
4. The way key constructs in this field of research are conceptualized is, in many senses, itself gendered. Thus, there is a need for greater self-reflection and critical analysis as a field in our approach to defining forms of gendered distress.

## SEX DIFFERENCES AND THE EPIDEMIOLOGY OF DEPRESSION

In discussions of gender and psychopathology, it is widely accepted that women are roughly twice as likely as men to be diagnosed with major depressive disorder (MDD). Among the most cited observations of sex differences in MDD is the National Comorbidity Survey Replication (NCS–R; Kessler et al., 2003). The NCS–R, which assessed the prevalence of MDD (among other mental disorders) in a sample of 9,090 Americans, found that women have a lifetime prevalence rate for depression that is about 1.7 times as high as that of men. Other cold-calling epidemiological research has reached similar conclusions, finding that women are approximately twice as likely as men to suffer from MDD (Angst et al., 2002; Bromet et al., 2011; Kuehner, 2003). Studies like the NCS–R present significant advantages over epidemiological research based on file reviews or other clinical data. As we discuss in this chapter, there are several reasons to assume that men might be particularly reluctant to seek professional help for depression; as a result, clinical data are poised to underestimate the prevalence of depression in men relative to women.

Sex differences in lifetime prevalence for depression have proved strikingly robust across large-scale epidemiological studies. The 2:1 difference between men's and women's lifetime prevalence holds up across ethnicities and national populations (Nolen-Hoeksema, 2001), with China proving to be one notable exception (Bromet et al., 2011). These rates also seem to hold steady over the past several decades (Kessler, McGonagle, Swartz, Blazer, & Nelson, 1993). Although the preceding studies generally used criteria from the third (text revision) and fourth editions of the *Diagnostic and Statistical Manual of Mental Disorders* (*DSM–III–TR* and *DSM–IV*), there is little theoretical rationale for expecting sex difference ratios to be any different if researchers were to use the current *DSM–5* criteria.

More broad-based exceptions to the pattern do emerge, however. During childhood, research has repeatedly demonstrated that boys and girls do not differ in their rates of depressive symptoms and that such differences tend to emerge only around ages 11 to 14 (Angold, Erkanli, Silberg, Eaves, & Costello, 2002; Kessler, 2003; Twenge & Nolen-Hoeksema, 2002). Research also indicates that the sex differences are much less pronounced for minor depression or dysthymia. Estimates of the sex difference ratio in the prevalence of subthreshold depression range from 1:1 to 1:1.25 (Angst et al., 2002; Kessler & Walters, 1998). One further qualification to the apparently robust difference between men and women's prevalence of depression relates to symptom frequency. One community study, for instance, suggests that whereas women tend to report a greater number of depressive symptoms than men, the severity of the symptoms they do report tends to be roughly equivalent to that of men's symptoms (Wilhelm, Roy, Mitchell, Brownhill, & Parker, 2002).

## CRITICAL CONSIDERATIONS IN ESTIMATING EPIDEMIOLOGY OF DEPRESSION IN MEN

In summary, the epidemiological literature shows that men are at less of a lifetime risk for MDD than women. On the one hand, interpretation of these findings is fairly straightforward; depression can be seen as an illness, relatively free from sociocultural influences that simply occurs more frequently in women than in men. On the other hand, there are reasons to question whether the 2:1 sex difference ratio is as reliable or universal as studies seem to suggest. Some of the issues have to do with potential gender-based biases in recognition and reporting of symptoms of emotional distress. Other considerations include the role gender may play in the diagnostic criteria themselves. Finally, there are reasons to question the utility of research focused exclusively on sex differences as the best way to understand depression in men. We take up each of these issues in turn.

First, the epidemiological research on men and depression is complicated by the role of gender norms in men's recognition and reporting of symptoms of distress, particularly those involving vulnerability such as grief, sadness, or tears (Addis, 2008; Cochran & Rabinowitz, 2000). Cold-calling research strategies such as those used in the NCS–R avoid biased prevalence estimates that may result from men's reluctance to seek help for depression. However, they still require that individual men respond "yes" to standard *DSM* diagnostic questions such as, "Have you had a period of time in the last six months where you felt depressed or down, most of the day, nearly every day?" Responding affirmatively to questions like this requires both awareness that one has in fact felt "depressed" and also the willingness to openly acknowledge this to another person. Masculine gender norms such as emotional control have been implicated in difficulty identifying and communicating vulnerable emotions and may lead to an underestimate of the true prevalence of depression in men.

Second, major depression as it is currently conceptualized can be considered a gendered construct. Because more women are diagnosed with MDD, it stands to reason that clinicians and researchers are more prepared to see it in women. At a broader cultural level, expression of vulnerable emotions is associated with enacting femininity, whereas denial of vulnerability and expression of hard emotions such as anger are associated with doing masculinity (West & Zimmerman, 1987). Historically, female experiences of distress formed the model for the development of scientific understandings of depression (Rousseau, 2000). Although it may be a stretch to conclude that sex differences in the epidemiology of depression are entirely an "artifact" of the social construction of gender, it seems plausible that the way we collectively construct the meanings of emotional distress along gendered lines affects our tendency to see various forms of distress and assign particular labels, depression or otherwise. Later in the chapter, we consider in greater detail a number of issues related to gender and sociocultural influences on defining psychopathology.

Finally, research on gender and mental health that focuses solely on sex differences carries several problematic assumptions that can stand in the way of a complete understanding of how masculinity affects the experience of depression (Addis, 2008; Addis & Mahalik, 2003). By treating sex (male/female) as a meaningful analytic category, a sex differences paradigm risks reifying men and women's gendered identities as essential properties of individuals. Decades of research and theory in sociology, critical theory, and anthropology, among other fields, have shown that gender identities are sociohistorically constructed, negotiated moment to moment, and continually shifting (Bederman, 2008; Butler, 1993; Connell & Messerschmidt, 2005; Haraway, 1989; Kimmel, 2004). Moreover, the focus on sex differences implies that the most important areas of research in men's mental health are those symptoms, coping strategies, or experiences of distress that are not shared by women (Addis, 2008). This is problematic because men's mental health may, in some domains, be quite similar to women's, yet nevertheless gendered. There are many ways to enact masculinity, and the diversity of masculinities suggests that men's experience of negative affect may differ as much as their performances of gender differ (Connell & Messerschmidt, 2005). An analysis centered on sex differences is not prepared to look at intersectional differences in men's experiences of depression.

## DEPRESSION AND MASCULINITY

In addition to research focused on sex differences, numerous studies have focused on individual differences in various masculinity constructs and their relationship to a variety of depression-related criteria. In this section, we summarize these findings and then consider some limitations of the research.

### Research Findings

One consistent finding is that individual differences in masculinity ideologies, norms, and role conflicts are frequently associated with distress, including symptoms of depression (Addis, 2008; Cochran & Rabinowitz, 2000; Magovcevic & Addis, 2008). Men who score higher on masculinity measures are also more likely to score higher on standardized measures of depression. Presumably, the contradictions inherent in predominant masculine norms are a uniquely gendered source of men's distress (Pleck, 1981). In the domain of mental health, gender role strains may increase men's risk for mental disorders like depression. This risk may become particularly acute when men make major life transitions (O'Neil, 2008). For instance, masculine norms of restrictive emotionality and self-reliance correlate highly with depression among men who have recently become unemployed (Syzdek & Addis, 2010).

Emotional distress related to hegemonic masculine gender norms can occur in multiple domains that may place individuals at risk for depression or related problems (O'Neil, 2008). This can occur interpersonally, when men are harassed or devalued by others for acting in a nonmasculine way, and also intrapersonally, when men feel shameful for not thinking, feeling, or behaving in a way that they think a "real" man should. For instance, Pollack (1998) noted that the injunction to exhibit masculine norms of aggression can cause boys and men to view themselves as cruel or malevolent, a self-image that may cause them considerable (but unexpressed) distress. The sort of self-loathing a man might experience by acting cruelly because he thinks masculinity requires it of him is particularly troublesome because of the double bind it places on him (Good & Wood, 1995)—norms of restrictive emotionality may prevent men from expressing their discomfort with adhering to norms of aggression and homophobia.

Young men must also negotiate the tenuous line between desiring intimacy with significant others and the notion that emotional closeness is not something that men should care about, that "girls [are] supposed to be emotional and relationship oriented; whereas guys [are] supposed to be detached and sex-oriented" (Gilmartin, 2007, p. 537). Again, a double bind amplifies the problematics of men's mental health; a relative de-emphasis on maintaining intimate relationships may both put men at greater risk of distress and potentially limit their ability to seek help informally when they experience significant episodes of distress. When there are fewer intimate supportive relationships in men's lives, this may also limit formal help-seeking; when men do not recognize depression in themselves, they may need the encouragement of their friends, family members, and significant others to visit a medical professional.

Compared with women, men appear to be reluctant to recognize or characterize themselves as being depressed and may have difficulty recognizing depression in other men (Swami, 2012). Men with and without depression express more self-stigma about depression than do women (Griffiths, Christensen, & Jorm, 2008) and hold more negative opinions about others who are depressed (Holzinger, Floris, Schomerus, Carta, & Angermeyer, 2012). Page and Bennesch (1993) found that changing the phrasing of the Beck Depression Inventory by eliminating the word *depression* and replacing it with *hassles in living* led men (but not women) to report a greater severity of depression. Other research has suggested that differences in the prevalence of depression between men and women appear much less pronounced when assessment instruments are not overtly or explicitly phrased as being about "depression" (Hunt, Auriemma, & Cashaw, 2003). Gender norms appear to play a key role in how men acknowledge or label depression; men who highly endorse masculine norms report higher levels of depression severity when assessment instruments are framed as being about "stress" instead of "depression" (Berger, Addis, Reilly, Syzdek, & Green, 2012). This research has also suggested that these effects of labeling might be influenced by further contextual factors, such as whether depression is framed as resulting from controllable versus uncontrollable factors (Berger et al., 2012). Research on the effect of labeling on men's acknowledgment of depression has been mixed in the significance and effect sizes of findings (Berger et al., 2012; Hunt et al., 2003), indicating that further research is needed in this area; additionally, the broader literature on stigma and depression suggests possible further directions for exploration (see Livingston & Boyd, 2010, for a review of research on self-stigma and mental disorders). For instance, biomedical models of depression may lead men high in endorsement of masculine norms to be less likely to self-report symptoms of depression. Determinist explanations of depression, compared with malleable, interactionist accounts of depression's biology, have been shown to cause both men and women to feel less control over their mood (Lebowitz, Ahn, & Nolen-Hoeksema, 2013); we might therefore expect men who value masculine norms of control in particular to eschew acknowledgment of depression-as-biological-disease when doing so causes such a diminution in self-perceptions of agency.

A growing body of research has assessed the gendered ways that men respond to, experience, and manifest depression and distress. Qualitative findings demonstrate that in men's own accounts of distress, externalizing behaviors such as anger and sexual promiscuity are part of a larger narrative that also includes aspects of depression (Chuick et al., 2009). Some researchers have hypothesized these externalizing behaviors to be part of a distinctly male form of depression and have developed scales such as the Gotland Scale of Male Depression (Zierau, Bille, Rutz, & Bech, 2002) and the Masculine Depression Scale (Magovcevic & Addis, 2008) to capture this atypical constellation of symptoms. Others have suggested that these same behaviors may be coping responses to negative affect more generally (Addis, 2008) or ways that men mask depression (Cochran & Rabinowitz, 2000; a more detailed outline of these three formulations of the relationship between masculinity and depression appears later in the chapter). In terms of how men present with depression, it is frequently asserted that typical masculine responses to depression include externalizing behaviors such as alcoholism, substance abuse, and anger (Cochran & Rabinowitz, 2003; Kilmartin, 2005; Mahalik & Rochlen, 2006; Möller-Leimkühler, 2003).

Outwardly expressed anger, as well as more stable trait anger and irritability, seems to accompany depression in men. However, research has been mixed on which of these two constructs—trait anger or angry outbursts—is a particularly salient correlate of depression among men who more strongly endorse masculine role norms. Winkler, Pjrek, and Kasper (2005) found that men reported triple the frequency of angry outbursts during their depressive episodes than did women. In terms of internal, trait anger, however, Winkler et al. (2005) detected no difference between men and women. In contrast, Genuchi and Valdez (2015) did find a relationship between trait anger and depression in a sample of college men but detected no correlation between outward anger and depression. Magovcevic and Addis (2008) found that men who more strongly endorsed hegemonic masculine norms were more likely to report externalizing behaviors, including irritability and anger; however, specific correlations with internal and external anger were not reported. Future research should aim to more clearly elucidate the relationship between typical depression symptoms, masculinity, and both inward and outward anger.

There is an extensive literature on the comorbidity of substance abuse and depression. Estimates of past year prevalence of combined alcohol abuse and dependence among individuals with depression range from 17% to 21% (Grant & Harford, 1995; Grant et al., 2004). Alcohol use disorders occur nearly 3 times as frequently among men with MDD compared with women with MDD (Grant & Harford, 1995). However, this sex difference ratio is actually less pronounced than the difference between men's and women's prevalence of alcohol use disorders without MDD. This suggests that when baseline use is taken into account, men with depression may be at a lower additional risk for comorbid alcohol disorders compared with women with depression. Moreover, the NCS found that women with alcohol abuse and dependence are at nearly twice the risk of depression than are men (Kessler & Walters, 1998). However, other research shows that men are more likely than women to respond to depression by consuming greater amounts of alcohol (Angst et al., 2002; Wilhelm et al., 2002). Such mixed results raise questions about whether alcoholism is a characteristic of depression in males. Further research might investigate the extent to which specific masculine role norms play a role in men's distress-related drinking.

Magovcevic and Addis (2008) proposed that depression in men may manifest with externalizing or distracting behaviors in addition to those already discussed, such as overworking, avoidance, or sexual promiscuity. Qualitative research does suggest that men may also turn to work when faced with depression as a way of avoiding feelings that would challenge their masculine identity (Brownhill, Wilhelm, Barclay, & Schmied, 2005). This theme of avoidance emerges repeatedly in qualitative research on depression with men (Chuick et al., 2009; Rochlen et al., 2010); however, to our knowledge, no quantitative research has looked at how avoidance and overfocusing on work or school relate to depression in men or how these avoidant behaviors covary with individual characteristics related to masculine socialization.

Sexual promiscuity has also emerged as a theme in qualitative studies of men's depression (Brownhill et al., 2005; Chuick et al., 2009). Clinical research indicates that a large proportion of patients with hypersexuality have trouble communicating their emotions, a tendency that may limit interpersonal, communicative help-seeking; moreover, current theory on hypersexuality indicates that such risk-taking behavior functions as an alternative interpersonal coping mechanism for negative affect (Kaplan & Krueger, 2010). While research on hypersexuality is still in its infancy, estimates of prevalence show that the condition is anywhere from 2 to 4 times as common in men as in women (Kafka, 2010; Kaplan & Krueger, 2010). These sex differences in the prevalence of hypersexuality and masculine "playboy" norms (Levant & Richmond, 2007; Mahalik et al., 2003; Pleck, Sonenstein, & Ku, 1993) suggest that sexuality might be another domain where men exhibit externalizing behaviors in conjunction with negative affect. Nevertheless, further empirical studies are needed to explicitly examine whether such sexual behaviors and compulsions correlate with both masculine role norms and negative affect.

As Whittle et al. (2015) noted, the large majority of studies investigating the way men respond to negative affect have tended to focus on dysfunctional coping mechanisms, such as the tendencies toward substance abuse and anger reviewed earlier. Moreover, Whittle et al. observed that in qualitative research on men's depression, there are often implicit parallels made between masculinity and maladaptive coping on the one hand, and femininity and adaptive coping on the other hand. Nevertheless, it stands to reason that specifically masculine gendered responses to depression do have *some* function, confer *some* benefits, or lead to successful coping in at least *some* instances. For instance, men's inclination toward distraction in contrast to rumination may serve as a buffer against depression (Nolen-Hoeksema & Morrow, 1993).

There are other gender differences in behavior and motivation that, although not typically positioned in the literature as gendered responses to depression, could serve as buffers against men's depression. In the area of physical activity men show a greater frequency of overall activity (Azevedo et al., 2007), and appear to be driven to exercise by motivations that focus more on revitalization and intrinsic factors instead of on appearance-management and extrinsic factors (Ryan, Frederick, Lepes, Rubio, & Sheldon, 1997). When faced with depression, men show a higher likelihood of turning to physical activity or sports as a means of coping (Angst et al., 2002). Conformity to masculine norms also predicts greater likelihood to turn to exercise in response to depression (Mahalik & Rochlen, 2006). One particular reason that such adaptive masculine strategies do not appear in the qualitative literature on coping is that men may not consider them as such. It is likely that there are other domains of men's behavior that, although not conceptualized by researchers or the public as coping, nevertheless do function as coping.

Just as Whittle et al. (2015) noted that masculine strategies are often equated with dysfunction, it may be that our scholarly language of "coping" is gendered in such a way that men's behavior in relation to negative affect is framed as either "maladaptive coping" or "not coping at all." Our scholarly discourse of "coping" is gendered in an even further sense in that men's coping is often viewed as extreme and women's coping is often viewed as mild. For example, although rigid emotional avoidance, alcoholism, and overworking are typically viewed as maladaptive and, stereotypically, as masculine, their milder forms—distraction, a glass of wine at dinner, and ego-investment in work—may serve as more functional responses to depressed mood. Similarly, although women's relative willingness to seek help and openness to sharing their emotional lives are seen as hallmarks of effective coping, when taken to their extremes of codependency or narcissistic oversharing, such behaviors would not appear particularly adaptive.

## Conceptual and Methodological Considerations

As the preceding summary makes clear, several consistent findings suggest that the social construction and learning of masculine gender norms play a role in the way men experience, express, and respond to depression. There is also evidence that masculine gender roles are associated with a greater likelihood of resistance to the label *depression*, as well as a greater likelihood of self-stigmatizing associated with the diagnosis (Berger et al., 2012; Griffiths et al., 2008; Hunt et al., 2003; Page & Bennesch, 1993).

Although there is intuitive appeal to the notion that masculinity, broadly conceived, plays a role in men's depression, research in this area is limited both by a proliferation of highly similar constructs and by overarching conceptual and methodological commitments that are rarely made explicit but nonetheless constrain the types of questions and answers considered. To put it succinctly, it is not always clear that one researcher's masculinity is another researcher's masculinity, nor even that particular studies are being guided by a single coherent conceptual framework. Yet despite this, the interpretation of research findings frequently boils down to the (greatly) oversimplified notion that "masculinity makes men do X." For these reasons, we first consider how psychological research has conceptualized masculinity and some of the effects this may have on our ability to understand depression in men. We give particular attention to the distinction between social learning/gender role versus social constructionist perspectives. This critique is relatively brief and underscores both the diversity of ways masculinity has been conceptualized and measured, and the comparative lack of coherence in framing the role of gender more broadly in the study of psychopathology. More detailed reviews with similar points can be found elsewhere (Addis, Reigeluth, & Schwab, 2016; Morawski, 2003).

The gendered social learning paradigm has broadly shaped much of the existing psychological research on men and depression. This paradigm begins with a rejection of biological essentialism (i.e., there is nothing inherent or essential about the male sex that necessarily gives rise to particular forms of masculinity) and instead focuses on socially constructed and enforced masculine norms, roles, and ideologies. For example, Pleck's (1981) gender role strain paradigm (see Chapter 1, this volume) does not view masculine traits and behaviors as determined by male genetics. Instead, Pleck argued that masculinity results from the dominant gender ideologies operating within a society. These ideologies contain numerous inconsistencies and contradictions, and the difficulty or "fragility" (Pascoe, 2011) of these norms is thought to negatively affect men's physical and mental health. In a similar vein, O'Neil's gender role conflict model (see Chapter 3, this volume) posits that normative masculine gender socialization leads to psychological conflict in particular domains related to emotional functioning and interpersonal relationships. Research using the conformity to masculine norms model (e.g., Mahalik et al., 2003; see also Chapter 5, this volume) follows a similar approach.

Whether focused on masculine roles, norms, ideologies, or psychological conflicts, each of these subparadigms begins with the assumption that masculinity is something "out there" in society that winds up "inside" individual men, largely through processes of social learning. Methodologically, this complex top-down social process is operationalized as individual differences in self-report measures of masculinity ideology, gender role conflict, norm conformity, and so on (Addis et al., 2016). These individual differences are then correlated with symptoms of depression, coping styles, attitudes toward help-seeking, and a host of other criteria. Although the majority of data from existing studies are correlational, interpretation of findings typically proceeds along the lines of "The results suggest that masculine (roles, norms, ideologies, etc.) appear to lead men to (express depression differently, resist help-seeking, cope through avoidance, restrict emotional expression, etc.)."

Several aspects of this research approach limit our understanding of the various ways gender may be involved in men's depression (for a more thorough consideration, see Addis, Mansfield, & Syzdek, 2010). Briefly, although these paradigms commit themselves to rejecting essentialism, the exclusive focus on presumably stable individual differences necessarily embraces a sort of quasi-psychological essentialism. Through the analysis of individual differences, governed by traditional psychometric logic, masculinity writ large is reduced to "men who . . . adhere more strongly to gender norms report more gender role conflict, are more masculine, etc." A productive analysis of contextual variability is a significant casualty of this approach. Addis et al. (2010) pointed out that, despite common gender stereotypes, in practice masculine gendered social learning is rarely about learning what men never do, or what they always do. Instead, boys and men learn to accommodate their actions to specific contexts to mark themselves as appropriately masculine depending on what is at stake. For example, although self-reliance is commonly thought of as a masculine norm, there are certain contexts in which men are taught to value cooperation—when playing on a sports team, for example. Similarly, crying after the loss of an important athletic event is typically not considered unmasculine (Walton, Coyle, & Lyons, 2004), whereas crying over the loss of a love interest is. With regard to depression, individual men may disclose vulnerable emotions or open up depending on who they are talking to and may even shift between the two stances within a single interaction, often in a matter of minutes (Schwab et al., 2015).[1]

A second limitation of the dominant paradigms for studying men and depression is that viewing masculinity only from a top-down social learning perspective obscures the roles of human agency and self-interest in constructing gender. This occurs alongside a significantly narrowed focus on hegemonic or "traditional" masculinity as opposed to exploring the diversity of masculinities that are constructed in relation to depression and mental health more broadly. For example, Connell and Messerschmidt (2005) observed that there exists a multiplicity of masculinities (both hegemonic and nonhegemonic) that intersect with distinct racial, sexual, religious, generational, and cultural identities, among others. Although the multiple masculinities approach has seen broad application in qualitative research, the area of men's mental health has typically focused only on hegemonic or traditional masculine role norms, with some notable exceptions (Fragoso & Kashubeck, 2000; Lane & Addis, 2005; Levant et al., 2003; Mahalik, Lagan, & Morrison, 2006; Szymanski & Carr, 2008; Vogel, Heimerdinger-Edwards, Hammer, & Hubbard, 2011). On the one hand, focusing only on hegemonic masculine norms has helped to clarify some of their restrictive effects on human functioning. Yet at the same time, it has perhaps inadvertently led to a common construction of men as passive recipients of gender socialization. In contrast, a more thorough-going constructionist perspective approaches masculinity as continually in the making, not only from the top down but also from the bottom up: Men (and people of all genders) produce masculinity through language and other symbolic practices in diverse settings, for example, in the military (Woodward, 2000), in boys versus girls school-ground play (Dyson, 1994), and in sports (Gorely, Holroyd, & Kirk, 2003). This sort of constructionist approach to masculinity follows more closely the nuanced understandings of gender that have emerged from sociology, gender studies, and related fields (Butler, 1993; Morawski, 2001).

---

[1]For a contrasting perspective on the question of whether the gendered social learning perspective is essentialistic, see the section titled "Assessment of the GRSP" in Chapter 1 of this volume.

## What About "Masculine Depression"?

Researchers and clinicians have repeatedly speculated about the possibility of a particularly "male" or "masculine" form of depression or of men's "masked" depression. The issues here are complex both conceptually and methodologically. For example, demonstrating that individual differences in masculinity are correlated with depression is not strong evidence of a particularly masculine form of depression; it may simply suggest that masculinity puts men at risk of prototypic depression. In a similar vein, findings that men who adhere more to hegemonic masculine norms are more likely to endorse externalizing symptoms following stressful life events (Magovcevic & Addis, 2008) does not indicate that these men are experiencing a masked form of depression; they may simply be engaging in higher rates of substance use, expression of anger, and impulsivity rather than experiencing some alternative form of depression per se. The challenge here is to define clearly what we mean by an alternative form of depression and the type of evidence that would lead us to conclude that it exists.

As a start, Addis (2008) identified three possible theoretical models of the relationship between masculinity and depression that can be differentiated by the degree to which gender is seen as playing a role in responses to depression, in the pattern of symptom expression, or in the social-cultural definition of what constitutes a psychiatric illness. In the first model, men's depression is assumed to sometimes present as masked (Brownhill et al., 2005; Cochran & Rabinowitz, 2000). The idea here is that nonprototypic depression symptoms such as impulsiveness, anger, and physical aches and pains sometimes really are depression "under the surface." However, men's coping mechanisms—avoidance, alcohol, and external attributions—may hide the correct diagnosis. These latter behaviors appear to correlate with the endorsement of traditional masculine norms—that is, the more men report adhering to hegemonic masculine norms, the more likely they are to exhibit externalizing behavior in conjunction with depression (Magovcevic & Addis, 2008).

A second model is that some men may not be so much masking "real depression," but rather presenting with a distinctly masculine set of depression symptoms (Magovcevic & Addis, 2008; Zierau et al., 2002). In other words, the masculine depression framework does not assume that men who, for example, present with anger, substance abuse, and passive suicidal ideation are "depressed underneath." Instead, the assumption is that this is precisely what depression looks like in some men; thus, the construct of masculine depression. The differences in symptoms of depression across both sexes support the notion that typical depression (as opposed to masculine depression under this schema) may be implicitly feminine-gendered. Analysis of epidemiological data reveals—in almost an exact reflection of the 1:2 sex difference ratio in the prevalence of depression—that men with depression present with crying at half the rate of women (Angst et al., 2002). Reanalysis of individuals in the NCS–R who met criteria for any psychiatric disorder demonstrated that men were more likely than women to experience symptoms of anger, risk-taking, and alcohol or substance abuse (Martin, Neighbors, & Griffith, 2013). Moreover, the sex difference in the prevalence of depression disappears when these alternative, masculine symptoms are considered alongside traditional symptoms to create a gender-neutral diagnostic criteria in an assessing the prevalence of depression (Martin et al., 2013). Whether these gender-neutral criteria are assessing masculine depression or simply the presence of externalizing symptoms and behaviors remains an open question.

A third model questions whether presumed psychiatric illnesses such as depression can really be meaningfully understood independent of the social construction and learning of gender. The assumption here is that psychiatric diagnoses are sociocultural products that have emerged to account for particular forms of gendered responding to more basic core negative affect. Core affect is an unfolding process roughly equivalent to "a neurophysiological barometer of the individual's relation to an environment at a given point in time" (Barrett, 2006, p. 31). Core negative affect is relatively undifferentiated and not cognitively elaborated. Put more colloquially, it can be thought of as the nervous system's basic sense that "things aren't right." In contrast, conceptual knowledge is the meanings that individuals attribute to core affect. This conceptual knowledge at once cues responses at the individual level and inheres in a repertoire of behavior that is socially distributed and continually reconstructed. Emotion arises out of the intersection between core affect and conceptual knowledge (Barrett, 2006).

It is important to note that conceptual knowledge is assumed to be learned, highly context specific, and heavily influenced by language. Moreover, there is ample evidence that gender plays a substantial role in structuring conceptual knowledge related to emotion and in shaping repertoires of behavioral responses to distress (Fischer, 2000; Kelly & Hutson-Comeaux, 1999; Wong & Rochlen, 2005). Thus, from this perspective, depression is neither a discrete illness nor a biological entity independent of the gendered social contexts in which it emerges. Instead, *depression* is the term we have come to use to describe a particular constellation of conceptual knowledge performed in the presence of core negative affect. When someone uses words such as *sad* and *down* to describe their private experience and reports having difficulty sleeping, fatigue, and loss of interest in things, we call this depression. In contrast, it has been widely noted in the literature on men and emotion that reporting vulnerability, grief, difficulty accomplishing goals, or low self-esteem is considered antithetical to marking oneself as appropriately masculine. Thus, men may be considerably less likely than women to "do depression" in the context of core negative affect not because they are masking the illness but because gendered conceptual knowledge (e.g., masculinities) in the presence of core negative affect produces something else. That "something else" could include anger, impulsiveness, external blame attributions, substance abuse, and other behaviors that draw on masculine conceptual knowledge. At present, we do not have a name for it because the field has assumed that such presentations are typically variations on depression. If we were to name this alternative, gendered performance of distress, rather than depression (to push down), it might plausibly be called "extension" (to push out).

Each of the three preceding models posits plausible relationships between the potential status of depression as a discrete illness and the social construction and learning of masculinity. Unfortunately, the relative utility of these models cannot be established with existing research findings. As long as the field continues to rely on standardized measures of depression and masculinity, correlational findings are likely to be consistent with any of the three perspectives. A major step forward would include the identification of men who are experiencing (or at risk of experiencing) negative affect. This would need to be accomplished with measures possessing construct validity indicating that they are not measuring prototypic depression, such as the PANAS (Watson, Clark, & Tellegen, 1988). These men could then be followed over time and assessed for patterns of distress that may or may not converge with what we now define as major depression.

## HELP-SEEKING, DEPRESSION, AND MASCULINITY

For the purposes of this chapter, we define help-seeking as consisting of both a behavioral component—going to a general practitioner, seeking a particular kind of treatment, or disclosing a particular worry to a health worker—as well as a cognitive and attitudinal component—that is, the opinions and understandings men have of various treatment options and sources of help. Comprehensive reviews on the subject of masculinity, help-seeking, and mental health are available elsewhere (Galdas, Cheater, & Marshall, 2005; Möller-Leimkühler, 2002; Vogel & Heath, 2016), and thus we present a brief account of the literature, with specific attention to men's help-seeking for depression. Reviewing this literature shows that although some differences between men and women in help-seeking behaviors and attitudes are evident, and there are some consistent correlations between masculinity and negative opinions about seeking help for depression, these differences are not consistent across different subgroups of men, types of problems for which help is sought, different kinds of help providers, and various forms of treatment.

On the whole, there is ample evidence that conformity to masculine norms correlates significantly with negative attitudes toward help-seeking behavior in general (Vogel et al., 2011). In terms of depression in particular, correlations between masculine role norms and negative opinions about seeking professional are consistently significant, albeit weak to moderate in size (Ang, Lim, Tan, & Yau, 2004; Good & Wood, 1995; McCusker & Galupo, 2011; Vogel & Heath, 2016). These correlations appear to be mediated by stigma (Vogel, Wade, & Hackler, 2007): One hypothesis might be that masculine role norms lead to greater stigma toward mental disorders, and this stigma then negatively influences help-seeking attitudes. The severity of depression also moderates the relationship between masculinity and help-seeking: Men who score higher on their endorsement of masculine norms will tend to look more favorably on help-seeking for depression when depression gets particularly severe, despite the putative stigma of help-seeking.

Despite reports that men are generally reluctant to seek help for depression, they do not appear to view all kinds of help-seeking for depression with the same degree of reservation. Instead, men's attitudes toward help-seeking might be expected to vary depending on beliefs about depression, that is, beliefs about the normality, controllability, and stigmatization of depression, as well as on beliefs about a help-giver's potential response and the broader social costs of seeking help (Addis & Mahalik, 2003; Mansfield, Addis, & Mahalik, 2003). Furthermore, help-seeking attitudes are likely to vary depending on treatment modality. Research comparing traditional therapy to executive coaching found that men high in self-reported masculine norm adherence preferred the latter to the former (McKelley & Rochlen, 2010). While researchers have observed that men tend to have more negative attitudes toward therapy than do women (Ang et al., 2004), Berger, Addis, Green, Mackowiak, and Goldberg (2013) observed that men have more positive attitudes toward psychotherapeutic treatment than taking medications for depression.

Men's preference for psychotherapy (Berger et al., 2013) appears theoretically congruent with masculine norms of self-reliance, which might predispose men to view psychotherapy as a more appealingly *active* or *effortful* treatment and medication as an abdication of agency. However, the preference seems more puzzling when considered in relation to masculine norms of emotional restrictiveness. If men are reluctant or unable to express vulnerable emotions, therapy should presumably be a form of treatment that is less congruent with gender norms, compared with medication. Part of the difference may have to do with what men picture when they think of psychotherapy—as, alternately, a goal-directed enterprise or a more reflective and open-ended process. Future research might address such ambiguities in how men differentially view psychotherapies by comparing attitudes toward therapies that emphasize homework and concrete modifications to cognitive structures and behaviors and more client-centered or interpersonally oriented psychotherapies.

Help-seeking behavior is not limited solely to professional contexts and treatment modalities like psychotherapy and depression. Individuals with depression may seek out help from a variety of nonprofessional sources, such as friends, family, religious counsel, and romantic partners, to name a few. Hegemonic masculine norms may be involved in men's reluctance to seek help or confide in close male friends, possibly because men fear that such disclosure risks their masculine identity (Lane & Addis, 2005). Similarly, Sears, Graham, and Campbell (2009) found that young boys are more willing to seek the help of female friends for emotional distress than they are of male friends.

There may be a large disjunction between actual help-seeking behavior and help-seeking attitudes. Such a disjunction is illustrated by Demyan and Anderson's (2012) findings in a study of attitudes toward seeking help versus intentions to seek help: Although men expressed more negative attitudes toward psychological help, they were more likely to report that they would seek out help if they started experiencing mental distress. If self-reported intentions and attitudes may differ, it is quite likely that attitudes and behaviors also differ. Research suggests that men and women differ significantly in terms of overall rates of help-seeking for mental health (Diala et al., 2000) and for depression specifically (Angst et al., 2002; Rickwood & Braithwaite, 1994). However, sex differences in global help-seeking behavior disappear when endorsement of masculine norms are controlled for, suggesting that differences in men and women's help-seeking behavior is largely determined by individual characteristics of masculine gender socialization (Yousaf, Popat, & Hunter, 2015). Furthermore, Vogel and Heath (2016) observed that these sex differences vary depending on the disorder for which help is being sought. Men are more likely to seek help during a manic episode of bipolar disorder than are women (Kawa et al., 2005) and are no less likely to seek help for recurrent depression (Angst et al., 2002). Research has found that men may also be more likely than women to seek help from mental health service providers (Wang et al., 2005), a finding that suggests that general differences in help-seeking are related to women's greater propensity to seek help from a general practitioner.

As Vogel and Heath (2016) noted, the idea that men eschew help is pervasive in society, with men depicted in "film, writing, and in the media as reluctant to seek out and ask for help" (p. 686). These societal norms are evident in research on masculinity and help-seeking attitudes; accumulated research demonstrates that masculine norms do, in general, stymie the acknowledgment of depression in men (Swami, 2012) and lead them to have more negative views toward help-seeking. These negative views appear to be weakly to moderately correlated with individual differences in masculine gender socialization, yet the research on actual behavioral differences between men and women's help-seeking behavior and how masculine gender norms affect help-seeking behavior is considerably more mixed and contradictory. Part of the problem is that research in this area has underarticulated the processes connecting help-seeking attitudes with behaviors (Vogel & Heath, 2016) and has underexplained the validity of using help-seeking attitudes as a means to understand men's actual on-the-ground decision making. Finally, it is particularly worth underscoring that both help-seeking behaviors and attitudes vary considerably by situational and contextual variables (Addis & Mahalik, 2003; Vogel & Heath, 2016). Although such situational and contextual variables are increasingly the focus of research on men's help-seeking, there are many domains that could benefit from further inquiry. For example, qualitative research on the decision-making processes and attributions of men actively involved in navigating treatment options (including not seeking help at all) would be a better use of resources than additional studies relying on self-reported attitudes toward help-seeking among college students.

## CONCLUSION

Although women are twice as likely as men to be diagnosed with major depression, there are many men who suffer from this disorder, and a significant number of both women and men never receive treatment. Despite considerable progress in the development of evidence-based psychotherapies and medications, there still seems to be a substantial stigma associated with the disorder. Common hegemonic masculine norms such as excessive emotional control and self-reliance may make it even more difficult for some men to recognize their own suffering, communicate it to others, and seek help when warranted.

It has been widely suggested in clinical and research literature that the social learning and social construction of gender may lead a significant number of men to mask symptoms of underlying depression with more externally oriented symptoms and behaviors such as anger, substance abuse, impulsiveness, hypersexuality, and somatic complaints. Such presentations of distress in men appear to be common, but it remains unclear whether they reflect masked depression, a more masculine variant of prototypic depression, or another disorder entirely. Part of the challenge here is that current research methods are not well designed to answer the question. In addition, gender is likely to play a significant role in our collective cultural sense of what constitutes a "mental health disorder." Thus, the question of whether angry, impulsive, and hard-drinking men are masking depression; experiencing some other, yet-to-be-named disorder; or simply enacting masculinities exists within a much larger societal context of comparative silence and ignorance about the diverse ways men experience and express vulnerability and emotional pain. Depression as we currently understand it is undoubtedly a significant public health concern. Yet professional discourse about men and depression seems, at times, on the verge of turning the construct into a procrustean bed in which any and all forms of distress linked to men and masculinity are reduced to undiagnosed or masked depression. As the first author observed on a recent blog for the Society for the Psychological Study of Men and Masculinity,

> the medical model is a powerful tool, but as mental health professionals and consumers we should not accept it uncritically because we can't see any other way to address the mental health of men. When men struggle with their well-being, the problems are real, de facto, regardless of what we call them. (see http://division51.net/homepage-slider/men-depression-and-the-medical-model)

## REFERENCES

Addis, M. E. (2008). Gender and depression in men. *Clinical Psychology: Science and Practice, 15*, 153–168. http://dx.doi.org/10.1111/j.1468-2850.2008.00125.x

Addis, M. E., & Mahalik, J. R. (2003). Men, masculinity, and the contexts of help seeking. *American Psychologist, 58*, 5–14. http://dx.doi.org/10.1037/0003-066X.58.1.5

Addis, M. E., Mansfield, A. K., & Syzdek, M. R. (2010). Is "masculinity" a problem? Framing the effects of gendered social learning in men. *Psychology of Men & Masculinity, 11*, 77–90. http://dx.doi.org/10.1037/a0018602

Addis, M. E., Reigeluth, C. S., & Schwab, J. R. (2016). Social norms, social construction, and the psychology of men and masculinity. In Y. J. Wong & S. R. Wester (Eds.), *APA handbook of men and masculinities* (pp. 81–104). http://dx.doi.org/10.1037/14594-004

Ang, R. P., Lim, K. M., Tan, A. G., & Yau, T. Y. (2004). Effects of gender and sex role orientation on help-seeking attitudes. *Current Psychology, 23*, 203–214. http://dx.doi.org/10.1007/s12144-004-1020-3

Angold, A., Erkanli, A., Silberg, J., Eaves, L., & Costello, E. J. (2002). Depression scale scores in 8–17-year-olds: Effects of age and gender. *Journal of Child Psychology and Psychiatry, and Allied Disciplines, 43*, 1052–1063. http://dx.doi.org/10.1111/1469-7610.00232

Angst, J., Gamma, A., Gastpar, M., Lépine, J. P., Mendlewicz, J., Tylee, A., & the Depression Research in European Society Study. (2002). Gender differences in depression. Epidemiological findings from the European DEPRES I and II studies. *European Archives of Psychiatry and Clinical Neuroscience, 252*, 201–209. http://dx.doi.org/10.1007/s00406-002-0381-6

Azevedo, M. R., Araújo, C. L. P., Reichert, F. F., Siqueira, F. V., da Silva, M. C., & Hallal, P. C. (2007). Gender differences in leisure-time physical activity. *International Journal of Public Health, 52*, 8–15. http://dx.doi.org/10.1007/s00038-006-5062-1

Barrett, L. F. (2006). Solving the emotion paradox: Categorization and the experience of emotion. *Personality and Social Psychology Review, 10*, 20–46. http://dx.doi.org/10.1207/s15327957pspr1001_2

Bederman, G. (2008). *Manliness and civilization: A cultural history of gender and race in the United States, 1880–1917.* Chicago, IL: University of Chicago Press.

Berger, J. L., Addis, M. E., Green, J. D., Mackowiak, C., & Goldberg, V. (2013). Men's reactions to mental health labels, forms of help-seeking, and sources of help-seeking advice. *Psychology of Men & Masculinity, 14*, 433–443. http://dx.doi.org/10.1037/a0030175

Berger, J. L., Addis, M. E., Reilly, E. D., Syzdek, M. R., & Green, J. D. (2012). Effects of gender, diagnostic labels, and causal theories on willingness to report symptoms of depression. *Journal of Social and Clinical Psychology, 31*, 439–457. http://dx.doi.org/10.1521/jscp.2012.31.5.439

Bromet, E., Andrade, L. H., Hwang, I., Sampson, N. A., Alonso, J., de Girolamo, G., . . . Kessler, R. C. (2011). Cross-national epidemiology of *DSM–IV* major depressive episode. *BMC Medicine, 9*, 90. http://dx.doi.org/10.1186/1741-7015-9-90

Brownhill, S., Wilhelm, K., Barclay, L., & Schmied, V. (2005). "Big build": Hidden depression in men. *Australian and New Zealand Journal of Psychiatry, 39*, 921–931.

Butler, J. (1993). *Bodies that matter: On the discursive limits of sex.* New York, NY: Routledge.

Chuick, C. D., Greenfeld, J. M., Greenberg, S. T., Shepard, S. J., Cochran, S. V., & Haley, J. T. (2009). A qualitative investigation of depression in men. *Psychology of Men & Masculinity, 10*, 302–313. http://dx.doi.org/10.1037/a0016672

Cochran, S. V., & Rabinowitz, F. E. (2000). *Men and depression: Clinical and empirical perspectives.* New York, NY: Academic Press.

Cochran, S. V., & Rabinowitz, F. E. (2003). Gender-sensitive recommendations for assessment and treatment of depression in men. *Professional Psychology: Research and Practice, 34*, 132–140. http://dx.doi.org/10.1037/0735-7028.34.2.132

Connell, R. W., & Messerschmidt, J. W. (2005). Hegemonic masculinity: Rethinking the concept. *Gender & Society, 19*, 829–859. http://dx.doi.org/10.1177/0891243205278639

Demyan, A. L., & Anderson, T. (2012). Effects of a brief media intervention on expectations, attitudes, and intentions of mental health help seeking. *Journal of Counseling Psychology, 59*, 222–229. http://dx.doi.org/10.1037/a0026541

Diala, C., Muntaner, C., Walrath, C., Nickerson, K. J., LaVeist, T. A., & Leaf, P. J. (2000). Racial differences in attitudes toward professional mental health care and in the use of services. *American Journal of Orthopsychiatry, 70*, 455–464. http://dx.doi.org/10.1037/h0087736

Dyson, A. H. (1994). The ninjas, the X-Men, and the ladies: Playing with power and identity in an urban primary school. *Teachers College Record, 96*, 219–239. Retrieved from http://www.tcrecord.org/library

Fischer, A. H. (Ed.). (2000). *Gender and emotion: Social psychological perspectives.* http://dx.doi.org/10.1017/CBO9780511628191

Fragoso, J. M., & Kashubeck, S. (2000). Machismo, gender role conflict, and mental health in Mexican American men. *Psychology of Men & Masculinity, 1*, 87–97. http://dx.doi.org/10.1037/1524-9220.1.2.87

Galdas, P. M., Cheater, F., & Marshall, P. (2005). Men and health help-seeking behaviour: Literature review. *Journal of Advanced Nursing, 49*, 616–623. http://dx.doi.org/10.1111/j.1365-2648.2004.03331.x

Genuchi, M. C., & Valdez, J. N. (2015). The role of anger as a component of a masculine variation of depression. *Psychology of Men & Masculinity, 16*, 149–159. http://dx.doi.org/10.1037/a0036155

Gilmartin, S. K. (2007). Crafting heterosexual masculine identities on campus: College men talk about romantic love. *Men and Masculinities, 9*, 530–539. http://dx.doi.org/10.1177/1097184X05284994

Good, G. E., & Wood, P. K. (1995). Male gender role conflict, depression, and help-seeking: Do college men face double jeopardy? *Journal of Counseling & Development, 74*, 70–75. http://dx.doi.org/10.1002/j.1556-6676.1995.tb01825.x

Gorely, T., Holroyd, R., & Kirk, D. (2003). Muscularity, the habitus and the social construction of gender: Towards a gender-relevant physical education. *British Journal of Sociology of Education, 24*, 429–448. http://dx.doi.org/10.1080/01425690301923

Grant, B. F., & Harford, T. C. (1995). Comorbidity between *DSM–IV* alcohol use disorders and major depression: Results of a national survey. *Drug and Alcohol Dependence, 39*, 197–206. http://dx.doi.org/10.1016/0376-8716(95)01160-4

Grant, B. F., Stinson, F. S., Dawson, D. A., Chou, S. P., Dufour, M. C., Compton, W., . . . Kaplan, K. (2004). Prevalence and co-occurrence of substance use disorders and independent mood and anxiety disorders: Results from the National Epidemiologic Survey on Alcohol and Related Conditions. *Archives of General Psychiatry, 61*, 807–816. http://dx.doi.org/10.1001/archpsyc.61.8.807

Griffiths, K. M., Christensen, H., & Jorm, A. F. (2008). Predictors of depression stigma. *BMC Psychiatry, 8*, 25. http://dx.doi.org/10.1186/1471-244X-8-25

Haraway, D. J. (1989). *Primate visions: Gender, race, and nature in the world of modern science.* New York, NY: Routledge.

Holzinger, A., Floris, F., Schomerus, G., Carta, M. G., & Angermeyer, M. C. (2012). Gender differences in public beliefs and attitudes about mental disorder in Western countries: A systematic review of population studies. *Epidemiology and Psychiatric Sciences, 21*, 73–85. http://dx.doi.org/10.1017/S2045796011000552

Hunt, M., Auriemma, J., & Cashaw, A. C. (2003). Self-report bias and underreporting of depression on the BDI–II. *Journal of Personality Assessment, 80*, 26–30. http://dx.doi.org/10.1207/S15327752JPA8001_10

Kafka, M. P. (2010). Hypersexual disorder: A proposed diagnosis for *DSM–5*. *Archives of Sexual Behavior, 39,* 377–400. http://dx.doi.org/10.1007/s10508-009-9574-7

Kaplan, M. S., & Krueger, R. B. (2010). Diagnosis, assessment, and treatment of hypersexuality. *Journal of Sex Research, 47,* 181–198. http://dx.doi.org/10.1080/00224491003592863

Kawa, I., Carter, J. D., Joyce, P. R., Doughty, C. J., Frampton, C. M., Wells, J. E., . . . Olds, R. J. (2005). Gender differences in bipolar disorder: Age of onset, course, comorbidity, and symptom presentation. *Bipolar Disorders, 7,* 119–125. http://dx.doi.org/10.1111/j.1399-5618.2004.00180.x

Kelly, J. R., & Hutson-Comeaux, S. L. (1999). Gender-emotion stereotypes are context specific. *Sex Roles, 40,* 107–120. http://dx.doi.org/10.1023/A:1018834501996

Kessler, R. C. (2003). Epidemiology of women and depression. *Journal of Affective Disorders, 74,* 5–13. http://dx.doi.org/10.1016/S0165-0327(02)00426-3

Kessler, R. C., Berglund, P., Demler, O., Jin, R., Koretz, D., Merikangas, K. R., . . . the National Comorbidity Survey Replication. (2003). The epidemiology of major depressive disorder: Results from the National Comorbidity Survey Replication (NCS–R). *JAMA, 289,* 3095–3105. http://dx.doi.org/10.1001/jama.289.23.3095

Kessler, R. C., McGonagle, K. A., Swartz, M., Blazer, D. G., & Nelson, C. B. (1993). Sex and depression in the National Comorbidity Survey. I. Lifetime prevalence, chronicity and recurrence. *Journal of Affective Disorders, 29,* 85–96. http://dx.doi.org/10.1016/0165-0327(93)90026-G

Kessler, R. C., & Walters, E. E. (1998). Epidemiology of *DSM–III–R* major depression and minor depression among adolescents and young adults in the National Comorbidity Survey. *Depression and Anxiety, 7,* 3–14. http://dx.doi.org/10.1002/(SICI)1520-6394(1998)7:1<3::AID-DA2>3.0.CO;2-F

Kilmartin, C. (2005). Depression in men: Communication, diagnosis and therapy. *Journal of Men's Health & Gender, 2,* 95–99. http://dx.doi.org/10.1016/j.jmhg.2004.10.010

Kimmel, M. S. (2004). Masculinity as homophobia: Fear, shame, and silence in the construction of gender identity. In P. S. Rothenberg (Ed.), *Race, class, and gender in the United States: An integrated study* (pp. 81–92). New York, NY: Worth.

Kuehner, C. (2003). Gender differences in unipolar depression: An update of epidemiological findings and possible explanations. *Acta Psychiatrica Scandinavica, 108,* 163–174. http://dx.doi.org/10.1034/j.1600-0447.2003.00204.x

Lane, J. M., & Addis, M. E. (2005). Male gender role conflict and patterns of help-seeking in Costa Rica and the United States. *Psychology of Men & Masculinity, 6,* 155–168. http://dx.doi.org/10.1037/1524-9220.6.3.155

Lebowitz, M. S., Ahn, W. K., & Nolen-Hoeksema, S. (2013). Fixable or fate? Perceptions of the biology of depression. *Journal of Consulting and Clinical Psychology, 81,* 518–527. http://dx.doi.org/10.1037/a0031730

Levant, R. F., & Richmond, K. (2007). A review of research on masculinity ideologies using the Male Role Norms Inventory. *The Journal of Men's Studies, 15,* 130–146. http://dx.doi.org/10.3149/jms.1502.130

Levant, R. F., Richmond, K., Majors, R. G., Inclan, J. E., Rossello, J. M., Heesacker, M., . . . Sellers, A. (2003). A multicultural investigation of masculinity ideology and alexithymia. *Psychology of Men & Masculinity*, *4*, 91–99. http://dx.doi.org/10.1037/1524-9220.4.2.91

Livingston, J. D., & Boyd, J. E. (2010). Correlates and consequences of internalized stigma for people living with mental illness: A systematic review and meta-analysis. *Social Science & Medicine*, *71*, 2150–2161. http://dx.doi.org/10.1016/j.socscimed.2010.09.030

Magovcevic, M., & Addis, M. E. (2008). The Masculine Depression Scale: Development and psychometric evaluation. *Psychology of Men & Masculinity*, *9*, 117–132. http://dx.doi.org/10.1037/1524-9220.9.3.117

Mahalik, J. R., Lagan, H. D., & Morrison, J. A. (2006). Health behaviors and masculinity in Kenyan and U.S. male college students. *Psychology of Men & Masculinity*, *7*, 191–202. http://dx.doi.org/10.1037/1524-9220.7.4.191

Mahalik, J. R., Locke, B. D., Ludlow, L. H., Diemer, M. A., Scott, R. P., Gottfried, M., & Freitas, G. (2003). Development of the Conformity to Masculine Norms Inventory. *Psychology of Men & Masculinity*, *4*, 3–25. http://dx.doi.org/10.1037/1524-9220.4.1.3

Mahalik, J. R., & Rochlen, A. B. (2006). Men's likely responses to clinical depression: What are they and do masculinity norms predict them? *Sex Roles*, *55*, 659–667. http://dx.doi.org/10.1007/s11199-006-9121-0

Mansfield, A. K., Addis, M. E., & Mahalik, J. R. (2003). "Why won't he go to the doctor?" The psychology of men's help-seeking. *International Journal of Men's Health*, *2*, 93–109. http://dx.doi.org/10.3149/jmh.0202.93

Martin, L. A., Neighbors, H. W., & Griffith, D. M. (2013). The experience of symptoms of depression in men vs. women: Analysis of the National Comorbidity Survey Replication. *JAMA Psychiatry*, *70*, 1100–1106. http://dx.doi.org/10.1001/jamapsychiatry.2013.1985

McCusker, M. G., & Galupo, M. P. (2011). The impact of men seeking help for depression on perceptions of masculine and feminine characteristics. *Psychology of Men & Masculinity*, *12*, 275–284. http://dx.doi.org/10.1037/a0021071

McKelley, R. A., & Rochlen, A. B. (2010). Conformity to masculine norms and preferences for therapy or executive coaching. *Psychology of Men & Masculinity*, *11*, 1–14. http://dx.doi.org/10.1037/a0017224

Möller-Leimkühler, A. M. (2002). Barriers to help-seeking by men: A review of sociocultural and clinical literature with particular reference to depression. *Journal of Affective Disorders*, *71*, 1–9. http://dx.doi.org/10.1016/S0165-0327(01)00379-2

Möller-Leimkühler, A. M. (2003). The gender gap in suicide and premature death or: Why are men so vulnerable? *European Archives of Psychiatry and Clinical Neuroscience*, *253*(1), 1–8. http://dx.doi.org/10.1007/s00406-003-0397-6

Morawski, J. G. (2001). Feminist research methods: Bringing culture to science. In D. L. Tolman & M. Brydon-Miller (Eds.), *From subjects to subjectivities: A handbook of interpretive and participatory methods* (pp. 57–75). New York, NY: NYU Press.

Morawski, J. G. (2003). Men crazy: Making theories of masculinity. In N. Stephenson, L. Radtke, R. Jorna, & H. Stam (Eds.), *Theoretical psychology: Critical contributions* (pp. 335–347). New York, NY: Captus Press.

Nolen-Hoeksema, S. (2001). Gender differences in depression. *Current Directions in Psychological Science, 10,* 173–176. http://dx.doi.org/10.1111/1467-8721.00142

Nolen-Hoeksema, S., & Morrow, J. (1993). Effects of rumination and distraction on naturally occurring depressed mood. *Cognition and Emotion, 7,* 561–570. http://dx.doi.org/10.1080/02699939308409206

O'Neil, J. M. (2008). Summarizing 25 years of research on men's gender role conflict using the Gender Role Conflict Scale: New research paradigms and clinical implications. *The Counseling Psychologist, 36,* 358–445. http://dx.doi.org/10.1177/0011000008317057

Page, S., & Bennesch, S. (1993). Gender and reporting differences in measures of depression. *Canadian Journal of Behavioural Science/Revue Canadienne des Sciences du Comportement, 25,* 579–589. Retrieved from http://psycnet.apa.org/journals/cbs/25/4/579.pdf

Pascoe, C. J. (2011). *Dude, you're a fag: Masculinity and sexuality in high school* (Rev. ed.). Berkeley: University of California Press.

Pleck, J. H. (1981). *The myth of masculinity.* Cambridge, MA: MIT Press.

Pleck, J. H., Sonenstein, F. L., & Ku, L. C. (1993). Masculinity ideology and its correlates. In S. Oskamp & M. Costanzo (Eds.), *Gender issues in contemporary society* (pp. 85–110). Thousand Oaks, CA: Sage.

Pollack, W. (1998). *Real boys: Rescuing our sons from the myth of boyhood.* New York, NY: Henry Holt.

Rickwood, D. J., & Braithwaite, V. A. (1994). Social-psychological factors affecting help-seeking for emotional problems. *Social Science & Medicine, 39,* 563–572. http://dx.doi.org/10.1016/0277-9536(94)90099-X

Rochlen, A. B., Paterniti, D. A., Epstein, R. M., Duberstein, P., Willeford, L., & Kravitz, R. L. (2010). Barriers in diagnosing and treating men with depression: A focus group report. *American Journal of Men's Health, 4,* 167–175. http://dx.doi.org/10.1177/1557988309335823

Rousseau, G. (2000). Depression's forgotten genealogy: Notes towards a history of depression. *History of Psychiatry, 11,* 71–106. http://dx.doi.org/10.1177/0957154X0001104104

Ryan, R. M., Frederick, C. M., Lepes, D., Rubio, N., & Sheldon, K. M. (1997). Intrinsic motivation and exercise adherence. *International Journal of Sport Psychology, 28,* 335–354. Retrieved from https://selfdeterminationtheory.org/SDT/documents/1997_RyanFrederickLepesRubioSheldon.pdf

Schwab, J. R., Addis, M. E., Reigeluth, C. S., & Berger, J. L. (2015). Silence and (in)visibility in men's accounts of coping with stressful life events. *Gender & Society, 30,* 289–311.

Sears, H. A., Graham, J., & Campbell, A. (2009). Adolescent boys' intentions of seeking help from male friends and female friends. *Journal of Applied Developmental Psychology, 30*, 738–748. http://dx.doi.org/10.1016/j.appdev.2009.02.004

Swami, V. (2012). Mental health literacy of depression: Gender differences and attitudinal antecedents in a representative British sample. *PLoS ONE, 7*, e49779. http://dx.doi.org/10.1371/journal.pone.0049779

Syzdek, M. R., & Addis, M. E. (2010). Adherence to masculine norms and attributional processes predict depressive symptoms in recently unemployed men. *Cognitive Therapy and Research, 34*, 533–543. http://dx.doi.org/10.1007/s10608-009-9290-6

Szymanski, D. M., & Carr, E. R. (2008). The roles of gender role conflict and internalized heterosexism in gay and bisexual men's psychological distress: Testing two mediation models. *Psychology of Men & Masculinity, 9*, 40–54. http://dx.doi.org/10.1037/1524-9220.9.1.40

Twenge, J. M., & Nolen-Hoeksema, S. (2002). Age, gender, race, socioeconomic status, and birth cohort differences on the children's depression inventory: A meta-analysis. *Journal of Abnormal Psychology, 111*, 578–588. http://dx.doi.org/10.1037/0021-843X.111.4.578

Vogel, D. L., & Heath, P. J. (2016). Men, masculinities, and help-seeking patterns. In Y. J. Wong & S. R. Wester (Eds.), *APA handbook of men and masculinities* (pp. 81–104). http://dx.doi.org/10.1037/14594-031

Vogel, D. L., Heimerdinger-Edwards, S. R., Hammer, J. H., & Hubbard, A. (2011). "Boys don't cry": Examination of the links between endorsement of masculine norms, self-stigma, and help-seeking attitudes for men from diverse backgrounds. *Journal of Counseling Psychology, 58*, 368–382. http://dx.doi.org/10.1037/a0023688

Vogel, D. L., Wade, N. G., & Hackler, A. H. (2007). Perceived public stigma and the willingness to seek counseling: The mediating roles of self-stigma and attitudes toward counseling. *Journal of Counseling Psychology, 54*, 40–50. http://dx.doi.org/10.1037/0022-0167.54.1.40

Walton, C., Coyle, A., & Lyons, E. (2004). Death and football: An analysis of men's talk about emotions. *British Journal of Social Psychology, 43*, 401–416. http://dx.doi.org/10.1348/0144666042038024

Wang, P. S., Lane, M., Olfson, M., Pincus, H. A., Wells, K. B., & Kessler, R. C. (2005). Twelve-month use of mental health services in the United States: Results from the National Comorbidity Survey Replication. *Archives of General Psychiatry, 62*, 629–640. http://dx.doi.org/10.1001/archpsyc.62.6.629

Watson, D., Clark, L. A., & Tellegen, A. (1988). Development and validation of brief measures of positive and negative affect: The PANAS scales. *Journal of Personality and Social Psychology, 54*, 1063–1070. http://dx.doi.org/10.1037/0022-3514.54.6.1063

West, C., & Zimmerman, D. H. (1987). Doing gender. *Gender & Society, 1*, 125–151. http://dx.doi.org/10.1177/0891243287001002002

Whittle, E. L., Fogarty, A. S., Tugendrajch, S., Player, M. J., Christensen, H., Wilhelm, K., . . . Proudfoot, J. (2015). Men, depression, and coping: Are we on the right path? *Psychology of Men & Masculinity, 16*, 426–438. http://dx.doi.org/10.1037/a0039024

Wilhelm, K., Roy, K., Mitchell, P., Brownhill, S., & Parker, G. (2002). Gender differences in depression risk and coping factors in a clinical sample. *Acta Psychiatrica Scandinavica, 106*, 45–53. http://dx.doi.org/10.1034/j.1600-0447.2002.02094.x

Winkler, D., Pjrek, E., & Kasper, S. (2005). Anger attacks in depression—Evidence for a male depressive syndrome. *Psychotherapy and Psychosomatics, 74*, 303–307. http://dx.doi.org/10.1159/000086321

Wong, Y. J., & Rochlen, A. B. (2005). Demystifying men's emotional behavior: New directions and implications for counseling and research. *Psychology of Men & Masculinity, 6*, 62–72. http://dx.doi.org/10.1037/1524-9220.6.1.62

Woodward, R. (2000). Warrior heroes and little green men: Soldiers, military training, and the construction of rural masculinities. *Rural Sociology, 65*, 640–657. http://dx.doi.org/10.1111/j.1549-0831.2000.tb00048.x

Yousaf, O., Popat, A., & Hunter, M. S. (2015). An investigation of masculinity attitudes, gender, and attitudes toward psychological help-seeking. *Psychology of Men & Masculinity, 16*, 234–237. http://dx.doi.org/10.1037/a0036241

Zierau, F., Bille, A., Rutz, W., & Bech, P. (2002). The Gotland Male Depression Scale: A validity study in patients with alcohol use disorder. *Nordic Journal of Psychiatry, 56*, 265–271. http://dx.doi.org/10.1080/08039480260242750

# 7

# A REVIEW OF RESEARCH ON MEN'S PHYSICAL HEALTH

BRENDAN GOUGH AND STEVE ROBERTSON

In this chapter, we present a critical overview of psychological theory and research on men's health. We focus in particular on "masculinity," or, more precisely, many different elements of masculinity, and spend some time explaining the key theoretical traditions here. Next we examine the evidence linking aspects of masculinity to specific health behaviors, incorporating a range of quantitative and qualitative studies. We emphasize U.S. work while also drawing on important work in other regions, including some work by scholars from outside the field of psychology. Recognizing that relationships between masculinity factors and health practices are complex and tied to race, social class, sexual orientation, and other social identities, we consider the importance of intersectionality, including literature on health disparities and on the health of men in non-Western regions. Our final section evaluates some recent approaches to men's health promotion and some recent policy initiatives in this area.

http://dx.doi.org/10.1037/0000023-008
*The Psychology of Men and Masculinities*, R. F. Levant and Y. J. Wong (Editors)

Men's health is a major issue that until relatively recently has been neglected by researchers, policymakers, and health professionals. Specifically, the role of gender (masculinity) in influencing men's health and well-being has received little attention in recent years; historically, men have been central to health-related research (e.g., new drugs tested on men but not women) but have not been understood as gendered beings. The significance of men's health is often underscored by one key fact: Men die younger than women in all developed countries (e.g., European Commission, 2011) and have done so for quite some time (Vos et al., 2015). Although male life expectancy is generally increasing, and at a greater rate than women's, this sex difference in mortality persists and in some contexts remains large (e.g., it is more than 11 years in Latvia); in many countries, the difference is about 6 years (European Commission, 2011; Vos et al., 2015); it is 5.2 years in the United States (Miniño, Heron, Murphy, & Kocharek, 2007). Male life expectancy also varies greatly within countries (and even within the same city), with men residing in multiply disadvantaged areas living up to 10 years less than more affluent peers (European Commission, 2011). This is an important point: Men's health is influenced by many social, economic and cultural factors, and we discuss these factors later in this chapter.

What are the major causes of premature male mortality? It is well established that forms of cardiovascular disease are more prominent in men than women, killing more than a third of men (see Mosca, Barret-Connor, & Wenger, 2011), with cancer also accounting for about a third of male deaths (White, Thomson, Forman, & Meryn, 2010). Men develop and die sooner from cancers that should affect men and women equally (White et al., 2010). Beyond disease, we know that men are 3 times more likely to die in road traffic accidents, account for approximately 95% of workplace accidents, are more prone to injury and death from violence, and are 3 or 4 times more likely to kill themselves than women in the United Kingdom (Department of Health, 2014) and the United States (Centers for Disease Control and Prevention [CDC], 2015), respectively; this difference is 5 times among 20-year-olds in the United Kingdom (Department of Health, 2014). The question remains: Why do more men die from these diseases, accidents, and violence-related episodes than women, especially when men on average continue to enjoy greater power, status, and privilege than women (in terms of income differentials, representation on high-level boards and committees, high-status professional occupations and positions, etc.)?

Within the health sciences, the present focus is very much on preventable health issues and health promotion (Ford, Zhao, Tsai, & Li, 2011). In other words, much attention is paid to individual health-related behaviors, often presented as "lifestyle risk factors." For example, excessive alcohol consumption and binge drinking are linked to various health problems, from obesity to liver disease and alcohol-fueled violence and injury (Alcohol and Public Policy Group, 2010), and we know that in general men consume more alcohol than women (and have more harmful alcohol consumption patterns, such as binge drinking) and are thereby more prone to medical conditions such as cirrhosis and alcohol-related deaths (CDC, 2013; Office for National Statistics, 2012). Smoking is another obvious cause of premature death through diseases such as lung cancer and cardiovascular disease, although sex differences in smoking are less clear-cut: There are slightly more male smokers than female smokers in the United States, whereas in the United Kingdom, there are no longer significant sex differences, and lung cancer rates are gradually equalizing (Office for National Statistics, 2009). In relation to diet, the evidence suggests that men's food preferences, portion control, and nutritional knowledge are inferior to women's and that poor diet, particularly greater intake of red meat and lower intake of fruit and vegetables, is more common among men and is associated with serious problems such as heart disease, diabetes, and obesity (Wardle et al., 2004). Another factor implicated in poor health and illness relates to sedentary behavior, and although men on average are more physically active than women (World Health Organization, 2012), the majority still do not engage in sufficient exercise to proffer health benefits (European Commission, 2011).

There is some evidence of the biological fragility (both genetic and hormonal; see Kraemer, 2000) of the male, leading to higher mortality than women from some of the major killers in the developed world, such as circulatory disease (Fazal et al., 2014) and cancers (Payne, 2001). However, to fully understand these differences, we must consider the greater influence of social and cultural factors on this phenomenon. One aspect of this concerns understanding the role that masculinity or masculinities might play in generating particular health practices and subsequent health outcomes.

## MASCULINITY AS HEALTH-DAMAGING

Early work implicated the "male sex role" in men's poor health (Harrison, 1978), with more recent work focusing on "masculinity" and its relation to health (Courtenay, 2000). Historically, men have been positioned as the stronger sex, which means that help-seeking, self-care, and health consciousness may be coded as feminine and weak (Courtenay, 2000). For instance, emotional expression is conventionally framed as feminine, meaning many men may prefer more action-oriented coping styles, some of which can include health-damaging behaviors, such as excessive alcohol consumption (Eisler, Skidmore, & Ward, 1988; Uy, Massoth, & Gottdiener, 2014), substance misuse, and even violence (Brownhill, Wilhelm, Barclay, & Schmied,

2005), whereas others can involve positively oriented coping activities such as those found within the men's shed movement, an initiative that has targeted older, isolated men to join a group who make things together that may then be used in their communities (Cordier & Wilson, 2014).

Within public health discourse, men (and masculinity) have often been presented as problematic (see Gough, 2006). The nature of "being a man," one's masculinity (whether seen as biologically driven or socially derived), means that men are generally seen as creating public health problems for themselves and for others (see Courtenay, 2000). As mentioned, men are more likely to engage in negative lifestyle practices (e.g., drinking, drug taking, violence, extreme sports, overworking) that are linked to traditional masculine ideals such as toughness, invulnerability, control, and risk-taking (Courtenay, 2000). In addition, these "masculine" practices also have public health implications for others who can be directly or indirectly affected by the impact of these actions—for example, female partners who may have to become caregivers after men's extreme sports accidents or the impact of male violence on those who are victims of such acts. This, in turn, leads some within the public health field to identify men as "their own worst enemy" (Taylor, Stewart, & Parker, 1998; Williamson, 1995) when it comes to their health and that of others. Linked to this is the idea that masculinity is also implicated in men's supposed poor uptake of services—that is, traditional masculine norms of being strong and stoical are said to mitigate against help-seeking and therefore lead to situations in which men are seen as irresponsible in presenting late and consequently suffering worse health outcomes associated with this late presentation (Robertson, 2007; Taylor et al., 1998).

Yet as well as being "their own worst enemies," men have also been presented as "victims" in terms of their health outcomes because of the pressure they are under to live up to conventional masculine ideals. For example, the traditional male breadwinner ideal may lead men from socioeconomically deprived communities to engage in criminal practices (e.g., drug supplying, gang violence) and men from more affluent communities to work excessively hard to purchase the symbols of such success (e.g., the right car, house, holiday). However, not being able to live up to these ideals may engender feelings of failure, which also has public health consequences (Robertson, 2007). For example, the centrality of work in men's lives has been said to account for men being more susceptible to work-related stress (and associated conditions such as cardiovascular disease) and to greater mental illness and suicide in times of economic recession and redundancy (Antonakakis & Collins, 2014). In addition, health services are widely regarded as "feminized" and lacking the necessary gender-sensitive approaches required to facilitate engagement with men. This, alongside the influence of masculinity on men's thinking about health care help-seeking, is also said to account for men's lower use of services and can form an alternative view to that of men taking an irresponsible approach to health service engagement (Banks, 2001; Banks & Baker 2013).

## WHAT IS "MASCULINITY"?

Before considering the evidence for links between masculinity and health, it is important to briefly review how masculinity has been conceptualized, assessed, and studied by psychologists (and others). Our focus here is on work emanating from sister disciplines such as sociology and the interdisciplinary field of men and masculinity studies; influential psychological perspectives are amply covered in other chapters of this volume. For example, Brannon's (1976) classic piece on the four canons of masculinity is described in Chapter 2, the gender role strain paradigm (GRSP; Pleck, 1981) is covered in Chapter 1, and the gender role conflict (O'Neil, 2008) approach is depicted in Chapter 3. In brief, U.S. psychologists have developed an understanding of masculinity that is multifaceted, socially situated, and linked to a repertoire of negative consequences, including unhealthy practices. Much of the U.S. psychological research on masculinity has used the normative measures associated with the GRSP and gender role conflict paradigms, although psychologists focusing on men and masculinity are increasingly using qualitative methods and mixed method designs (e.g., Silverstein, Auerbach, & Levant, 2002; Sloan, Gough, & Conner, 2010). This greater openness to methodological diversity, the plurality of masculinity, and the complexity of the relationships between specific masculinity dimensions and health practices chimes with the work conducted outside U.S. psychology (but see the featured article by Wetherell & Edley, 2014, plus responses that debate the extent of any commonalities in theory and methodology).

## CRITICAL STUDIES OF MEN AND MASCULINITY

In the interdisciplinary field of critical studies of men and masculinity, an explicitly social constructionist approach has prevailed; it considers what men do in practice and how this influences (and is influenced by) self, others, and society. Writers such as Lohan (2007), Robertson (2007), Oliffe and Phillips (2008), and Robertson and Williams (2012) have highlighted how men's health research should embrace insights from contemporary masculinity theories that situate masculinity and gender within sets of interpersonal (intersubjective) relationships that become embedded within social structures in ways that have a significant impact on public health. The most influential concept in this literature is *hegemonic masculinity* (Carrigan, Connell, & Lee, 1985; Connell, 1995; Connell & Messerschmidt, 2005).

Hegemonic masculinity concerns the gender order more widely—it is not (only) about men or masculinity but encompasses gender identities, relations, and conflicts. As originally formulated, it referred to "the currently most honored way of being a man, it required all other men to position themselves in relation to it, and it ideologically legitimated the global subordination of women to men" (Connell & Messerschmidt, 2005, p. 832). A pluralistic and hierarchical perspective is presented in which multiple masculinities (and femininities) exist and operate in relation to each other. Specifically, Connell highlighted the operation of power through masculinities, which are best understood as "configurations of practice"; at a given moment in a given context, some men will enact and be privileged by locally "hegemonic" masculinities, whereas women and other men will be marginalized or subordinated by these hegemonic practices. Opposition to and oppression of women and gay men (among others) are built into hegemonic masculinities. Disabled men may be marginalized by having limited access to material resources and valued masculinities. Similarly, gay men, oppressed by heterosexism and homophobia and judged to fall short of "masculine" standards, are subordinated in both representational and material terms. The discrimination, prejudice, and oppression faced by disempowered, alienated men will inevitably have an impact on health. We know, for example, that the health of economically disadvantaged men, racial and ethnic minority men, and gay and bisexual men tends to be worse than that of more privileged groups of men (Griffith, Allen, & Gunter, 2011). We must consider, then, how masculinity intersects with issues of class, ethnicity, sexual orientation, among other factors, to explain the health of particular groups of men, and we return to this issue shortly. An individual man will experience a range of situations and relationships and in some contexts will take up (or be assigned) more powerful positions but then be placed in subordinated or marginalized positions in other contexts. For example, a manager may assume more power within an organization compared with a security guard, but this could be reversed in other circumstances (e.g., drinking or sporting scenarios). So individuals may embody aspects of hegemonic masculinity in a particular setting but may nonetheless be relatively disempowered through their positioning in other social contexts and structures. Thus, material and cultural constraints often influence men's capacity to occupy hegemonic status; that is, engaging in particular configurations is not a matter of free choice. The embedding of gender within social structures is significant here as it is this that often facilitates or restricts access to a range of possible subject positions and access to material resources (Robertson & Williams, 2012).

Connell also made the point that many men may be "complicit" with hegemonic masculinities—that is, they may embody or concur with key features in particular contexts while not actively promoting or consciously subscribing to these hegemonic values. Connell (1995, p. 41) also used the term *patriarchal dividend* to suggest that all men gain in some way from the benefits that the structural embedding of hegemonic norms confers. So Connell's theory of masculinity is relational as it concerns social comparisons, relative status, and competition. Central to Connell's approach is relations between men and women because configurations of masculinities impact on women as well as men. For example, if masculinity has been defined around paid work outside the home (the traditional "breadwinner" role), then women have been positioned, representationally and materially, within the household and as responsible for child care and domestic labor. Another feature of hegemonic masculinity is fluidity: What counts as hegemonic in one time or setting can and does shift, and there may be tensions and conflicts between different masculinities in competition for hegemonic status. For example, for increasing numbers of men, an investment in appearance is important and beneficial in an image-conscious consumer society (e.g., for success at work, in relationships, for well-being), and all manner of grooming and beauty practices may be marshaled—activities unthinkable even a generation ago (moisturizing, self-tanning, applying cosmetics; see Gough, Hall, & Seymour-Smith, 2014). Thus, changing societal norms will mean that men may well have to be vigilant and responsive to change to secure and hold on to a hegemonic position, and dealing with such shifts affects health practices. This (new hegemonic) requirement for men to invest in appearance, for example, has increased men's engagement in gym exercise but has also been linked to increases in steroid abuse and eating disorders among young men (Grogan, 2008).

Some theorists highlight the flexibility of contemporary masculinities, whereby men can deploy, rework, and resist specific masculinities as appropriate such that "masculinity" can be conceived of as "hybrid" (Bridges & Pascoe, 2014), "inclusive" (Anderson, 2005), or "pastiche" (Atkinson, 2010). In general, it is argued that boys and men are embracing skills, practices, and values once assigned to women and femininity. For example, Anderson's work points to a softening of (heterosexual) masculinity in which young men are comfortable in expressing affection for male peers and enjoy the company of women and gay friends. How far inclusive masculinity is enacted outside a particular milieu (most of Anderson's research participants have been university "jocks") remains to be seen, however. Some argue that by taking on practices conventionally associated with marginalized others (women, gay men, and ethnic minorities), hegemonic masculinity is simply being repackaged by elite men to maintain power and privilege in a changing world (see Bridges & Pascoe, 2014).

In sum, theories of masculinity have become more sophisticated in recent years, both in the field of the psychology of men and masculinity in the United States and in the interdisciplinary field of critical studies of men and masculinities. However, there is little cross-fertilization of ideas between these two fields, which is a shame. One reason perhaps is methodological: The psychological research is dominated by quantitative survey-based work, whereas outside psychology masculinity scholars have generally preferred qualitative methods. However, this situation is changing: Some psychologists researching men's health are now using qualitative methods (see Gough, 2013), and GRSP work in the United States is increasingly being referenced in men's health and masculinities work in other countries (e.g., Sloan, Conner, & Gough, 2015). We now turn to consider the research base on men's health and masculinity.

## MASCULINITY AND MEN'S HEALTH: THE EVIDENCE

### Psychological Studies of Masculinity and Health in the United States

Psychologists in the United States have produced a wealth of evidence linking both general and specific aspects of masculinity to health behaviors, mostly using normative scales (e.g., Conformity to Masculine Norms Inventory [CMNI]—Mahalik et al., 2003; Male Role Norms Inventory—Revised [MRNI–R]) and measures of gendered stress (e.g., Gender Role Conflict Scale [GRCS]; O'Neil, Helms, Gable, David, & Wrightsman, 1986), although some studies have used trait measures (e.g., Bem Sex Role Inventory [BSRI]—Bem, 1974; Extended Personal Attributes Questionnaire [EPAQ]—Spence, Helmreich, & Holahan, 1979), or a mix of trait, ideology, and stress measures. A review of 12 studies by Levant, Wimer, Williams, Smalley, and Noronha (2009) indicated that endorsement of masculinity norms (MRNI–R), conformity to masculinity norms (CMNI), masculine gender role stress (Masculine Gender Role Stress Scale [MGRSS]; Eisler et al., 1988) and gender role conflict (GRCS) are all associated with engagement in various risky health behaviors. Early quantitative studies tended to examine substance misuse (McCreary, Newcomb, & Sadava, 1999; Monk & Ricciardelli, 2003; Snell, Belk, & Hawkins, 1987), particularly alcohol. A study by McCreary et al. (1999), using the Male Role Norms Scale (MRNS; Thompson & Pleck, 1986), found a direct relationship between high alcohol consumption and men who believed that achieving status and demonstrating toughness and antifemininity was important. The MGRSS (Eisler et al., 1988) measures stress resulting from threats to male role competence in areas such as Emotional

Expression, Subordination to Women, and Physical Inadequacy. McCreary et al.'s (1999) study also found that higher ratings on this scale were related to "problematic alcohol behavior" for men. Conversely, the same study found that socially desirable and stereotypical masculine traits (assertiveness, confidence), as measured by Spence and Helmreich's (1978) Agency Factor of the Extended Personal Attributes Questionnaire (EPAQ), were inversely related to alcohol problems for men.

More recent quantitative studies have examined a wider variety of health behaviors in relation to diverse groups of men, including gay men (Hamilton & Mahalik, 2009), American and Kenyan men (Mahalik, Lagan, & Morrison, 2006), African American men (Wade, 2009), older males (Tannenbaum & Frank, 2011), men with alcohol dependency (Uy et al., 2014) and Australian men (Mahalik, Levi-Minzi, & Walker, 2007). One interesting finding is that if healthy behaviors are perceived as normative for men (i.e., if men notice lots of other men looking after their health), then individual men are more likely to adopt healthier practices (Mahalik, Burns, & Syzdek, 2007).

For example, with regard to diet, Mahalik, Levi-Minzi, and Walker (2007) found that Australian men who scored higher on the CMNI reported consuming less fiber and fruit. Furthermore, Rothgerber (2012) reported that masculinity as measured by the MRNS was related to increased meat consumption for both men and women. In addition, Helgeson (1995) found that socially undesirable traits (Unmitigated Agency on the EPAQ) were predictive of smoking status after myocardial infarction. Masculinity measured using the BSRI (Bem, 1981) has also been found to be predictive of smoking (Emslie, Hunt, & Macintyre, 2002). Conversely, femininity measured using the BSRI has also been found to be predictive of smoking status in older men (Hunt, Hannah, & West, 2004). Regarding physical activity, there is little quantitative research that has addressed the relationship with masculinity factors, although Helgeson (1995) found that more positive masculine traits (Agency) were related to problem-focused coping and increased physical activity levels after myocardial infarction. A recent study by Iwamoto, Corbin, Lejuez, and MacPherson (2014) found that some factors on the CMNI–45 (Parent & Moradi, 2011) in U.S. culture, in particular, the Playboy and Risk-Taking factors, were directly predictive of increased alcohol use, whereas other CMNI–45 factors (i.e., Emotional Control and Heterosexual Presentation) were related to less alcohol use. These results show that not all masculinity scale factors are predictive of negative health behaviors and emphasize the utility of examining specific masculinity subscales and not just using whole scale scores. Another recent study with a sample of men and women from the United Kingdom

(Sloan et al., 2015) found that the Toughness factor of the MRNS was predictive of poorer diet (e.g., high saturated fat consumption and low fruit intake) especially for men. Conversely, Agency (EPAQ) traits were predictive of increased physical activity levels and, for men, less saturated fat consumption. McCreary et al. (1999) argued that perhaps those who develop more Agency-type traits such as mastery and instrumentality may feel that they are meeting societal prescriptions of masculinity and that this is health protective.

The work of Courtenay, McCreary, and colleagues has used a multidimensional health measure, the Health Risks Inventory (HRI), which assesses six factors, including a "beliefs about masculinity" factor (Courtenay, McCreary, & Merighi, 2002). However, this scale has been critiqued by Levant and colleagues on issues of validity, item phrasing, and the needless inclusion of masculinity items; subsequently, the scale has been substantially revised, renamed (Health Behavior Inventory, or HBI–20), and found to have good validity and reliability (see Levant, Wimer, & Williams, 2011). The HBI–20 covers five factors: diet, preventative care, and medical compliance (health-promoting behaviors), and anger and stress and substance use (health-risk behaviors). In the Levant et al. (2011) study, specific masculinity factors were correlated with specific health risk behaviors; for example, CMNI Dominance and Self-Reliance scales were associated with less avoidance of anger and stress, while CMNI Risk-Taking, Playboy, and GRCS Restrictive Emotionality were associated with less appropriate use of health care resources. Conversely, some masculinity factors were linked to health promoting behaviors; for example, CMNI Dominance and Primacy of Work scales were related to Preventative Self-Care, whereas the CMNI Winning scale was associated with avoidance of substance use. As Levant et al. (2011) concluded, "the relationship between health behavior and masculinity depends on which dimension of health behavior one is interested in predicting, and which facets of masculinity one is using as predictors" (p. 38). To complicate matters further, some masculinity scales were associated with both risky and health-promoting behaviors; for example, CMNI Dominance is related to less avoidance of anger and stress and substance use, but also to preventative health care. The links between masculinity norms and health behavior and outcomes have been at least partly replicated with a larger, more diverse sample (see Levant & Wimer, 2014), although another recent study focusing on energy drinks suggests that age and race moderate the association between masculinity ideology and the consumption and health consequences (e.g., sleep disturbance) of energy drink use (Levant, Parent, McCurdy, & Bradstreet, 2015). Clearly, there is more work to be done with both larger and more diverse samples of men, employing specific measures of masculinity and specific indicators of health and well-being.

## Men's Health Research From Europe

What contemporary psychological research means for men's health is clear: We should not assume that men are poor at engaging in positive health practices and looking after themselves. Rather, we should acknowledge that men do prioritize their health and adopt "salutogenic masculinities" (MacDonald, 2011) or at least adopt some health-promoting behaviors (see Gough & Robertson, 2009) in specific contexts and settings. We must move away from generalizing (negatively) about all men and consider how, when, where, and why individual and subgroups of men orient to health-related issues so that more informed and tailored interventions can be devised. In seminal work in this area, Robertson (2007) showed how men face a dilemma in relation to engaging in healthy practices and with health services. On the one hand, men are expected not to care about health and well-being because these are "feminine" concerns, yet simultaneously, on the other hand, as "morally good" citizens, we are all (men included) expected to show care and concern for our health. Robertson called this the "don't care/should care" dilemma that men face and went on to show how men (more so than women) therefore have to find ways to legitimize their engagement in health practices and with health services. We suggest that qualitative research methods are well placed to help us to examine how men actually invoke particular masculinity constructs when accounting for health-related practices, as some recent studies have demonstrated.

For example, a qualitative interview study with men provides an example of such legitimation showing how the men drew on masculine-relevant themes of "autonomy" and "independence" (valued masculine subject positions) to reject poor health practices and legitimize their pursuit of healthier lifestyles (Sloan et al., 2010). In addition, in a study comprising focus group discussions with middle-aged Scottish men, Emslie, Hunt, and Lyons (2013) found that drinking alcohol with other males facilitated friendships and provided a gender-relevant context for the discussion of emotions that may not have been sanctioned in other environments—the association between heavy drinking and ill health was rejected, and the socially beneficial aspects of drinking and the concomitant positive influence on well-being were emphasized. Other qualitative research on men and alcohol (de Visser & Smith, 2007) demonstrates that men who had accrued sufficient masculine "capital" in other areas of their life (in other social practices, e.g., through sporting roles and achievements) were able to resist pressures toward drunkenness in pubs and clubs. This concept of masculinity capital has been used by others (e.g., Hunt, McCann, Gray, Mutrie, & Wyke, 2013) and could transfer to other studies. For example, Calzo, Corliss, Blood, Field, and Austin (2013) focused on sexual orientation and muscularity: Clearly, having a muscular physique carries masculine capital for certain straight and gay men, but it is also worth pointing out that any behavior could be imbued with masculine capital. For example, help-seeking, particularly for mental health concerns, is traditionally avoided by men but could be reframed as a brave or courageous choice and therefore be congruent with valued masculinities (rather than be feminized as weakness; see Emslie, Ridge, Ziebland, & Hunt, 2006; Oliffe, Ogrodniczuk, Bottorff, Johnson, & Hoyak, 2012). Which behaviors are furnished with capital depends on a number of factors and changes with context. For example, Calasanti, Pietilä, Ojala, and King (2013) presented interview data based on older men living in the United States and Finland, highlighting both sources of masculine capital (e.g., professional status, self-discipline) and challenges to securing previously accessed capital (e.g., physical decline).

As well as highlighting the complexity associated with men's health-related practices such as drinking and diet, the topic of medical help-seeking also requires consideration (Addis and Hoffman cover men's help-seeking regarding mental health in Chapter 6 of this volume). The conventional view, often repeated in lay and health professional discourse, is that men use health services less than women and delay seeking help for symptoms for longer than do women. However, a great deal of recent work shows the situation is far more complicated than this. There is some evidence from the United Kingdom and Ireland that men are diagnosed at a later stage for certain cancers (Banks & Baker, 2013), yet this does not necessarily mean men present later (i.e., there may be other reasons for this later diagnosis, such as physiological sex differences in cancer progression or gendered differences in how and when health professionals make referral into diagnosis pathways). Several studies over the past 2 decades coming from the Medical Research Council Unit in Glasgow suggest that sex differences in presentation (apart from the area of mental health and psychosocial concerns) are rarely significant across major condition types (Hunt, Ford, Harkins, & Wyke, 1999): for back pain and headaches (Hunt, Adamson, Hewitt, & Nazareth, 2011), for three non–sex-specific cancers (Wang, Freemantle, Nazareth, & Hunt, 2014), and for general primary care consultations (Wang, Hunt, Nazareth, Freemantle, & Petersen, 2013). This work is further supported by a review of gender-comparative studies, which concluded that men experiencing ill health were no less likely to seek help than women (Galdas, Cheater, & Marshall, 2005). What seems to be the case is that sex differences in primary care consultation rates (only apparent in the 16- to 60-year age range) seem more linked to women's use of reproductive and female-specific screening services and differences in consultation for psychosocial concerns than they are to masculinity-linked fears of being seen as weak when symptoms present (Robertson & Williams, 2009). Indeed, a study in Australia showed that men actively engage in self-monitoring their health before seeking help (Smith

& Robertson, 2008). Sex differences in health-related help-seeking, then, are primarily linked to differences in service use for prevention and for psychosocial (mental health) concerns, not to differences once physical symptoms arise.

The evidence to date linking masculinity and health behaviors paints a complex picture. Conventional assumptions that men are reluctant to seek help or eschew healthy lifestyles are unfounded. A wide range of research by psychologists and others working in the field of men's health highlights the importance of studying particular groups of men in particular settings, focusing on specific masculinity factors and their relationship to specific health practices and outcomes. But work linking masculinities to the health of marginalized groups of men is in its infancy, and researchers are increasingly aware of the importance of intersectionality, which we now consider.

## INTERSECTIONALITY AND MEN'S HEALTH

### Health Disparities Between Groups of Men

Men's health-related practices and outcomes are not shaped solely by (changing) masculinities. As well as gathering data about sex differences in mortality and morbidity, it is also important to investigate health differences between groups of men because health and well-being are affected by a host of intersecting social, cultural, and economic factors (e.g., Griffith et al., 2011; Treadwell & Young, 2013). A careful examination of aggregated data reveals substantial differences between categories of men. Most obviously, mortality and morbidity are heavily influenced by social (dis)advantage, with men from the lower occupational classes having poorer health outcomes and experiencing significantly higher mortality rates for the five major causes of death (White, De Sousa, et al., 2011). Indeed, as socioeconomic circumstances worsen, men's life expectancy falls dramatically, with the rate of premature death increasing across the spectrum of health conditions. Academic, policy, and public discourses have been attuned to such inequalities or disparities in health outcomes and practices for some years now; in the United Kingdom (see http://www.nice.org.uk/advice/lgb4/chapter/What-can-local-authorities-achieve-by-tackling-health-inequalities), the debate has focused mainly on comparisons between higher and lower socioeconomic groups, whereas in the United States the main focus has been on comparisons between racial and ethnic groups (see http://www.healthypeople.gov/2020/about/foundation-health-measures/Disparities). In these and other countries, however, there is increasing recognition of health disparities between groups based on a range of identifiers, including sexual orientation, age, and disability versus ability (Parent and Bradstreet consider masculinities and well-being for gay, bisexual, and transgender men in Chapter 10 of this volume).

With regard to socioeconomic status, what is particularly noteworthy is that the magnitude of the differential in mortality is greater among men than it is among women, suggesting that men's death rates, including premature death rates, appear to be more strongly influenced by socioeconomic factors (White, McKee, et al., 2011). Furthermore, compared with women and men from more affluent backgrounds, men who live in poorer material and social conditions, including unemployed men (Institute of Public Health in Ireland, 2011), ethnic minority men (Fésüs, Östlin, McKee, & Ádány, 2012), prisoners (Binswanger et al., 2007), homeless men (Morrison, 2009), and those with lower educational attainment (Huisman et al., 2005), are less likely to eat healthily or engage in adequate physical activity; more likely to be overweight or obese, engage in harmful drinking, smoke, or use illicit drugs; and less likely to engage in routine or preventative health checks. The category "men" is not a homogenous group, and it is important to understand gender and health issues in the wider sociocultural context of men's lives and to consider how gender interacts with factors such as social class, education, age, employment status, race, ethnicity, sexual orientation, and disability and how particular men's health outcomes and practices are affected by specific mutually interacting factors. In particular, it is important to examine health disparities in context (Watkins & Griffith, 2013), without reducing complex relationships between social and cultural ideals and practices to factors that operate independently or additively (Warner & Brown, 2011).

Ethnic minority groups are disproportionately distributed within deprived communities, meaning that social class and race/ethnicity interact and contribute to health inequalities between men (Warner & Brown, 2011; Watkins & Griffith, 2013). The concept of *intersectionality* describes how social identities, positions, and discourses are enmeshed in a complex of mutual influence (Cole, 2009). It can be simplistic and reductionist to separate out a particular dimension (e.g., masculinity) and link it to health variables when that dimension will always be partly shaped and constrained by other forces (e.g., class position, occupational status, sexual orientation). The form(s) of masculinities that prevail in one particular community will not necessarily gain influence in other communities; for example, in neighborhoods where gangs are dominant, tough and violent masculinities may hold sway, with obvious implications for the health of boys and men within the locale (Chong et al., 2009). However, the embedding of hegemonic configurations of masculinity in social structures, what many recognize as patriarchy, does continue to influence how local masculinities are enacted and the opportunities and constraints that exist for engaging in various configurations at the local level (Scott-Samuel, 2009).

In the United States in particular, a body of work has emerged that focuses on the health of men of color (Watkins & Griffith, 2013; see also Wong, Liu, &, Klann, Chapter 9, this volume, for a fuller discussion of intersectionality with a particular focus on race). Ethnic minority men in general have a worse health profile than their White counterparts (Griffith, 2012; Thorpe, Richard, Bowie, Lavesit, & Gaskin, 2013). These disparities are dramatically evidenced in life expectancy trends: African American males consistently experience life expectancy approximately 8 years shorter (70.7 years) than Hispanic males (78.7 years) and about 6 years shorter than White males (76.3 years; Kochanek, Xu, Murphy, Miniño, & Kung, 2011). Hispanic and African American men have a significantly higher incidence of end-stage renal disease than White men (Karter et al., 2002). African American men, in contrast to White men, are more likely to present clinically with more advanced stages of prostate cancer and with higher grade tumors (Diaz, 2006). Moreover, African American men tend to have a higher incidence for conditions such as hypertension, heart disease, diabetes, and lung, colorectal, and prostate cancers than White men (Harvey & Alston, 2011). African American men also have a shorter lifespan than any other group in the United States (Harvey & Alston, 2011).

## Men's Health in the Global South

So far this chapter has focused on men and public health in a developed, global North context. Men and masculinity scholars, as well as health researchers, are beginning to examine men's health issues in the global South, where the gender inequalities in life expectancy noted at the start of this chapter are also present. In countries classified as least or less developed, adult mortality has fallen faster among women than among men over the past 20 years, and in the region with lowest life expectancy at birth, sub-Saharan Africa, men are living 5.3 years less than women (Jamison et al., 2013), which is interesting because this difference mirrors that in some Western countries, including the United States (Miniño et al., 2007). The impact of social structures (rather than individual behaviors) as factors creating inequitable health outcomes among different groups of men (as well as between men and women) has been recognized in the Asian continent context, leading to a call for a public health approach to addressing Asian men's health needs (Tong & Low, 2012). In the wake of HIV and wider concerns about sexual and reproductive health, a significant amount of work has now been undertaken considering the role of masculinity in gender equality and public health in Africa and in South America. Across several African countries, adherence to certain aspects of hegemonic masculinity has been associated with increased risk of HIV infection, inhibition in seeking HIV testing, and difficulty dealing with

HIV diagnosis (Skovdal et al., 2011) and accessing antiretroviral therapy (Cornell, McIntyre, & Myer, 2011).

Much of this epidemiological data has generated interest in how gender and masculinity might be addressed to create better outcomes not only in HIV rates and treatment but also in other areas of reproductive health and in wider public health issues such as men's involvement as parents and male violence. Taking a lead from the women's movement and emerging from the Beijing Declaration, particular attention has been paid to how taking a gender relations approach and engaging male partners can lead to more successful interventions across a range of public health issues. Consequently, programs based on more equitable gender relations have been implemented across a range of public health contexts in the global South. These programs have often been aimed at transforming hegemonic masculinity views and associated practices. For example, the "One Man Can" program in South Africa (now replicated across other African countries), which seeks to reduce the spread of HIV and reduce male violence, was successful in reconfiguring ideas about hegemonic masculinity and shifting participants' beliefs and practices regarding relationships, household division of labor, and women's rights (Dworkin, Hatcher, Colvin, & Peacock, 2013). Indeed, a significant piece of work reviewing 58 public health programs with men and boys, the majority of which were in the developing world context (Barker, Ricardo, Nascimento, Olukoya, & Santos, 2010), shows that those incorporating a gender-transformative approach and promoting gender-equitable relationships, were more effective in producing behavior change among men than those that were gender-neutral or gender-sensitive. *Gender-neutral* programs have been defined as those that distinguish little between the needs of men and women and neither reinforce nor question gender roles. *Gender-sensitive* programs are said to be those that recognize the specific needs and realities of men based on the social construction of gender roles, and *gender-transformative* approaches are those that seek to transform gender roles and promote more gender-equitable relationships (WHO, 2007). It would be timely to consider whether inserting gender-transformative elements into men and public health interventions in the global North could deliver similar results and help move beyond the mainly individual behavior–oriented interventions that form the current men's public health arena.

What we can see from the growing literature on intersectionality is that the relevant masculinity and health issues for men will vary according to community, cultural, and social contexts. The distinction between regions within the Northern and Southern hemispheres is especially important to bear in mind here because factors such as extreme poverty, rapid urbanization and displacement, and poor access to health care clearly have an impact on men's (and women's and children's) health across regions such as Latin

America, sub-Saharan Africa, and India. Attention to diverse cultural contexts is to be welcomed, but there is huge scope for investigating the health concerns of men in marginalized locations both within and beyond Western metropolitan environments. Clearly, greater understanding of local men's health needs can inform dedicated health promotion interventions, a topic we turn to now.

## HEALTH PROMOTION WITH MEN

Health has been viewed as a feminized domain, with primary health care and health promotion advice being dominated by women-friendly discourse and practice (with the more prestigious acute, secondary care services dominated by men)—so much so that men can be regarded (by themselves and health professionals alike) as interlopers in a female land (see Seymour-Smith, Wetherell, & Phoenix, 2002). Indeed, health information and support relevant to men and boys has often traditionally been addressed to women (wives and mothers). For example, Lyons and Willott (1999) analyzed an extended U.K. newspaper feature, "A Woman's Guide to Men's Health," and found that women were positioned as responsible for men's health (without taking control), which was portrayed as "in crisis" because of men's risk-taking, work immersion, and childlike ignorance of health and health care. A few years later, Gough (2006) examined another U.K. newspaper supplement devoted to men's health, this time addressing men more directly. Although pointing to a number of health problems associated with men, reinforcing the notion of a crisis in men's health, Gough (2006) noted that a preoccupation with stereotyped portrayals of men and masculinity (e.g., as naive about health and well-being, unwilling to seek help, risk-taking) means that the focus shifts away from (fixed) gender ideals to the development of "male-friendly" services. What is missing is recognition of the complexity of masculinities, including evidence that men can and do engage in health promoting practices and the context-specific nature of such engagement.

In light of the Western concern around rising obesity levels and the (presumed) links to ill health and disease (see Gard & Wright, 2005), much health promotion in recent years has prioritized weight management, specifically diet- and exercise-based programs. Because men tend not to access traditional corporate weight management groups and services, with "dieting" perceived as feminized and women-centered (Bye, Avery, & Lavin, 2005), some recent initiatives have developed to encourage more men to adopt healthier lifestyles. For example, a series of men's health "manuals" has been produced in the United Kingdom, sponsored by the Men's Health Forum and styled in the format of a well-known car maintenance manual (e.g., Banks,

2005). One such manual, which targeted overweight and obese men and promoted healthy eating and exercise activities, was analyzed by Gough (2009). As with the previous studies of men's health promotion in U.K. newspapers cited earlier, Gough noted, somewhat ironically, that (overweight) male bodies were presented as machine-like, requiring regular maintenance (as a car would), that men were presented as disembodied thinkers who could use mental strength and logic to lose weight and that their masculinity-related practices (e.g., eating red meat, drinking beer) should remain intact. Thus, men's health promotion becomes caught in a tension between providing dedicated advice and reinforcing aspects of masculinity associated with unhealthy lifestyles and poor health outcomes. The possible negative impact of reinforcing particular aspects of masculinity on public health more broadly has been highlighted elsewhere (Smith & Robertson, 2008).

Beyond health promotion advice in print media, some initiatives have attempted to recruit men into programs using more nuanced understandings of masculinity within these processes, such as drawing on the popularity and power of sport for many men (Gray et al., 2009). A recent health promotion intervention designed specifically for men, Football (i.e., soccer) Fans in Training, has proved successful with overweight men in Scotland (Hunt, McCann, Gray, Mutrie, & Wyke, 2013). This program was supported by professional football clubs who offered their stadiums as sites for group-based work with overweight men; another strand of the program entailed pedometer-based walking and physical activity sessions on the soccer field facilitated by club coaches. Qualitative interviews with the men after weight loss highlighted an appreciation of the pedometers as a tool for self-monitoring, a valuing of enhanced fitness within a male-friendly soccer space, and the associated masculine capital accrued (Hunt et al., 2013). Likewise, men's health promotion work within English football, the Premier League Health program, showed significant changes in a range of lifestyle "risk" factors (smoking, alcohol consumption, exercise, and diet) and likewise showed the importance of male camaraderie and "fun" in the success of the work (Robertson et al., 2013; Zwolinsky et al., 2013). It is worth noting that sport-based interventions are now being applied to a wide range of health issues, including men's mental health (e.g., Darongkamas, Scott, & Taylor, 2011; McElroy, Evans, & Pringle, 2008). Sport-based health-focused programs are examples of community initiatives through which health care is delivered outside clinical contexts in settings that target groups are familiar with and value and where medical language is avoided or at least minimized in favor of locally meaningful terms and values.

Beyond the design and delivery of male-friendly health interventions, at the health policy level there have been moves to build a *gender mainstreaming* approach (Walby, 2005): a strategy that promotes the integration

of gender concerns into the formulation, monitoring, and analysis of policies, programs and projects, with the objective of ensuring that women
and men achieve the highest health status (Commission on the Social
Determinants of Health, 2008). Gender mainstreaming has historically
emerged out of a feminist discourse examining inequities between men and
women (Woodford-Berger, 2004) but can now be deployed to tackle gendered inequalities that affect men and women; this has been taking place
in both the global North and global South and is linked into the intersectionality agenda discussed earlier (see Tolhurst et al., 2012). Furthermore,
Williams, Robertson, and Hewison (2009) advised that approaches in which
there is a political commitment to social and economic policies that promote
equity and social justice (e.g., redistributive taxation; greater increases in the
national minimum wage; increases in benefit levels; policies committed to
drive down unemployment and underemployment; investment in affordable,
good-quality housing and child care) are likely to be the most appropriate
and effective ways to improve the health of men (and, relatedly, of women
and children).

It is only in relatively recent times that men have been identified as a
specific population group for the strategic planning of health, with the emergence of policy responses in countries such as Ireland (Department of Health
and Children, 2009), Australia (Department of Health and Ageing, 2009),
and Brazil (Ministério da Saúde, 2009). In Ireland, for example, the policy has
been translated into some promising workplace-based men's health promotion initiatives and the expansion of community-based men's health initiatives targeted at vulnerable groups of men (Richardson, 2013). In Australia,
the implementation of the policy has led to funding and expansion of the
men's shed movement, which eases the significant problems of social isolation for aging and retired men and providing them with a new, valued sense
of male identity (Cordier & Wilson, 2014).

Health promotion initiatives then can take a variety of forms, and there
is growing evidence that community-based programs that incorporate aspects
of conventional masculinized ideals and practices (e.g., around sport) can be
appealing to men, although Gough (2009) cautioned against reproducing
masculinity norms that can also help reinforce risky practices. Because sport
will not appeal to all men, it is important to provide alterative interventions, and some health benefits have been associated with other activities,
including walking, making things in sheds, and music groups (e.g., Cordier
& Wilson, 2014). To this end, researchers and health professionals need to
work more with local communities of men to establish preferred activities
and, goals and targets. At the policy level, dedicated men's health policies
can help raise awareness of prevailing health issues for men and could lead to
funded interventions. But given that men's health issues also affect women

and children and because it is now widely recognized that other sociodemographic variables, such as socioeconomic status, race, and sexual orientation,
intersect with masculinity factors and affect the health and well-being of
men, we also need wide-ranging policies that address gender relations and
inequalities between groups of men.

## CONCLUSION

In this chapter, we have argued that simplistic associations between
"masculinity" and indices of ill health should be replaced by more sophisticated conceptions of masculinities and more nuanced links drawn with
different health-related practices, including health-promoting activities.
Traditionally, most of the evidence from U.S. GRSP-inspired work has linked
global and specific scores on conventional masculinity norms to health
behaviors, emphasizing the negative health behaviors that ensue. As noted
in this chapter, more recent work has begun to delve into the links between
specific masculinity factors, measured by normative (e.g., CMNI, MRNI–R)
and stress/conflict scales (e.g., MGRSS, GRCS), and specific health practices
(both risky and protective behaviors), as measured by the HBI–20. It is important that both quantitative and qualitative research on masculinity and men's
health are now encompassing health-promoting as well as health-defeating
practices. For example, various CMNI factors (e.g., Winning, Emotional
Control) have been related to preventative health care, such as lower alcohol
consumption (e.g., Iwamoto et al., 2014), and qualitative interview research
similarly suggests that masculinized ideals such as independence and self-
control are used by some men to account for their healthy lifestyle choices
(e.g., Sloan et al., 2010). Some themes are common between quantitative
and qualitative work (e.g., control), and thus more mixed methods research
is required to further test and develop emerging hypotheses about healthy
masculinities.

Although researchers are now producing lots of evidence in relation
to masculinities and the health status of marginalized groups of men, there
is still more work to be done here. In light of the increased policy and media
attention to health disparities and the currency of the intersectionality concept, we need to develop more research that is designed to understand the
health-related practices of specific communities in diverse settings to more
effectively deliver health interventions informed by gender-sensitive and
gender-transformative health policy. There are encouraging signs, including
Levant et al.'s (2015) consideration of age and race in their study of masculinity factors and energy drink use, and Bowleg, Heckert, Brown, and Massie's
(2015) qualitative work with African American men and condom use, but

both qualitative and quantitative researchers could do more in this regard. When all the possible intersections of masculinity with other social categories are considered, as well as the sheer number of behaviors related to health, illness, and well-being, there is much more potential to explore and explicate the associations between masculinities and health for clearly defined groups of men. We have come a long way since the 1970s declaration that "masculinity" was bad for men's health (Harrison, 1978), and the increased sophistication of current research projects points to an exciting future ahead.

## REFERENCES

Anderson, E. (2005). Orthodox and inclusive masculinity: Competing masculinities among heterosexual men in feminized terrain. *Sociological Perspectives, 48,* 337–355. http://dx.doi.org/10.1525/sop.2005.48.3.337

Alcohol and Public Policy Group. (2010). [Summary of the book *Alcohol: No ordinary commodity* (2nd ed.), by T. Babor, R. Caetano, S. Casswell, G. Edwards, N. Giesbrecht, K. Graham, . . . I. Rossow]. *Addiction, 105,* 769–779.

Antonakakis, N., & Collins, A. (2014). The impact of fiscal austerity on suicide: On the empirics of a modern Greek tragedy. *Social Science & Medicine, 112,* 39–50. http://dx.doi.org/10.1016/j.socscimed.2014.04.019

Atkinson, M. (2010). *Deconstructing men and masculinities.* Toronto, Ontario, Canada: Oxford University Press.

Banks, I. (2001). No man's land: Men, illness, and the NHS. *British Medical Journal, 323,* 1058–1060. http://dx.doi.org/10.1136/bmj.323.7320.1058

Banks, I. (2005). *The HGV Man manual.* Somerset, England: Haynes.

Banks, I., & Baker, P. (2013). Men and primary care: Improving access and outcomes. *Trends in Urology & Men's Health, 4,* 39–41. http://dx.doi.org/10.1002/tre.357

Barker, G., Ricardo, C., Nascimento, M., Olukoya, A., & Santos, C. (2010). Questioning gender norms with men to improve health outcomes: Evidence of impact. *Global Public Health: An International Journal for Research, Policy and Practice, 5,* 539–553. http://dx.doi.org/10.1080/17441690902942464

Bem, S. L. (1974). The measurement of psychological androgyny. *Journal of Consulting and Clinical Psychology, 42,* 155–162.

Bem, S. L. (1981). Gender schema theory: A cognitive account of sex typing. *Psychological Review, 88,* 354–364. http://dx.doi.org/10.1037/0033-295X.88.4.354

Binswanger, I. A., Stern, M. F., Deyo, R. A., Heagerty, P. J., Cheadle, A., Elmore, J. G., & Koepsell, T. D. (2007). Release from prison—A high risk of death for former inmates. *The New England Journal of Medicine, 356,* 157–165. http://dx.doi.org/10.1056/NEJMsa064115

Bowleg, L., Heckert, A. L., Brown, T. L., & Massie, J. S. (2015). Responsible men, blameworthy women: Black heterosexual men's discursive constructions of safer sex and masculinity. *Health Psychology, 34,* 314–327. http://dx.doi.org/10.1037/hea0000216

Brannon, D. (1976). The male sex role: Our culture's blueprint for manhood and what it's done for us lately. In D. S. David & R. Brannon (Eds.), *The forty-nine percent majority: The male sex role* (pp. 1–49). Reading, MA: Addison-Wesley.

Bridges, T., & Pascoe, C. J. (2014). Hybrid masculinities: New directions in the sociology of men and masculinities. *Social Compass, 8,* 246–258. http://dx.doi.org/10.1111/soc4.12134

Brownhill, S., Wilhelm, K., Barclay, L., & Schmied, V. (2005). "Big build": Hidden depression in men. *Australian and New Zealand Journal of Psychiatry, 39,* 921–931.

Bye, C., Avery, A., & Lavin, J. (2005). Tackling obesity in men—Preliminary evaluation of men-only groups within a commercial slimming organization. *Journal of Human Nutrition and Dietetics, 18,* 391–394. http://dx.doi.org/10.1111/j.1365-277X.2005.00642.x

Calasanti, T., Pietilä, I., Ojala, H., & King, N. (2013). Men, bodily control, and health behaviors: The importance of age. *Health Psychology, 32,* 15–23. http://dx.doi.org/10.1037/a0029300

Calzo, J. P., Corliss, H. L., Blood, E. A., Field, A. E., & Austin, S. B. (2013). Development of muscularity and weight concerns in heterosexual and sexual minority males. *Health Psychology, 32,* 42–51. http://dx.doi.org/10.1037/a0028964

Carrigan, T., Connell, R. W., & Lee, J. (1985). Toward a new sociology of masculinity. *Theory and Society, 14,* 551–604. http://dx.doi.org/10.1007/BF00160017

Centers for Disease Control and Prevention. (2013). *Fact sheets: Excessive alcohol use and risks to men's health.* Retrieved from http://www.cdc.gov/alcohol/fact-sheets/mens-health.htm

Centers for Disease Control and Prevention. (2015). *National suicide statistics at a glance.* Retrieved from http://www.cdc.gov/violenceprevention/pdf/suicide-datasheet.a.pdf

Chong, V., Um, K., Hahn, M., Pheng, D., Yee, C., & Auerswald, C. (2009). Toward an intersectional understanding of violence and resilience: An exploratory study of young Southeast Asian men in Alameda and Contra Costa County, California. *Aggression and Violent Behavior, 14,* 461–469. http://dx.doi.org/10.1016/j.avb.2009.07.001

Cole, E. R. (2009). Intersectionality and research in psychology. *American Psychologist, 64,* 170–180. http://dx.doi.org/10.1037/a0014564

Connell, R. W. (1995). *Masculinities.* Cambridge, England: Polity.

Connell, R. W., & Messerschmidt, J. W. (2005). Hegemonic masculinity: Rethinking the concept. *Gender & Society, 19,* 829–859. http://dx.doi.org/10.1177/0891243205278639

Cornell, M., McIntyre, J., & Myer, L. (2011). Men and antiretroviral therapy in Africa: Our blind spot. *Tropical Medicine & International Health, 16,* 828–829. http://dx.doi.org/10.1111/j.1365-3156.2011.02767.x

Cordier, R., & Wilson, N. J. (2014). Community-based Men's Sheds: Promoting male health, wellbeing and social inclusion in an international context. *Health Promotion International, 29*, 483–493. http://dx.doi.org/10.1093/heapro/dat033

Courtenay, W. H. (2000). Constructions of masculinity and their influence on men's well-being: A theory of gender and health. *Social Science & Medicine, 50*, 1385–1401. http://dx.doi.org/10.1016/S0277-9536(99)00390-1

Courtenay, W. H., McCreary, D. R., & Merighi, J. R. (2002). Gender and ethnic differences in health beliefs and behaviors. *Journal of Health Psychology, 7*, 219–231. http://dx.doi.org/10.1177/1359105302007003216

Commission on the Social Determinants of Health. (2008). *Closing the gap in a generation: Health equity through action on the social determinants of health* [final report]. Geneva, Switzerland: World Health Organization.

Darongkamas, J., Scott, H., & Taylor, E. (2011). Kick-starting men's mental health: An evaluation of the effect of playing football on mental health service users' well-being. *International Journal of Mental Health Promotion, 13*, 14–21. http://dx.doi.org/10.1080/14623730.2011.9715658

Department of Health. (2014). *Statistical update on suicide.* Retrieved from http://www.gov.uk/government/uploads/system/uploads/attachment_data/file/278120/Suicide_update_Jan_2014_FINAL_revised.pdf

Department of Health and Ageing. (2009). *Building a 21st century primary health care system: A draft of Australia's first national primary health care strategy.* Canberra: Commonwealth of Australia.

Department of Health and Children. (2009). *National Men's Health Policy: Working with men in Ireland to achieve optimum health and wellbeing.* Dublin, Ireland: Hawkins House.

de Visser, R., & Smith, J. (2007). Alcohol consumption and masculine identity among young men. *Psychology & Health, 22*, 595–614. http://dx.doi.org/10.1080/14768320600941772

Diaz, V. A., Jr. (2006). Hispanic male health disparities. *Primary Care, 33*, 45–60, viii. http://dx.doi.org/10.1016/j.pop.2005.11.013

Dworkin, S. L., Hatcher, A. M., Colvin, C., & Peacock, D. (2013). Impact of a gender-transformative HIV and antiviolence program on gender ideologies and masculinities in two rural South African communities. *Men & Masculinities, 16*, 181–202.

Eisler, R. M., Skidmore, J. R., & Ward, C. H. (1988). Masculine gender-role stress: Predictor of anger, anxiety, and health-risk behaviors. *Journal of Personality Assessment, 52*, 133–141. http://dx.doi.org/10.1207/s15327752jpa5201_12

Emslie, C., Hunt, K., & Lyons, A. (2013). The role of alcohol in forging and maintaining friendships amongst Scottish men in midlife. *Health Psychology, 32*, 33–41. http://dx.doi.org/10.1037/a0029874

Emslie, C., Hunt, K., & Macintyre, S. (2002). How similar are the smoking and drinking habits of men and women in non-manual jobs? *European Journal of Public Health, 12*, 22–28. http://dx.doi.org/10.1093/eurpub/12.1.22

Emslie, C., Ridge, D., Ziebland, S., & Hunt, K. (2006). Men's accounts of depression: Reconstructing or resisting hegemonic masculinity? *Social Science & Medicine*, 62, 2246–2257. http://dx.doi.org/10.1016/j.socscimed.2005.10.017

European Commission. (2011). *The state of men's health in Europe* (Report). Brussels, Belgium: Author.

Fazal, L., Azibani, F., Vodovar, N., Cohen Solal, A., Delcayre, C., & Samuel, J. L. (2014). Effects of biological sex on the pathophysiology of the heart. *British Journal of Pharmacology*, 171, 555–566. http://dx.doi.org/10.1111/bph.12279

Fésüs, G., Östlin, P., McKee, M., & Ádány, R. (2012). Policies to improve the health and well-being of Roma people: The European experience. *Health Policy*, 105, 25–32. http://dx.doi.org/10.1016/j.healthpol.2011.12.003

Ford, E. S., Zhao, G., Tsai, J., & Li, C. (2011). Low-risk lifestyle behaviors and all-cause mortality: Findings from the National Health and Nutrition Examination Survey III Mortality Study. *American Journal of Public Health*, 101, 1922–1929. http://dx.doi.org/10.2105/AJPH.2011.300167

Galdas, P. M., Cheater, F., & Marshall, P. (2005). Men and health help-seeking behaviour: Literature review. *Journal of Advanced Nursing*, 49, 616–623. http://dx.doi.org/10.1111/j.1365-2648.2004.03331.x

Gard, M., & Wright, J. (2005). *The obesity epidemic: Science, morality & ideology*. London, England: Routledge.

Gough, B. (2006). Try to be healthy, but don't forgo your masculinity: Deconstructing men's health discourse in the media. *Social Science & Medicine*, 63, 2476–2488. http://dx.doi.org/10.1016/j.socscimed.2006.06.004

Gough, B. (2009). Promoting "masculinity" over health: A critical analysis of men's health promotion with particular reference to an obesity reduction manual. In B. Gough & S. Robertson (Eds.), *Men, masculinities and health: Critical perspectives* (pp. 125–143). Basingstoke, England: Palgrave.

Gough, B. (2013). The psychology of men's health: Maximizing masculine capital. *Health Psychology*, 32, 1–4. http://dx.doi.org/10.1037/a0030424

Gough, B., Hall, M., & Seymour-Smith, S. (2014). Straight guys do wear make-up: Contemporary masculinities and investment in appearance. In S. Roberts (Ed.), *Debating modern masculinities: Change, continuity, crisis?* (pp. 106–124). http://dx.doi.org/10.1057/9781137394842_7

Gough, B., & Robertson, S. (2009). *Men, masculinities and health: Critical perspectives*. Basingstoke, England: Palgrave.

Gray, C. M., Anderson, A. S., Dalziel, A., Hunt, K., Leishman, J., & Wyke, S. (2009). Addressing male obesity: An evaluation of a group-based weight management intervention for Scottish men. *Journal of Men's Health & Gender*, 6, 70–81. http://dx.doi.org/10.1016/j.jomh.2008.11.002

Griffith, D. M. (2012). An intersectional approach to men's health. *Journal of Men's Health, 9,* 106–112. http://dx.doi.org/10.1016/j.jomh.2012.03.003

Griffith, D. M., Allen, J. O., & Gunter, K. (2011). Social and cultural factors influence African American men's medical help seeking. *Research on Social Work Practice, 21,* 337–347. http://dx.doi.org/10.1177/1049731510388669

Grogan, S. (2008). *Body image: Understanding body dissatisfaction in men, women, and children.* London, England: Routledge.

Hamilton, C. J., & Mahalik, J. R. (2009). Minority stress, masculinity, and social norms predicting gay men's health risk behaviors. *Journal of Counseling Psychology, 56,* 132–141. http://dx.doi.org/10.1037/a0014440

Harrison, J. (1978). Warning: The male sex role may be dangerous to your health. *Journal of Social Issues, 34,* 65–86. http://dx.doi.org/10.1111/j.1540-4560.1978.tb02541.x

Harvey, I. S., & Alston, R. J. (2011). Understanding preventive behaviors among mid-Western African-American men: A pilot qualitative study of prostate screening. *The Journal of Men's Health, 8,* 140–151. http://dx.doi.org/10.1016/j.jomh.2011.03.005

Helgeson, V. (1995). Masculinity, men's roles, and coronary heart disease. In D. Sabo & D. F. Gordon (Eds.), *Men's health and illness: Gender power and the body* (pp. 68–97). Thousand Oaks, CA: Sage.

Huisman, M., Kunst, A. E., Bopp, M., Borgan, J. K., Borrell, C., Costa, G., . . . Mackenbach, J. P. (2005). Educational inequalities in cause-specific mortality in middle-aged and older men and women in eight western European populations. *The Lancet, 365,* 493–500. http://dx.doi.org/10.1016/S0140-6736(05)70273-7

Hunt, K., Adamson, J., Hewitt, C., & Nazareth, I. (2011). Do women consult more than men? A review of gender and consultation for back pain and headache. *Journal of Health Services Research & Policy, 16,* 108–117. http://dx.doi.org/10.1258/jhsrp.2010.009131

Hunt, K., Ford, G., Harkins, L., & Wyke, S. (1999). Are women more ready to consult than men? Gender differences in family practitioner consultation for common chronic conditions. *Journal of Health Services Research & Policy, 4,* 96–100.

Hunt, K., Hannah, M. K., & West, P. (2004). Contextualizing smoking: Masculinity, femininity and class differences in smoking in men and women from three generations in the west of Scotland. *Health Education Research, 19,* 239–249. http://dx.doi.org/10.1093/her/cyg061

Hunt, K., McCann, C., Gray, C. M., Mutrie, N., & Wyke, S. (2013). "You've got to walk before you run": Positive evaluations of a walking program as part of a gender-sensitized, weight-management program delivered to men through professional football clubs. *Health Psychology, 32,* 57–65. http://dx.doi.org/10.1037/a0029537

Institute of Public Health in Ireland. (2011). *Facing the challenge: The impact of recession and unemployment on men's health in Ireland.* Dublin: Author.

Iwamoto, D. K., Corbin, W., Lejuez, C., & MacPherson, L. (2014). College men and alcohol use: Positive alcohol expectancies as a mediator between distinct masculine norms and alcohol use. *Psychology of Men & Masculinity, 15,* 29–39. http://dx.doi.org/10.1037/a0031594

Jamison, D. T., Summers, L. H., Alleyne, G., Arrow, K. J., Berkley, S., Binagwaho, A., . . . Yamey, G. (2013). Global health 2035: A world converging within a generation [correction appears in *The Lancet* (2014), *383,* 218]. *The Lancet, 382,* 1898–1955. http://dx.doi.org/10.1016/S0140-6736(13)62105-4

Karter, A. J., Ferrara, A., Liu, J. Y., Moffet, H. H., Ackerson, L. M., & Selby, J. V. (2002). Ethnic disparities in diabetic complications in an insured population. *JAMA, 287,* 2519–2527. http://dx.doi.org/10.1001/jama.287.19.2519

Kochanek, K. D., Xu, J., Murphy, S. L., Miniño, A. M., & Kung, H.-C. (2011). Deaths: Final data for 2009. *National Vital Statistics Reports, 60,* 1–116.

Kraemer, S. (2000). The fragile male. *British Medical Journal, 321,* 1609–1612. http://dx.doi.org/10.1136/bmj.321.7276.1609

Levant, R. F., Parent, M. C., McCurdy, E. R., & Bradstreet, T. C. (2015). Moderated mediation of the relationships between masculinity ideology, outcome expectations, and energy drink use. *Health Psychology, 34,* 1100–1106. http://dx.doi.org/10.1037/hea0000214

Levant, R. F., & Wimer, D. J. (2014). Masculinity constructs as protective buffers and risk factors for men's health. *American Journal of Men's Health, 8,* 110–120. http://dx.doi.org/10.1177/1557988313494408

Levant, R. F., Wimer, D. J., & Williams, C. M. (2011). An evaluation of the Health Behavior Inventory—20 (HBI–20) and its relationships to masculinity and attitudes towards seeking psychological help among college men. *Psychology of Men & Masculinity, 11,* 26–41. http://dx.doi.org/10.1037/a0021014

Levant, R. F., Wimer, D. J., Williams, C., Smalley, K. B., & Noronha, D. (2009). The relationships between masculinity variables, health risk behaviors and attitudes toward seeking psychological help. *International Journal of Men's Health, 8,* 3–21.

Lohan, M. (2007). How might we understand men's health better? Integrating explanations from critical studies on men and inequalities in health. *Social Science & Medicine, 65,* 493–504. http://dx.doi.org/10.1016/j.socscimed.2007.04.020

Lyons, A., & Willott, S. (1999). From suet pudding to superhero: Representations on men's health for women. *Health, 3,* 283–303. http://dx.doi.org/10.1177/136345939900300303

MacDonald, J. (2011). Building on the strength of Australian males. *International Journal of Men's Health, 10,* 82–96. http://dx.doi.org/10.3149/jmh.1001.82

Mahalik, J. R., Burns, S. M., & Syzdek, M. (2007). Masculinity and perceived normative health behaviors as predictors of men's health behaviors. *Social Science & Medicine, 64,* 2201–2209. http://dx.doi.org/10.1016/j.socscimed.2007.02.035

Mahalik, J. R., Lagan, H., & Morrison, J. A. (2006). Health behaviors and masculinity in Kenyan and U.S. male college students. *Psychology of Men & Masculinity*, 7, 191–202. http://dx.doi.org/10.1037/1524-9220.7.4.191

Mahalik, J. R., Levi-Minzi, M., & Walker, G. (2007). Masculinity and health behaviors in Australian men. *Psychology of Men & Masculinity*, 8, 240–249. http://dx.doi.org/10.1037/1524-9220.8.4.240

Mahalik, J. R., Locke, B. D., Ludlow, L. H., Diemer, M. A., Scott, R. P. J., Gottfried, M., & Freitas, G. (2003). Development of the Conformity to Masculine Norms Inventory. *Psychology of Men & Masculinity*, 4, 3–25. http://dx.doi.org/10.1037/1524-9220.4.1.3

McCreary, D. R., Newcomb, M. D., & Sadava, S. W. (1999). The male role, alcohol use, and alcohol problems: A structural modeling examination in adult men and women. *Journal of Counseling Psychology*, 46, 109–124. http://dx.doi.org/10.1037/0022-0167.46.1.109

McElroy, P., Evans, P., & Pringle, A. (2008). Sick as a parrot or over the moon: An evaluation of the impact of playing regular matches in a football league on mental health service users. *Practice Development in Health Care*, 7, 40–48. http://dx.doi.org/10.1002/pdh.245

Miniño, A. M., Heron, M. P., Murphy, S. L., & Kochanek, K. D. (2007). Deaths: Final data for 2004. *National Vital Statistics Reports*, 55, 1–119.

Ministério da Saúde [Ministry of Health]. (2009). *Gabinete do Ministro* [Minister's office]. (Portaria No. 1.944 [Portfolio No. 1.944]). *Institui no âmbito do Sistema Único de Saúde (SUS), a Política Nacional de Atenção Integral à Saúde do Homem* [Institute within the framework of the Single Health (SUS), the National Policy of Comprehensive Health Care for Man]. Brazil: Diário Oficial da União.

Monk, D., & Ricciardelli, L. A. (2003). Three dimensions of the male gender role as correlates of alcohol and cannabis involvement in young Australian men. *Psychology of Men & Masculinity*, 4, 57–69. http://dx.doi.org/10.1037/1524-9220.4.1.57

Morrison, D. S. (2009). Homelessness as an independent risk factor for mortality: Results from a retrospective cohort study. *International Journal of Epidemiology*, 38, 877–883. http://dx.doi.org/10.1093/ije/dyp160

Mosca, L., Barrett-Connor, E., & Wenger, N. K. (2011). Sex/gender differences in cardiovascular disease prevention: What a difference a decade makes. *Circulation*, 124, 2145–2154. http://dx.doi.org/10.1161/circulationaha.110.968792

Office for National Statistics. (2009). *Smoking and drinking among adults 2009: A report on the 2009 General Lifestyle Survey*. Retrieved from http://www.ons.gov.uk/ons/rel/ghs/general-lifestyle-survey/2009-report/index.html

Office for National Statistics. (2012). *Drinking habits amongst adults, 2012*. Retrieved from http://www.ons.gov.uk/ons/rel/ghs/opinions-and-lifestyle-survey/drinking-habits-amongst-adults--2012/stb-opn-drinking-2012.html

Oliffe, J. L., Ogrodniczuk, J. S., Bottorff, J. L., Johnson, J. L., & Hoyak, K. (2012). "You feel like you can't live anymore": Suicide from the perspectives of

Canadian men who experience depression. *Social Science & Medicine, 74*, 506–514. http://dx.doi.org/10.1016/j.socscimed.2010.03.057

Oliffe, J. L., & Phillips, M. (2008). Men, depression, and masculinities: A review and recommendations. *The Journal of Men's Health, 5*, 194–202. http://dx.doi.org/10.1016/j.jomh.2008.03.016

O'Neil, J. M. (2008). Summarizing 25 years of research on men's gender role conflict using the Gender Role Conflict Scale: New research paradigms and clinical implications. *The Counseling Psychologist, 36*, 358–445. http://dx.doi.org/10.1177/0011000008317057

O'Neil, J. M., Helms, B., Gable, R., David, L., & Wrightsman, L. (1986). Gender Role Conflict Scale (GRCS): College men's fears of femininity. *Sex Roles, 14*, 335–350.

Parent, M. C., & Moradi, B. (2011). An abbreviated tool for assessing feminine norm conformity: Psychometric properties of the Conformity to Feminine Norms Inventory–45. *Psychological Assessment, 23*, 958–969. http://dx.doi.org/10.1037/a0024082

Payne, S. (2001). "Smoke like a man, die like a man"?: A review of the relationship between gender, sex and lung cancer. *Social Science & Medicine, 53*, 1067–1080. http://dx.doi.org/10.1016/S0277-9536(00)00402-0

Pleck, J. (1981). *The myth of masculinity*. Cambridge, MA: MIT Press.

Richardson, N. (2013). Building momentum, gaining traction: Ireland's National Men's Health Policy—5 years on. *New Male Studies, 2*, 93–103.

Robertson, S. (2007). *Understanding men and health: Masculinities, identity and well-being*. Buckingham, England: Open University Press.

Robertson, S., & Williams, R. (2009). Men: Showing willing. *Community Practitioner, 82*, 34–35.

Robertson, S., & Williams, R. (2012). The importance of retaining a focus on masculinities in future studies on men and health. In G. Tremblay & F. Bernard (Eds.), *Future perspectives for intervention, policy and research on men and masculinities: An international forum*. Harriman, TN: Men's Studies Press.

Robertson, S., Zwolinsky, S., Pringle, A., McKenna, J., Daly-Smith, A., & White, A. (2013). "It is fun, fitness and football really": A process evaluation of a football based health intervention for men. *Qualitative Research in Sport, Exercise and Health, 5*, 419–439. http://dx.doi.org/10.1080/2159676X.2013.831372

Rothgerber, H. (2012). Real men don't eat (vegetable) quiche: Masculinity and the justification of meat consumption. *Psychology of Men & Masculinity, 13*, 1–13.

Scott-Samuel, A. (2009). Patriarchy, masculinities and health inequalities. *Gaceta Sanitaria, 23*, 159–160. http://dx.doi.org/10.1016/j.gaceta.2008.11.007

Seymour-Smith, S., Wetherell, M., & Phoenix, A. (2002). "My wife ordered me to come!": A discursive analysis of doctors' and nurses' accounts of men's use of general practitioners. *Journal of Health Psychology, 7*, 253–267. http://dx.doi.org/10.1177/1359105302007003220

Silverstein, L. B., Auerbach, C. F., & Levant, R. F. (2002). Contemporary fathers reconstructing masculinity: Clinical implications of gender role strain. *Profes-*

*sional Psychology: Research and Practice, 33,* 361–369. http://dx.doi.org/10.1037/0735-7028.33.4.361

Skovdal, M., Campbell, C., Madanhire, C., Mupambireyi, Z., Nyamukapa, C., & Gregson, S. (2011). Masculinity as a barrier to men's use of HIV services in Zimbabwe. *Globalization and Health, 7,* 13. http://dx.doi.org/10.1186/1744-8603-7-13

Sloan, C., Conner, M. T., & Gough, B. (2015). How does masculinity impact on health? A quantitative study of masculinity and health behavior in a sample of UK men and women. *Psychology of Men & Masculinity, 16,* 206–217. http://dx.doi.org/10.1037/a0037261

Sloan, C., Gough, B., & Conner, M. (2010). Healthy masculinities? How ostensibly healthy men talk about lifestyle, health and gender. *Psychology & Health, 25,* 783–803. http://dx.doi.org/10.1080/08870440902883204

Smith, J. A., & Robertson, S. (2008). Men's health promotion: A new frontier in Australia and the UK? *Health Promotion International, 23,* 283–289. http://dx.doi.org/10.1093/heapro/dan019

Snell, W. E., Jr., Belk, S., & Hawkins, R. C., II. (1987). Alcohol and drug use in stressful times: The influence of the masculine role and sex-related personality attributes. *Sex Roles, 16,* 359–373. http://dx.doi.org/10.1007/BF00289548

Spence, J. T., & Helmreich, R. L. (1978). *Masculinity and femininity. Their psychological dimensions, correlates, and antecedents.* Austin: University of Texas Press.

Spence, J. T., Helmreich, R. L., & Holahan, C. C. (1979). Negative and positive components of psychological masculinity and femininity and their relationships to neurotic and acting-out behaviors. *Journal of Personality and Social Psychology, 37,* 1631–1644.

Tannenbaum, C., & Frank, B. (2011). Masculinity and health in late life men. *American Journal of Men's Health, 5,* 243–254. http://dx.doi.org/10.1177/1557988310384609

Taylor, C., Stewart, A., & Parker, R. (1998). "Machismo" as a barrier to health promotion in Australian males. In T. Laws (Ed.), *Promoting men's health: An essential text book for nurses* (pp. 15–30). Ascot Vale, Australia: Ausmed.

Thompson, E. H., & Pleck, J. H. (1986). The structure of male role norms. *American Behavioral Scientist, 29,* 531–543. http://dx.doi.org/10.1177/000276486029005003

Thorpe, R. J., Richard, P., Bowie, J., Lavesit, T., & Gaskin, D. (2013). Economic burden of men's health disparities in the United States. *International Journal of Men's Health, 12,* 195–213. http://dx.doi.org/10.3149/jmh.1203.195

Tolhurst, R., Leach, B., Price, J., Robinson, J., Ettore, E., Scott-Samuel, A., . . . Theobald, S. (2012). Intersectionality and gender mainstreaming in international health: Using a feminist participatory action research process to analyse voices and debates from the global south and north. *Social Science & Medicine, 74,* 1825–1832. http://dx.doi.org/10.1016/j.socscimed.2011.08.025

Tong, S. F., & Low, W. Y. (2012). Public health strategies to address Asian men's health needs. *Asia-Pacific Journal of Public Health, 24,* 543–555. http://dx.doi.org/10.1177/1010539512452756

Treadwell, H. M., & Young, A. M. W. (2013). The right U.S. men's health report: High time to adjust priorities and attack disparities. *American Journal of Public Health, 103*, 5–6. http://dx.doi.org/10.2105/AJPH.2012.300895

Uy, P. J., Massoth, N. A., & Gottdiener, W. H. (2014). Rethinking male drinking: Traditional masculine ideologies, gender-role conflict, and drinking motives. *Psychology of Men & Masculinity, 15*, 121–128. http://dx.doi.org/10.1037/a0032239

Vos, T., Barber, R. M., Bell, B., Bertozzi-Villa, A., Biryukov, S., Bolliger, I., . . . Murray, C. J. L. (2015). Global, regional, and national incidence, prevalence, and years lived with disability for 301 acute and chronic diseases and injuries in 188 countries, 1990–2013: A systematic analysis for the Global Burden of Disease Study 2013. *The Lancet, 386*, 743–800.

Wade, J. C. (2009). Traditional masculinity and African American men's health-related attitudes and behaviors. *American Journal of Men's Health, 3*, 165–172. http://dx.doi.org/10.1177/1557988308320180

Walby, S. (2005). Gender mainstreaming: Productive tensions in theory and practice. *Social Politics, 12*, 321–343. http://dx.doi.org/10.1093/sp/jxi018

Wang, Y., Freemantle, N., Nazareth, I., & Hunt, K. (2014). Gender differences in survival and the use of primary care prior to diagnosis of three cancers: An analysis of routinely collected UK general practice data. *PLoS ONE, 9*, e101562. http://dx.doi.org/10.1371/journal.pone.0101562

Wang, Y., Hunt, K., Nazareth, I., Freemantle, N., & Petersen, I. (2013). Do men consult less than women? An analysis of routinely collected UK general practice data. *BMJ Open, 3*, e003320. http://dx.doi.org/10.1136/bmjopen-2013-003320

Wardle, J., Haase, A. M., Steptoe, A., Nillapun, M., Jonwutiwes, K., & Bellisle, F. (2004). Gender differences in food choice: The contribution of health beliefs and dieting. *Annals of Behavioral Medicine, 27*, 107–116. http://dx.doi.org/10.1207/s15324796abm2702_5

Warner, D. F., & Brown, T. H. (2011). Understanding how race/ethnicity and gender define age-trajectories of disability: An intersectionality approach. *Social Science & Medicine, 72*, 1236–1248. http://dx.doi.org/10.1016/j.socscimed.2011.02.034

Watkins, D. C., & Griffith, D. M. (2013). Practical solutions to addressing men's health disparities. *International Journal of Men's Health, 12*, 187–195. http://dx.doi.org/10.3149/jmh.1203.187

Wetherell, M., & Edley, N. (2014). A discursive psychological framework for analyzing men and masculinities, *Psychology of Men & Masculinities*, 355–365.

White, A., De Sousa, B., De Visser, R., Hogston, R., Madsen, S. A., Makara, P., . . . Zatonski, W. (2011). Men's health in Europe. *Journal of Men's Health, 8*, 192–201. http://dx.doi.org/10.1016/j.jomh.2011.08.113

White, A., McKee, M., Richardson, N., Visser, R., Madsen, S. A., Sousa, B. C., . . . Makara, P. (2011). Europe's men need their own health strategy. *BMJ, 343*, d7397. http://dx.doi.org/10.1136/bmj.d7397

White, A., Thomson, C. S., Forman, D., & Meryn, S. (2010). Men's health and the excess burden of cancer in men. *European Urology Supplements, 9,* 467–470. http://dx.doi.org/10.1016/j.eursup.2010.03.003

Williams, R., Robertson, S., & Hewison, A. (2009). Men's health, inequalities, and policy: Contradictions, masculinities, and public health in England. *Critical Public Health, 19,* 475–488. http://dx.doi.org/10.1080/09581590802668457

Williamson, P. (1995). Men's health. Their own worst enemy. *Nursing Times, 91,* 24–26.

Woodford-Berger, P. (2004). Gender mainstreaming: What is it (about) and should we continue doing it? *International Development Studies Bulletin, 35,* 65–72. http://dx.doi.org/10.1111/j.1759-5436.2004.tb00157.x

World Health Organization. (2007). *Engaging men and boys in changing gender-based inequity in health: Evidence from programme interventions.* Geneva, Switzerland: Author.

World Health Organization. (2012). *The European health report 2012: Charting the way to well-being.* Retrieved from http://www.euro.who.int/__data/assets/pdf_file/0004/197113/EHR2012-Eng.pdf

Zwolinsky, S., McKenna, J., Pringle, A., Daly-Smith, A., Robertson, S., & White, A. (2013). Optimizing lifestyles for men regarded as "hard-to-reach" through top-flight football/soccer clubs. *Health Education Research, 28,* 405–413. http://dx.doi.org/10.1093/her/cys108

# 8

# A REVIEW OF RESEARCH ON MEN'S BODY IMAGE AND DRIVE FOR MUSCULARITY

SARAH K. MURNEN AND BRYAN T. KARAZSIA

*Body image* is a multidimensional construct that encompasses attitudes, feelings, and perceptions of body size, shape, and other dimensions (e.g., Banfield & McCabe, 2002). Body satisfaction used to be stereotyped as a female concern, and early research focused on women and girls nearly exclusively. This made sense because researchers were trying to understand the impact of increasingly thin images of "ideal" women presented in the media (e.g., Garner, Garfinkel, Schwartz, & Thompson, 1980; Rubinstein & Caballero, 2000), which covaried with heightened levels of body dissatisfaction and eating disorders among women in North American culture (e.g., Stice & Shaw, 2002). The intense research focus on women's body issues could signify that women fare worse than men in terms of body satisfaction and that men have few body concerns. Indeed, when men were included in early research on body satisfaction, their self-reported rates were better than women's (e.g., Fallon & Rozin, 1985; Feingold & Mazzella, 1998).

http://dx.doi.org/10.1037/0000023-009
*The Psychology of Men and Masculinities*, R. F. Levant and Y. J. Wong (Editors)

Recent large-scale studies have found small gender differences in body satisfaction in a variety of age groups (e.g., Austin, Haines, & Veugelers, 2009; Frederick, Forbes, Grigorian, & Jarcho, 2007; Frederick, Peplau, & Lever, 2006; Neumark-Sztainer, Paxton, Hannan, Haines, & Story, 2006) and have also revealed an important finding when examining the relationship between body mass index (BMI) and body dissatisfaction by gender. Among females, there is a linear association between these variables such that the larger the BMI, the greater the amount of dissatisfaction. This is consistent with the idea that thinness is valued in women who try to model a thin ideal. Among males, however, the relationship between BMI and body dissatisfaction is curvilinear such that those with a relatively small BMI or a relatively large BMI are the most dissatisfied (e.g., Austin et al., 2009; Frederick, Forbes, et al., 2007). Thus, male body image issues are perhaps more nuanced than those found among females, which has led researchers to go beyond scales developed and tested on women to develop measures specific to the concerns of men.

The purpose of the present chapter is to review research on male body image, especially research published after 2000 that seeks to understand male body image as an important topic in its own right, not just in comparison with females' body concerns. Researchers have charted the existence of a muscular ideal in popular culture that is proposed to pressure men to adopt muscularity motives, which can be measured by a variety of scales we review. Theories have been tested to understand the correlates and consequences of men's body image dissatisfaction measured by these scales. Earlier theoretical work adapted theories developed to understand women's concerns to understand men's issues (with varying success); more recently, male-centric theories have been developed and tested. These theories are reviewed, as is research on subgroups of men with heightened body concerns and research on the potentially serious consequences of male body dissatisfaction.

## THE MUSCULAR IDEAL

Researchers have gathered evidence that there is a "muscular ideal" male body advertised in the culture, similar to the thin ideal for women. There is both an increased portrayal of the male body as an object of emulation and an increased portrayal of unrealistic levels of muscularity as attractive. For example, across the years 1975 to 2005 in *Sports Illustrated*, men's bodies were increasingly portrayed in fragmented ways and with greater nudity, suggesting objectification (Farquhar & Wasylkiw, 2007). Similarly, the "erotic male" was the most common depiction of men in five mainstream magazines, representing 37.8% of 1987 and 38.5% of 1997 depictions (Rohlinger, 2002).

This portrayal involves placing men on "display," emphasizing their physical attractiveness. The magazines *Men's Health* and *Men's Fitness* were launched in the late 1980s, and both have been found to have a strong focus on body appearance in their ads and articles (Labre, 2005).

In addition to an increase in the objectification of men, the body displayed has become more muscular, lean, and V-shaped, which is what men consider ideal (Ridgeway & Tylka, 2005). For instance, BMI values of *Playgirl* centerfold models between 1973 and 1997 were positively correlated with date of publication ($r = .29$) and negatively with body fat ($r = -.34$; Leit, Pope, & Gray, 2001). A comparison of the original version of various action figures (e.g., Batman) with their contemporary versions revealed significantly larger necks, chests, arms, forearms, thighs, and calves (but not waists) to the point that they now represent grossly unrealistic proportions (Baghurst, Hollander, Nardella, & Haff, 2006). H. G. Pope and colleagues noted that the most recent depictions of action figures such as GI Joe are so unrealistic that "if extrapolated to 70 in. in height, the (1990's-version of) GI Joe Extreme would sport larger biceps than any bodybuilder in history" (H. G. Pope, Olivardia, Gruber, & Borowiecki, 1999, p. 68).

Given this evidence of muscular images of men in the media, it is not surprising that many males express concerns about muscularity. In one study, it was found that more than 90% of men from four regions of the United States desired greater muscularity (Frederick, Buchanan, et al., 2007). A study of adolescents found that although girls expressed less body satisfaction than boys, perceived more media pressure to lose weight, and engaged in more eating and exercise strategies to lose weight, boys felt more pressure from the media to increase muscle tone and engaged in more eating and exercise strategies to increase muscles (McCabe, Ricciardelli, & Finemore, 2002). In a study of nearly 3,000 adolescents, it was found that 34.7% used protein powders or shakes, and 5.9% used steroids (Eisenberg, Wall, & Neumark-Sztainer, 2012). Rates were higher among boys than girls and suggested a fair degree of muscularity concern among boys.

## MEASURING MEN'S BODY CONCERNS

Given evidence of an emphasis on muscularity for men in popular culture, there was also interest in measuring men's muscularity concerns with valid and reliable scales. In 2004, Cafri and Thompson reviewed measures used to assess male body image and concluded that it was important to focus on muscularity. One of the measures they suggested, currently the most widely cited in the literature, is McCreary and Sasse's (2000) Drive for Muscularity Scale (DMS).

Items for the 15-item DMS were developed by talking to those who engage in weight training and by looking at weight-training magazines. Some items measure muscularity attitudes (*I wish that I were more muscular*) and some behavior (*I lift weights to build muscle*). In the original study where it was administered to high school students, responses were negatively correlated with self-esteem and positively correlated with depression (McCreary & Sasse, 2000). In a subsequent validity study with participants in high school and college, it was concluded through factor analysis that the attitudinal and behavioral items could be used as two separate scales or combined in a total score for men; but for women, it was deemed appropriate to use the total score (McCreary, Sasse, Saucier, & Dorsch, 2004).

The DMS has now been administered in many other countries, and the two-factor structure was upheld in Brazil (Campana, Tavares, Swami, & da Silva, 2013), Italy (Dakanalis et al., 2015), Scotland (McPherson, McCarthy, McCreary, & McMillan, 2010), and Mexico (where a three-factor solution also worked; Escoto et al., 2013). In a sample of Asian American men, three items had to be removed from the scale for the two-factor model to fit the data (Keum, Wong, DeBlaere, & Brewster, 2015). Cafri and Thompson (2004) used the DMS Body Image (BI) scale, along with several body contour measures, to try to predict DMS muscularity behavior, and the DMS BI was the best predictor. In other validity work associated with the DMS, the behavioral scale predicted the use of performance-enhancing substances and weight-lifting behavior across a 6-week time period in undergraduate men, controlling for previous indices of these behaviors (Litt & Dodge, 2008).

During the same year the DMS was published, Edwards and Launder (2000) reported on the development of their Swansea Muscularity Attitudes Questionnaire (SMAQ). They administered items to 112 male participants in their initial study, but there were no other scales administered to determine construct validity. The authors developed subscales based on the factors of drive for muscularity (*I want to be more muscular than I am now*) and positive attributes of muscularity (*I feel more masculine when I am more muscular*). The two subscales were confirmed in a second sample of 303 men.

T. G. Morrison, Morrison, Hopkins, and Rowan (2004) critiqued the DMS and the SMAQ for not having any reverse-scored items, the DMS for containing both attitudinal and behavioral items, and the SMAQ for insufficient validity information. Thus, they argued for researchers to adopt their Drive for Muscularity Attitudes Questionnaire (DMAQ). Out of an initial pool of 42 items, eight formed an internally consistent one-factor scale with items such as *Muscularity is important to me*. Support for the validity of the scale includes positive correlations with protein supplement use and weight-lifting behavior and a negative correlation with self-esteem. Athletes scored higher than nonathletes, as expected ($d = .87$). In another study, T. G. Morrison and Harriman (2005) lauded the brief nature of the DMAQ and confirmed its unitary construct using another sample.

Tod, Morrison, and Edwards (2012) further evaluated the validity, as well as test–retest reliability, of these three drive-for-muscularity questionnaires, along with one developed by Yelland and Tiggemann (2003; Yelland and Tiggemann's DMS [DMS–YT]). The DMS–YT was published in a study as part of one measure in a model, so the authors did not provide much testing of its validity. Correlations between scores on these four scales were high, ranging from .59 to .82, which indicates a fair degree of overlap in measurement, as approximately 36% to 65% of variance among measures was shared. The behavioral scale of the DMS had the lowest correlations with other scales, which makes sense because it measures behaviors, whereas the rest concern attitudes. All of the scales showed good temporal consistency. Both the DMAQ and the DMS–YT are unidimensional, which should be factored into their use.

The exclusive focus on muscularity with the scales just reviewed might be leading researchers and clinicians to miss out on important body image issues among some men, as indicated previously by the curvilinear function between BMI and body dissatisfaction. Tylka, Bergeron and Schwartz (2005) developed the Male Body Attitudes Scale (MBAS) to measure men's attitudes about muscularity, leanness, and height. The items measure both satisfaction and preoccupation, and explicitly separate out different dimensions of men's body concerns. The item *I think my body should be leaner* is associated with thinness, whereas *I wish my arms were stronger* is associated with muscularity, and *I am satisfied with my height* with height. In the initial three samples tested for the scale, good construct validity was established. For example, they measured the uniqueness of body dissatisfaction with respect to muscularity, body fat, and height, assessing relationships with psychological well-being. They found that it was important to measure muscularity dissatisfaction in addition to drive for muscularity because it uniquely predicted lower self-esteem and worse coping. They also found that body fat dissatisfaction was associated with higher psychological distress and depressive symptoms and lower self-esteem and hardiness, which was not true of drive for muscularity.

Among the scales reviewed, the most well-validated and widely used is the DMS. The measure uniquely concerns both attitudes and behaviors related to muscularity. It has been used in many samples, so much comparison data are available. If one wants a scale that measures attitudes in a concise way, the DMAQ might be considered. For a more comprehensive examination of men's body issues, the MBAS should be considered.

# THEORETICAL PERSPECTIVES

Some of the research conducted with muscularity measures reveals a high level of discontent. Where does it come from? Three general theoretical perspectives have been used to explain male body image dissatisfaction and its correlates and consequences. First, we review the growing body of research on sociocultural theory. This theory was originally developed to explain female body concerns but has been successfully used to understand male body concerns. Second, we examine objectification theory, which was also developed to understand women's body concerns. There has been some success applying this to understand men's body image issues, but some of the proposed relationships do not translate well in men. Third, we review a group of hypotheses concerning the influence of masculinity on the body, particularly relationships between masculinity and muscularity.

## Sociocultural Theory

Sociocultural theory is one of the first models used to try to understand the body concerns of men and boys. (This theory is sometimes referred to as the *tripartite model of social influence*.) As outlined earlier, sociocultural theories highlight the importance of pressure from parents, peers, and the media on body image dissatisfaction, mediated by internalization of ideals and the process of social comparison (e.g., Thompson, Heinberg, Altabe, & Tantleff-Dunn, 1999). Body image dissatisfaction is then proposed to result in eating problems or other problematic behavior, such as excessive exercise. This model has been successful in predicting eating disordered attitudes among girls and women (e.g., Keery, van den Berg, & Thompson, 2004; Thompson & Stice, 2001).

This model has been applied to study men and boys, sometimes using measures developed for females, sometimes using measures developed for males, and sometimes using a mixture of both. If boys and girls are compared in terms of this model, a typical finding is that girls will report more pressure to lose weight, greater body dissatisfaction, internalization of media ideals, and peer comparison than boys, but that these variables will predict body concerns in the same pattern (e.g., Halliwell & Harvey, 2006). Model variables have been used to successfully predict muscle-building techniques in adolescent boys (Smolak, Murnen, & Thompson, 2005); muscularity dissatisfaction and excessive exercise in college men (Karazsia & Crowther, 2009); and risky body change behaviors, including substance use to increase muscle in college men (Karazsia & Crowther, 2010). Some studies have examined dual pathway models that differentiate leanness from muscularity (e.g., McCabe & Ricciardelli, 2004; Rodgers, Ganchou, Franko, & Chabrol, 2012; Tylka, 2011).

When studying boys and men, it is important to examine all of the scales used for gender appropriateness. Sometimes this means changing the wording of a scale. For example, researchers have modified internalization scales to be more appropriate for men and boys by measuring muscularity concerns (e.g., Karazsia & Crowther, 2008). Additionally, a meta-analytic review of bivariate associations between sociocultural constructs (i.e., internalization, awareness of pressures, and experienced pressures) and body dissatisfaction revealed that the strength of the correlations varied as a function of assessment. When measures included muscularity components, then the correlations were stronger (Karazsia & Peiper, 2011). Further testing of the validity of scales should be conducted because many scales that have been adapted for use with men have not undergone rigorous psychometric evaluations.

*Media Effects*

In addition to the research that has tested sociocultural variable influences in models with multiple variables, there have also been studies of specific pressures and their influence. For example, the media have been the focus of a sufficient number of studies that meta-analytic reviews have been conducted. In a meta-analysis of the research on experimental exposure to depictions of men with ideal bodies on subsequent body dissatisfaction, the largest effects were found for measures of "body part dissatisfaction," $d = .66$, based on eight samples (Blond, 2008). In another meta-analysis, it was found that the effect size for correlational studies was smaller than that for experimental studies: $d = -.22$ and $d = -.40$, respectively (Barlett, Vowels, & Saucier, 2008). These effect sizes are similar to one that emerged compiling data on correlational and experimental studies in women: $d = .28$, based on 90 samples (Grabe, Ward, & Hyde, 2008).

More recent research on media is considering more nuanced relationships between media exposure and body satisfaction, sometimes with surprising findings. For example, portraying men's bodies in motion rather than in an objectified way led to worse satisfaction with appearance in one study (Mulgrew, Johnson, Lane, & Katsikitis, 2014). In another, men who were not exercisers reported more negative affect in response to images of muscular male models than men from a gym, which led the authors to conclude that muscular ideal images might be aspirational to some groups of men (Halliwell, Dittmar, & Orsborn, 2007).

There are few developmental studies on the effects of exposure to media, and these would be helpful to determine possible long-term relationships. One such study of elementary school boys was conducted by Harrison and Bond (2007). They studied exposure to a variety of types of magazines, including gaming magazines because they are thought to idealize the muscular body. Exposure to gaming magazines, but not other magazines, predicted an increase in drive for muscularity among White boys but not Black boys, perhaps because of White models.

*Peer Pressures*

Peer pressures are another element of sociocultural models that have received some focused attention among men. Although females have been studied to a greater degree than males with respect to the experience of weight-related teasing, there were sufficient data on this topic to conduct a meta-analysis (Menzel et al., 2010). It was found that teasing about being overweight had a smaller association with male body dissatisfaction ($r = .24$) than female body dissatisfaction ($r = .37$), but more general appearance teasing had similar associations, with $r = .35$ for males, and $r = .33$ for females. These are moderate-sized associations that warrant more research attention.

One of the peer pressures that females experience that is associated with body dissatisfaction is "fat talk" in which female peers disparage their bodies, in part for social approval (e.g., Clarke, Murnen, & Smolak, 2010). Recently it was found then men also engage in negative body talk (Engeln, Sladek, & Waldron, 2013), and the frequency of engaging in negative body talk was associated with drive for muscularity scores. Sladek, Engeln, and Miller (2014) developed a body talk scale for men with subscales of muscle talk and fat talk. Scores on the muscle talk scale were correlated with DMS scores, and scores on the fat talk scale were moderately correlated with eating disordered attitudes.

## Objectification Theory

Another theory that is not incompatible with sociocultural theory but incorporates a wider view of societal influence as well as multiple domains of impaired functioning as a result, is objectification theory (Fredrickson & Roberts, 1997). This theory was first developed to explain women's high level of body concerns. It was argued that the pervasive sexual objectification of women leads women to internalize the objectification. As a result, women survey their bodies, comparing them with others. Because the comparison is often unrealistic, this can lead to body shame, and potentially to eating disorders, sexual disorders, depression, and decreased experiences of "flow." This model has been tested in women and has generally been found to be supported (e.g., Calogero, Tantleff-Dunn, & Thompson, 2011).

Moradi and Huang (2008) reviewed research on objectification theory, including its use with men and concluded that although rates of constructs such as surveillance and body shame were lower among men than women, they still predicted eating disordered attitudes and appearance-focused muscularity concerns in the expected direction. There were not many studies on men at the time of the review, however, and a few recent studies call into question some of the paths in the model for men.

For example, Daniel and Bridges (2010) looked at a path model that included objectification theory variables, attempting to link them with drive for muscularity. They did not find that objectification theory variables were significant mediators between media internalization and drive for muscularity. In another study, Parent and Moradi (2011) acknowledged that men are not objectified to the degree that women are but still hypothesized that internalization and self-objectification would predict steroid use intention. Although internalization and surveillance related to body shame, body shame did not relate to drive for muscularity and steroid use intention. Interestingly and quite importantly, these associations may vary across men with different sexual orientations. For example, Martins, Tiggemann, and Kirkbride (2007) reported results from two investigations (one correlational and one experimental) that supported the salience of body shame as an important construct in gay men's experiences with objectifying societal messages.

These data suggest that objectification theory variables might not always operate in (heterosexual) men in relation to predicting muscularity attitudes and behaviors the same way they predict eating attitudes and behaviors in females. Women are judged by their bodies to a greater degree than heterosexual men because thinness concerns and caring for appearance are central aspects of feminine gender role norms (Mahalik et al., 2005). Thus, if women fail to attain thinness, it could lead to negative feelings in the form of body shame. In men muscularity is viewed positively, associated with dominance and attractiveness (e.g., Swami et al., 2013), and a lack of muscularity might arouse concerns, but perhaps not in the form of body shame. Instead, it is possible that muscularity concerns might heighten emotions more central to men's gender role norms, such as competitiveness or aggression (Mahalik et al., 2003). We turn next to theories that focus more specifically on masculine norms.

## Masculinity Models

Several researchers have proposed that increased muscularity concerns among men in the culture are related to masculinity concerns. In the theory of threatened masculinity, it is proposed that men are focusing on increasing muscularity today because other avenues of exerting masculinity have been thwarted. A shift from "an occupational to physical identity has encouraged males to seek a lean, muscular, mesomorphic body type to distinguish themselves from women," according to Baghurst and Lirgg (2009, p. 221). In one experiment where men's masculinity was threatened, men perceived themselves as less muscular and weaker than the control group men, providing some support for this idea (Mills & D'Alfonso, 2007).

There has been a sufficient number of studies examining links between masculinity and body image that a meta-analysis was conducted (Blashill, 2011). In the studies reviewed, masculinity was measured in a variety of manners, including older, trait-based measures such as the Bem Sex-Role Inventory (Bem, 1974), as well as more recent measures that conceptualize masculinity as multidimensional such as the Conformity to Masculine Norms Inventory (CMNI; Mahalik et al., 2003). Body dissatisfaction was also operationalized in a variety of ways, including scales that measure thinness concerns and scales that measure muscularity concerns. A small relationship was found between masculinity and muscle dissatisfaction ($r = -.03$), although the relationship was significantly different and opposite in direction using trait-based measures of muscularity ($r = -.20$) compared with multidimensional ones ($r = .18$). The extent to which men were higher in trait-based masculinity, the less muscle dissatisfaction they reported, but the higher in multidimensional masculinity, the more muscle dissatisfaction. It is likely that trait-based measures that measure adherence to socially desirable personality traits associated with masculinity (e.g., assertiveness) do not capture the conflicts associated with the masculine role.

In some recent research measures related to less socially desirable aspects of masculinity, or conflicts associated with masculinity, have been examined. For example, McCreary, Saucier, and Courtenay (2005) found that the success, power, and competition dimensions of gender role conflict predicted drive for muscularity in a sample of young men. Smolak and Stein (2006) found that the importance middle school boys placed on athletic and appearance superiority (measured by a scale they developed) predicted drive for muscularity scores. Other researchers have measured conformity to masculine norms such as *winning* and *power over women* using the CMNI (Mahalik et al., 2003) and have been able to predict muscularity concerns in young men (Griffiths, Murray, & Touyz, 2015; Smolak & Murnen, 2008).

Two other studies worth mention relate to masculinity concerns that have not been examined previously. Swami and Voracek (2013) tested a feminist hypothesis that the increased participation of women in the workforce might lead men to focus on power and strength as a way to maintain patriarchal values. They recruited heterosexual men from the community in London and found that DMS scores were correlated with the objectification of women, ambivalent sexism endorsement, and attitudes indicative of hostility toward women. In another study of heterosexual community men in London, having a sociosexual orientation (valuing sexual variety), higher sexual sensation-seeking, and higher sexual assertiveness scores were related to DMS scores (Swami, Diwell, & McCreary, 2014).

These data suggest it might be productive to develop a masculinity model with predictions about specific norms or constructs that should relate to muscularity concerns. Men who are not secure in various aspects of masculinity might seek a muscular body to try to affirm masculinity. Men who believe men and women are very different from one another and value some of the less socially desirable aspects of masculinity such as aggression and power over women might be particularly likely to value muscularity.

**Group Differences**

There are some groups of men who experience heightened body dissatisfaction, and these data are reviewed briefly with an attempt to explain the differences with the reviewed theories. First, gay men are overrepresented in men with classically defined eating disorders (Feldman & Meyer, 2007), so they have been the subject of focused study. A meta-analysis of the data comparing gay men with heterosexual men in terms of body satisfaction found a small effect size of $d = .29$, based on 35 samples (M. A. Morrison, Morrison, & Sager, 2004).

Most researchers conceptualize gay men's body issues with respect to objectification theory in that aspects of gay male culture might put more pressure on men with respect to appearance, including pressures that are unique to this subculture of men. For example, gay men might be more likely to be objectified by romantic partners than heterosexual men, and gay-oriented magazines have been found to have thinner models than magazines directed at heterosexual men (Lanzieri & Cook, 2013). There is some support for using objectification theory to conceptualize gay men's body concerns (e.g., Wiseman & Moradi, 2010), especially if a dual-pathway model is used (Calzo, Corliss, Blood, Field, & Austin, 2013; Tylka & Andorka, 2012).

A couple of studies examined gay men using masculinity models with some success (Blashill & Vander Wal, 2009; Kimmel & Mahalik, 2005). More specifically, Kimmel and Mahalik (2005) desired to predict scores on their newly developed Masculine Body Ideal Distress Scale (Kimmel & Mahalik, 2004), as well as scores on a more general body image dissatisfaction scale in a sample of gay men. They were better able to predict body ideal distress than body image dissatisfaction (16% of the variability vs. 6%), and distress was associated with minority stress variables such as stigma and internalized homophobia, as well as conformity to masculine norms.

Therefore, evidence is emerging that suggests gay male culture might pose specific risks for body image concerns and eating disorders (Russell & Keel, 2002). The possibility that gay men are exposed to higher levels of sexual objectification (e.g., Martins et al., 2007), as well as the possibility that minority stress contributes to problematic outcomes, should be studied further. Perhaps a blending of variables derived from several theoretical models would help us understand the somewhat greater risk for body dissatisfaction that has been found among gay men. It seems particularly important when studying gay men to examine a dual-pathway model.

Another group that would seem to be at risk for body concerns associated with muscularity is men who value muscularity for athletic pursuits. Some of the scales reviewed were developed by comparing athletes with nonathletes, and athletes had higher concerns with muscularity. Some research findings support the idea that sport participation may offer a unique sociocultural context (Karazsia, Crowther, & Galioto, 2013) that increases risk of anabolic steroid use (Dodge & Jaccard, 2006). Some studies of weight lifters have shown heightened levels of muscularity concerns in certain groups (e.g., Hale, Roth, DeLong, & Briggs, 2010).

Future research might examine sports contexts in more detail and determine which variables from the various models might be influential, such as peer pressure, heightened self-objectification, and perhaps masculinity norms. In a study of Division II football players, it was found that the importance of athletic identity was a significant predictor of DMS scores along with adherence to many of the masculine norms measured by the CMNI (Steinfeldt, Gilchrist, Halterman, Gomory, & Steinfeldt, 2011). When all of the variables were entered into a multiple regression equation, the significant predictors were emotional control, risk taking, and primacy of work.

Other men who might be at risk for body-related concerns are men who are representative of ethnic and racial minorities. Ricciardelli, McCabe, Williams, and Thompson (2007) reviewed research on the role of ethnicity and culture in predicting body image concerns among men in American culture. They compared White Americans with other groups. Black American men appeared to have more positive body image, despite rating a larger body size as ideal. Hispanic men did not seem to differ too much in terms of body image, although they might engage in more extreme weight loss behaviors and binge eating. The data on Asian American men were inconsistent, and the authors suggested that not all Asian groups should be grouped together for comparison. Pacific Islanders have larger ideal body sizes than Whites. There were few studies of Native American men to examine, but data suggested greater body image concerns. It has been proposed that minority men might be at greater risk for manipulating their bodies as a means to deal with cultural conflict issues.

Ricciardelli et al. (2007) compared Black, Asian American, and White college men on a number of different variables. Asian American men had significantly higher levels of binge eating than the other two groups of men, as well as higher levels of internalization of cultural ideals and drive for muscularity scores (and other measures of body dissatisfaction). This pattern of results was explained with the idea that putting on muscle mass might be difficult for Asian American men because of their genetic body type, and they might be perceived as low in masculinity relative to other men, which could motivate a drive for muscularity. Despite having the largest BMI of the three groups, Black men expressed the highest level of body satisfaction, consistent with other research.

Gattario et al. (2015) examined conformity to masculine norms and drive for muscularity in four Western cultures and looked at specific masculine norms, arguing that certain norms would be more evident in some cultures than others. They found that college men in the United States had the highest drive for muscularity scores, followed by men in Australia, the United Kingdom, and Sweden. In all four countries, adherence to the norms explained about 20% of the variability in DMS scores, but the pattern of which particular norms were the best predictors varied by country. In the United States, the best predictors were subscribing to a playboy norm and having disdain for homosexuality; in Australia, the playboy norm and risk-taking were the best predictors; in the United Kingdom, it was acceptance of violence and primacy of work; and in Sweden, it was primacy of work, the importance of winning, and self-reliance. The meaning of muscularity by country and how it relates to the expression of masculinity should be studied further.

One other cross-cultural study examined images of male bodies portrayed in magazines in Taiwan, and also examined body image dissatisfaction of a sample of heterosexual men from Taiwan (of Chinese descent; Yang, Gray, & Pope, 2005). These data were compared with some previously collected from men in the United States, France, and Austria. Taiwanese men reported the least amount of discrepancy between their body size and the size perceived to be ideal to women in their culture. Furthermore, in Taiwanese magazines, it was rare to portray the bodies of Asian men in an objectified way, suggesting support for a sociocultural model or objectification theory that Taiwanese men might be less dissatisfied with their bodies due to low exposure to bodies that idealize muscularity. In addition, it is common in Chinese culture to emphasize male intelligence over appearance as important to self-definition.

The data on group differences suggest that each of the three theoretical models reviewed could be relevant to understanding difference. Sociocultural theory can be used to hypothesize that there will be country and cultural differences in body dissatisfaction due to varying exposure to unrealistic body ideals. Objectification theory can be used to predict that any individual exposed to high levels of objectification might engage in self-objectification if appearance is important to self-definition. Masculinity models have been used to help explain country differences and could also be used to try to explain within-country group differences. Masculinity models could be studied in more detail, perhaps making predictions about the specific norms that might predict muscularity concerns in particular groups of men, including possible mediating and moderating variables, and measurement of possible outcomes.

## CORRELATES AND CONSEQUENCES

As demonstrated, there are various theories that explain why men develop body dissatisfaction. A commonality among all of these theories is that they include similar maladaptive outcomes. A general term that has been applied to all of these outcomes collectively is *maladaptive body change behaviors*. They include the following specific outcomes: anabolic-androgenic steroids (AAS), unhealthy eating, excessive weight training, cosmetic surgery, and muscle dysmorphia. The data related to these outcomes are reviewed next.

### Anabolic-Androgenic Steroids

Approximately 2.6% to 3.5% of adolescent males report the use of AAS (Cafri, van den Berg, & Thompson, 2006; Johnston, O'Malley, & Bachman, 2002). There is some evidence that men who use AAS follow a progression from licit substance use to illicit muscle-building substances. Specifically, Karazsia and colleagues (2013) found that among individuals reporting illicit substance use, nearly all of them (96.2%) also reported a history of protein use, and 84.6% reported a history of creatine use. Importantly, the age of onset of protein and creatine use preceded age of onset of illicit substance use. Previous substance use also predicted AAS use, even after controlling for various constructs drawn from sociocultural theories (e.g., drive for muscularity, pressures from peers). Goldberg and colleagues (e.g., Goldberg et al., 1996) have developed gender-specific steroid prevention programs that target adolescents. These programs, part of the Adolescents Training and Learning to Avoid Steroids (ATLAS) project, seek to prevent adolescent adoption of AAS by promoting healthy, legal, and effective weight-training and exercise programs.

### Unhealthy Eating

It is well documented that rates of overweight and obesity, as defined by BMI cutoffs, are steadily increasing, with no significant differences in obesity prevalence between boys and girls as of 2011–2012 (e.g., Ogden, Carroll, Kit, & Flegal, 2014). In adults, approximately one third of the adult population currently meets or exceeds the BMI cutoff for obesity, again with comparable rates for men and women (Ogden et al., 2014). Although the causes of obesity are complex and multifaceted (e.g., Wright & Aronne, 2012), research clearly indicates that caloric intake is associated with BMI (e.g., Guyenet & Schwartz, 2012). Perhaps counterintuitively, body image concerns are associated with maladaptive eating patterns for weight loss among men (e.g., Kaminski, Chapman, Haynes, & Own, 2005) as well as weight gain. In a longitudinal study of more than 1,000 adolescent males spanning 5 years, Neumark-Sztainer and colleagues (2006) reported that lower body satisfaction at Time 1 predicted more frequent dieting (defined as changing eating patterns to lose weight) and binge eating. This pattern of results is particularly interesting when interpreted in the context of sociocultural theories, which posit primarily that body dissatisfaction leads to maladaptive strategies to attain an ideal image. However, empirical investigations indicate that body dissatisfaction can lead to a complex constellation of unhealthy eating patterns that for some individuals result in weight loss, but for others can result in weight gain.

## Excessive Weight Training

Given the cultural context of increasing rates of obesity (e.g., Ogden et al., 2014), many recent efforts have been devoted to increasing exercise. In fact, healthy weight-training programs have been shown to improve not only muscularity but also self-evaluations of appearance and body satisfaction (Williams & Cash, 2001). However, men with significant body image concerns can also resort to unhealthy exercise strategies, such as weight training that induces injury (e.g., McCreary, Hildebrandt, Heinberg, Boroughs, & Thompson, 2007). Although a substantial body of literature exists regarding the link between body image constructs and body change behaviors (e.g., McCabe & Ricciardelli, 2003, 2004), a current challenge for the field is distinguishing between healthy and unhealthy weight-training behaviors (and exercise more generally). On the basis of existing assessment practices, it appears that at least two dimensions associated with exercise may differentiate healthy versus unhealthy weight training: exercising to the point of injury (Mayville, Williamson, White, Netemeyer, & Drab, 2002) and exercising to the point that it interferes with daily life due to amount of time spent exercising or preoccupation with exercise (e.g., Hildebrandt, Langenbucher, & Schlundt, 2004). Research does indicate that men who report more body dissatisfaction also report more functional impairment related to exercise and exercising to the point of injury (e.g., Hildebrandt et al., 2004; Karazsia & Crowther, 2008).

## Cosmetic Surgery

According to the American Society of Plastic Surgeons (2014), even though male patients are recipients of less than 10% of all cosmetic surgeries, plastic surgery is increasing in popularity among men. For example, rates of breast augmentation among males increased 11% from 2012 to 2013. The following surgeries are those in which men represent more than half of the total cosmetic procedures: pectoral implants (100%), hair transplantation (71%), calf augmentation (56%), and chin augmentation (51%). As is evidenced in these figures, men resort to cosmetic surgery for various appearance-oriented reasons, including concerns with hair, face, and musculature. Empirical evidence supports applications of theories developed to explain eating disorders (e.g., sociocultural theories) to men seeking cosmetic surgery (e.g., Menzel et al., 2011), suggesting that cosmetic surgery is an important body change behavior with similar precursors as other, more often-studied behaviors.

## Muscle Dysmorphia

After more than a decade of scholarly work proposing muscle dysmorphia as a clinical disorder (e.g., C. G. Pope et al., 2005), the *Diagnostic and Statistical Manual of Mental Disorders* (fifth edition; DSM–5; American Psychiatric Association, 2013) included "with muscle dysmorphia" as a specifier for body dysmorphic disorder. According to the DSM–5, this specifier applies to individuals who are "preoccupied with the idea that his or her body build is too small or insufficiently muscular. This specifier is used even if the individual is preoccupied with other body areas, which is often the case" (p. 243). As reported by C. G. Pope and colleagues (2005), individuals with muscle dysmorphia resemble patients with body dysmorphic disorder in many respects, including symptoms of delusionality, number of body parts that are concerning, and severity of symptomatology. However, C. G. Pope et al. also noted that patients with muscle dysmorphia were more likely to have attempted suicide, abuse substances (including AAS, among others), and report a lower quality of life. Thus, it appears that individuals with muscle dysmorphia experience a high degree of psychopathology and clinical impairment. At its core, muscle dysmorphia represents a severe dissatisfaction with appearance, and thus not surprisingly, several measures of body dissatisfaction among men correlate with symptoms of muscle dysmorphia (e.g., Robert, Munroe-Chandler, & Gammage, 2009).

## IMPLICATIONS FOR PREVENTION AND INTERVENTION

Given the link among men's body image, drive for muscularity, and clinically relevant behavioral patterns such as risky exercise behavior, unhealthy eating, and steroid use, it is critical that the reviewed literature translate to effective intervention and prevention programs. To some extent, such programs do exist for at least some of the maladaptive outcomes reviewed. For example, the aforementioned ATLAS program was developed 2 decades ago. To our knowledge, this gender-specific, team-based program that targets athletes in high school should be considered a prevention program because empirical research indicates that it significantly prevents onset of steroid use, as well as use of other illicit substances (e.g., Goldberg et al., 2000). Interestingly, the mediators of the ATLAS program do not align with the sociocultural influences reviewed in this chapter. They include constructs very specific to use of anabolic steroids, such as knowledge of effects of steroids, reasons for not using steroids, and perceived severity of steroid use (MacKinnon et al., 2001).

Dissonance-based prevention programs have had success in preventing body image concerns and depression among young women (e.g., Stice, Rohde, Gau, & Shaw, 2009). These programs are based in the sociocultural perspective that the media are an important source of information about body ideals. By training young women to be critical of the body ideals displayed in various media sources, the programs are effective in decreasing body dissatisfaction, preventing future body image concerns, and decreasing internalization of sociocultural ideals (e.g., Stice et al., 2009). There are at least two reasons to believe that this approach to prevention could be effective among men. First, as reviewed in this chapter, the sociocultural models developed initially for women (and that were the basis of the dissonance-based prevention programs) are relevant for men as well. That is, we know that men use sources of societal influence for obtaining information about body ideals and that internalization of these ideals is linked with body image dissatisfaction, drive for muscularity, and maladaptive outcomes (e.g., Karazsia & Crowther, 2010). Second, young men with a positive body image report that they are critical of body ideals displayed in the media (Holmqvist & Frisén, 2012). Therefore, if young men can be trained to become more critical of their media consumption, it seems plausible that they will be less likely to develop unrealistic expectations for their bodies (Yager & O'Dea, 2008). Therefore, although efforts to prevent steroid use among young men have been successful, much less attention has focused on constructs that are broader, such as drive for muscularity, that may broaden the impact of prevention programs.

## SUGGESTIONS FOR FUTURE RESEARCH

Reflecting on this body of work, we see various directions for fruitful lines of research. First, there should be additional development of scales to measure body concerns specific to men. Drive for muscularity seems to be a well-measured construct, but some researchers are examining other issues associated with muscularity, such as distress associated with this issue (e.g., Kimmel & Mahalik, 2004). The existence of different measures will allow researchers to hone in on the specific aspects of muscularity that might predict problematic behaviors. For example, data suggest that some men have a functional view of muscularity that might motivate behavior to increase muscularity, and some men seem to be motivated by distress. Is distress about muscularity important in predicting maladaptive body change behaviors? Is there a difference between functional concern (i.e., wanting to increase muscularity for specific functional purposes, such as athletics or manual labor duties), appearance concern (i.e., wanting to increase muscularity for aesthetic purposes), and health concern (i.e., wanting to increase muscularity for health purposes), and if so, do these constructs differentially predict healthy versus unhealthy exercise behaviors? The existence of different scales related to muscularity will allow us to test specific hypotheses in this regard.

Knowledge of the correlates and consequences of men's body dissatisfaction should be used to develop effective prevention and intervention strategies. More information on group differences would be helpful to inform these efforts. For example, more study of specific sports cultures that might put men at risk is needed, as is more study of cultural and sexual minority groups. It will also be interesting to learn more about men's body talk (e.g., Engeln et al., 2013) and how that might relate to body concerns. Body-related teasing was a relatively strong predictor of body concerns (Menzel et al., 2010) that should be studied further.

We also feel that it is important to focus attention on theoretical grounding. When this field was in its infancy, most scholars applied theoretical models that were originally developed to explain eating disorders among women. As the field matured, scholars developed revisions of these models (e.g., Tylka, 2011) and models specific to men, although they often shared components with the early theories developed for women (e.g., Cafri et al., 2006). To our knowledge, few scholars have integrated components of various theories, and this may be important, particularly given the fact that most empirical studies do not explain all observed variation in measured outcome variables. Furthermore, there is empirical support for a broad range of constructs from different theories. For example, some studies include social comparison as an important predictor of outcomes, but others do not. By integrating constructs from sociocultural, objectification, and masculinity theories, scholars may be able to build more comprehensive models with more predictive utility. These integrated theories could then form a comprehensive foundation for prevention programs that have broad impacts across a variety of hypothesized mediators, such as internalization, and maladaptive outcomes, such as unhealthy exercise patterns or steroid use.

As an example, Karazsia, Crowther, and Galioto (2013) integrated a theory of drug use (The Gateway Hypothesis; Kandel, 2002) with sociocultural theories and concluded that both sociocultural theories and previous supplement use predicted men's anabolic supplementation, which increases variance explained. Thus, by integrating sociocultural theories, self-objectification theory, and theories of masculinity, scholars will be able to develop and then test more comprehensive models that may enhance prediction of important outcomes. Such integration would then translate into more comprehensive prevention and intervention programs.

There might be ways to link the body image research on women with that on men to develop more comprehensive theories related to how men's and women's gender roles work together to support unrealistic body image ideals (Murnen, 2011; Murnen & Don, 2012). Consistent with a future emphasis on integration across theories, we see potential for developmental perspectives to play an important role in future research. Historically in this field, the term *development* has been applied predominantly to children and adolescents. Once again, this may simply be an extension of previous research demonstrating that puberty and adolescence are developmental periods of risk for many women (e.g., Mendle, Turkheimer, & Emery, 2007). However, there may be other developmental periods that are risky for men. Biologically, many men grow closer to the mesomorphic ideal during puberty instead of away from it, which is an important difference between men and women. From this perspective, a developmental period during which men grow away from the ideal may be an important period to study. For men, this may be later in life. This notion is supported by research indicating that most users of nonmedical AAS are nonathletes, with a mean age of onset of 25.81 years (Cohen, Collins, Darkes, & Gwartney, 2007).

## CONCLUSION

In sum, the body of work that examines male body image concerns has grown a great deal in the past 15 years. This work has revealed that socio-cultural pressures can encourage men to obtain and maintain muscular and lean bodies. Research using several theoretical models and accompanying measures has found that men are influenced by cultural variables to adopt both thinness and muscular ideals, with some men particularly at risk for adopting maladaptive body change behaviors. Scholars and clinicians should be concerned about high rates of body dissatisfaction in men and boys, similar to concern shown for women and girls. Increased pressures from the commercial culture to purchase products for "body work" are affecting females and males, and some believe that our vulnerability to such products has increased. In her 2009 book *Bodies*, informed by her clinical experiences, Orbach (2009) opined that men and women in commercial cultures are experiencing "body instability" in part because many of us no longer use our bodies to make things. In fact, instead of making things with our bodies, we might be making our bodies into things.

## REFERENCES

American Psychiatric Association. (2013). *Diagnostic and statistical manual of mental disorders* (5th ed.). Arlington, VA: Author.

American Society of Plastic Surgeons. (2014). *2013 Plastic surgery statistics report.* Retrieved from https://d2wirczt3b6wjm.cloudfront.net/News/Statistics/2013/plastic-surgery-statistics-full-report-2013.pdf

Austin, S. B., Haines, J., & Veugelers, P. J. (2009). Body satisfaction and body weight: Gender differences and sociodemographic determinants. *BMC Public Health, 9,* 313–320. http://dx.doi.org/10.1186/1471-2458-9-313

Baghurst, T., Hollander, D. B., Nardella, B., & Haff, G. G. (2006). Change in sociocultural ideal male physique: An examination of past and present action figures. *Body Image, 3,* 87–91. http://dx.doi.org/10.1016/j.bodyim.2005.11.001

Baghurst, T., & Lirgg, C. (2009). Characteristics of muscle dysmorphia in male football, weight training, and competitive natural and non-natural bodybuilding samples. *Body Image, 6,* 221–227. http://dx.doi.org/10.1016/j.bodyim.2009.03.002

Banfield, S. S., & McCabe, M. P. (2002). An evaluation of the construct of body image. *Adolescence, 37,* 373–393.

Barlett, C. P., Vowels, C. L., & Saucier, D. A. (2008). Meta-analyses of the effects of media images on men's body-image concerns. *Journal of Social and Clinical Psychology, 27,* 279–310. http://dx.doi.org/10.1521/jscp.2008.27.3.279

Bem, S. L. (1974). The measurement of psychological androgyny. *Journal of Consulting and Clinical Psychology, 42,* 155–162. http://dx.doi.org/10.1037/h0036215

Blashill, A. J. (2011). Gender roles, eating pathology, and body dissatisfaction in men: A meta-analysis. *Body Image, 8,* 1–11. http://dx.doi.org/10.1016/j.bodyim.2010.09.002

Blashill, A. J., & Vander Wal, J. S. (2009). Mediation of gender role conflict and eating pathology in gay men. *Psychology of Men & Masculinity, 10,* 204–217. http://dx.doi.org/10.1037/a0016000

Blond, A. (2008). Impacts of exposure to images of ideal bodies on male body dissatisfaction: A review. *Body Image, 5,* 244–250. http://dx.doi.org/10.1016/j.bodyim.2008.02.003

Cafri, G., & Thompson, K. (2004). Measuring male body image: A review of the current methodology. *Psychology of Men & Masculinity, 5,* 18–29. http://dx.doi.org/10.1037/1524-9220.5.1.18

Cafri, G., van den Berg, P., & Thompson, J. K. (2006). Pursuit of muscularity in adolescent boys: Relations among biopsychosocial variables and clinical outcomes. *Journal of Clinical Child and Adolescent Psychology, 35*, 283–291. http://dx.doi.org/10.1207/s15374424jccp3502_12

Calogero, R. M., Tantleff-Dunn, S., & Thompson, J. K. (Eds.). (2011). *Self-objectification in women: Causes, consequences, and counteractions.* Washington, DC: American Psychological Association.

Calzo, J. P., Corliss, H. L., Blood, E. A., Field, A. E., & Austin, S. B. (2013). Development of muscularity and weight concerns in heterosexual and sexual minority males. *Health Psychology, 32*, 42–51. http://dx.doi.org/10.1037/a0028964

Campana, A., Tavares, M., Swami, V., & da Silva, D. (2013). An examination of the psychometric properties of Brazilian Portuguese translations of the Drive for Muscularity Scale, the Swansea Muscularity Attitudes Questionnaire, and the Masculine Body Ideal Distress Scale. *Psychology of Men & Masculinity, 14*, 376–388. http://dx.doi.org/10.1037/a0030087

Clarke, P., Murnen, S. K., & Smolak, L. (2010). Development and psychometric evaluation of a quantitative measure of "fat talk." *Body Image, 7*, 1–7. http://dx.doi.org/10.1016/j.bodyim.2009.09.006

Cohen, J., Collins, R., Darkes, J., & Gwartney, D. (2007). A league of their own: Demographics, motivations and patterns of use of 1,955 male adult non-medical anabolic steroid users in the United States. *Journal of the International Society of Sports Nutrition, 4*, 12. http://dx.doi.org/10.1186/1550-2783-4-12

Dakanalis, A., Zanetti, A. M., Riva, G., Colmegna, F., Volpato, C., Madeddu, F., & Clerici, M. (2015). Male body dissatisfaction and eating disorder symptomatology: Moderating variables among men. *Journal of Health Psychology, 20*, 80–90. http://dx.doi.org/10.1177/1359105313499198

Daniel, S., & Bridges, S. K. (2010). The drive for muscularity in men: Media influences and objectification theory. *Body Image, 7*, 32–38. http://dx.doi.org/10.1016/j.bodyim.2009.08.003

Dodge, T. L., & Jaccard, J. J. (2006). The effect of high school sports participation on the use of performance-enhancing substances in young adulthood. *Journal of Adolescent Health, 39*, 367–373. http://dx.doi.org/10.1016/j.jadohealth.2005.12.025

Edwards, S., & Launder, C. (2000). Investigating muscularity concerns in male body image: Development of the Swansea Muscularity Attitudes Questionnaire. *International Journal of Eating Disorders, 28*, 120–124. http://dx.doi.org/10.1002/(SICI)1098-108X(200007)28:1<120::AID-EAT15>3.0.CO;2-H

Eisenberg, M. E., Wall, M., & Neumark-Sztainer, D. (2012). Muscle-enhancing behaviors among adolescent girls and boys. *Pediatrics, 130*, 1019–1026. http://dx.doi.org/10.1542/peds.2012-0095

Engeln, R., Sladek, M. R., & Waldron, H. (2013). Body talk among college men: Content, correlates, and effects. *Body Image, 10*, 300–308. http://dx.doi.org/10.1016/j.bodyim.2013.02.001

Escoto, C., Alvarez-Rayón, G., Mancilla-Díaz, J. M., Camacho Ruiz, E. J., Franco Paredes, K., & Juárez Lugo, C. S. (2013). Psychometric properties of the drive for muscularity scale in Mexican males. *Eating and Weight Disorders, 18*, 23–28. http://dx.doi.org/10.1007/s40519-013-0010-6

Fallon, A. E., & Rozin, P. (1985). Sex differences in perceptions of desirable body shape. *Journal of Abnormal Psychology, 94*, 102–105. http://dx.doi.org/10.1037/0021-843X.94.1.102

Farquhar, H. J., & Wasylkiw, L. (2007). Media images of men: Trends and consequences of body conceptualization. *Psychology of Men & Masculinity, 8*, 145–160. http://dx.doi.org/10.1037/1524-9220.8.3.145

Feingold, A., & Mazzella, R. (1998). Gender differences in body image are increasing. *Psychological Science, 9*, 190–195. http://dx.doi.org/10.1111/1467-9280.00036

Feldman, M. B., & Meyer, I. H. (2007). Eating disorders in diverse lesbian, gay, and bisexual populations. *International Journal of Eating Disorders, 40*, 218–226. http://dx.doi.org/10.1002/eat.20360

Frederick, D. A., Buchanan, G. M., Sadehgi-Azar, L., Peplau, L. A., Haselton, M. G., Berezovskaya, A., & Lipinski, R. E. (2007). Desiring the muscular ideal: Men's body satisfaction in the United States, Ukraine, and Ghana. *Psychology of Men & Masculinity, 8*, 103–117. http://dx.doi.org/10.1037/1524-9220.8.2.103

Frederick, D. A., Forbes, G. B., Grigorian, K. E., & Jarcho, J. M. (2007). The UCLA Body Project I: Gender and ethnic differences in self-objectification and body satisfaction among 2,206 undergraduates. *Sex Roles, 57*, 317–327. http://dx.doi.org/10.1007/s11199-007-9251-z

Frederick, D. A., Peplau, L. A., & Lever, J. (2006). The swimsuit issue: Correlates of body image in a sample of 52,677 heterosexual adults. *Body Image, 3*, 413–419. http://dx.doi.org/10.1016/j.bodyim.2006.08.002

Fredrickson, B. L., & Roberts, T. A. (1997). Objectification theory: Toward understanding women's lived experiences and mental health risks. *Psychology of Women Quarterly, 21*, 173–206. http://dx.doi.org/10.1111/j.1471-6402.1997.tb00108.x

Garner, D. M., Garfinkel, P. E., Schwartz, D., & Thompson, M. (1980). Cultural expectations of thinness in women. *Psychological Reports, 47*, 483–491. http://dx.doi.org/10.2466/pr0.1980.47.2.483

Gattario, K. H., Frisén, A., Fuller-Tyszkiewicz, M., Ricciardelli, L. A., Diedrichs, P. C., Yager, Z., . . . Smolak, L. (2015, January 19). How is men's conformity to masculine norms related to their body image? Masculinity and muscularity across Western countries. *Psychology of Men & Masculinity, 16*, 337–347. http://dx.doi.org/10.1037/a0038494

Goldberg, L., Elliot, D., Clarke, G. N., MacKinnon, D. P., Moe, E., Zoref, L., . . . Lapin, A. (1996). Effects of a multidimensional anabolic steroid prevention intervention. The Adolescents Training and Learning to Avoid Steroids (ATLAS) program. *JAMA, 276*, 1555–1562. http://dx.doi.org/10.1001/jama.1996.03540190027025

Goldberg, L., MacKinnon, D. P., Elliot, D. L., Moe, E. L., Clarke, G., & Cheong, J. (2000). The Adolescents Training and Learning to Avoid Steroids program: Preventing drug use and promoting health behaviors. *Archives of Pediatrics & Adolescent Medicine, 154,* 332–338. http://dx.doi.org/10.1001/archpedi.154.4.332

Grabe, S., Ward, L. M., & Hyde, J. S. (2008). The role of the media in body image concerns among women: A meta-analysis of experimental and correlational studies. *Psychological Bulletin, 134,* 460–476. http://dx.doi.org/10.1037/0033-2909.134.3.460

Griffiths, S., Murray, S. B., & Touyz, S. B. (2015). Extending the masculinity hypothesis: An investigation of gender role conformity, body dissatisfaction, and disordered eating in young heterosexual men. *Psychology of Men & Masculinity, 16,* 108–114. http://dx.doi.org/10.1037/a0035958

Guyenet, S. J., & Schwartz, M. W. (2012). Clinical review: Regulation of food intake, energy balance, and body fat mass: Implications for the pathogenesis and treatment of obesity. *The Journal of Clinical Endocrinology and Metabolism, 97,* 745–755. http://dx.doi.org/10.1210/jc.2011-2525

Hale, B. D., Roth, A. D., DeLong, R. E., & Briggs, M. S. (2010). Exercise dependence and the drive for muscularity in male bodybuilders, power lifters, and fitness lifters. *Body Image, 7,* 234–239. http://dx.doi.org/10.1016/j.bodyim.2010.02.001

Halliwell, E., Dittmar, H., & Orsborn, A. (2007). The effects of exposure to muscular male models among men: Exploring the moderating role of gym use and exercise motivation. *Body Image, 4,* 278–287. http://dx.doi.org/10.1016/j.bodyim.2007.04.006

Halliwell, E., & Harvey, M. (2006). Examination of a sociocultural model of disordered eating among male and female adolescents. *British Journal of Health Psychology, 11,* 235–248. http://dx.doi.org/10.1348/135910705X39214

Harrison, K., & Bond, B. J. (2007). Gaming magazines and the drive for muscularity in preadolescent boys: A longitudinal examination. *Body Image, 4,* 269–277. http://dx.doi.org/10.1016/j.bodyim.2007.03.003

Hildebrandt, T., Langenbucher, J., & Schlundt, D. G. (2004). Muscularity concerns among men: Development of attitudinal and perceptual measures. *Body Image, 1,* 169–181. http://dx.doi.org/10.1016/j.bodyim.2004.01.001

Holmqvist, K., & Frisén, A. (2012). "I bet they aren't that perfect in reality:" Appearance ideals viewed from the perspective of adolescents with a positive body image. *Body Image, 9,* 388–395. http://dx.doi.org/10.1016/j.bodyim.2012.03.007

Johnston, L. D., O'Malley, P. M., & Bachman, J. G. (2002). Ecstasy use among American teens drops for the first time in recent years, and overall drug and alcohol use also decline in year after 9/11 [press release]. Retrieved from http://monitoringthefuture.org/pressreleases/02drugpr.pdf

Kaminski, P. L., Chapman, B. P., Haynes, S. D., & Own, L. (2005). Body image, eating behaviors, and attitudes toward exercise among gay and straight men. *Eating Behaviors, 6,* 179–187. http://dx.doi.org/10.1016/j.eatbeh.2004.11.003

Kandel, D. B. (2002). Stages and pathways of drug involvement: Examining the gateway hypothesis. In D. B. Kandel & R. Jessor (Eds.), *Examining the gateway hypothesis: Stages and pathways of drug involvement* (pp. 3–16). http://dx.doi.org/10.1017/CBO9780511499777.003

Karazsia, B. T., & Crowther, J. H. (2008). Psychological and behavioral correlates of the SATAQ-3 with males. *Body Image, 5,* 109–115. http://dx.doi.org/10.1016/j.bodyim.2007.08.004

Karazsia, B. T., & Crowther, J. H. (2009). Social body comparison and internalization: Mediators of social influences on men's muscularity-oriented body dissatisfaction. *Body Image, 6,* 105–112. http://dx.doi.org/10.1016/j.bodyim.2008.12.003

Karazsia, B. T., & Crowther, J. H. (2010). Sociocultural and psychological links to men's engagement in risky body change behaviors. *Sex Roles, 63,* 747–756. http://dx.doi.org/10.1007/s11199-010-9802-6

Karazsia, B. T., Crowther, J. H., & Galioto, R. (2013). Undergraduate men's use of performance- and appearance-enhancing substances: An examination of the gateway hypothesis. *Psychology of Men & Masculinity, 14,* 129–137. http://dx.doi.org/10.1037/a0027810

Karazsia, B. T., & Peiper, K. (2011). A meta-analytic review of sociocultural influences on male body image. In S. B. Greene (Ed.), *Body image: Perceptions, attitudes and interpretations* (pp. 153–172). Hauppauge, NY: NOVA Science.

Keery, H., van den Berg, P., & Thompson, J. K. (2004). An evaluation of the tripartite influence model of body dissatisfaction and eating disturbance with adolescent girls. *Body Image, 1,* 237–251. http://dx.doi.org/10.1016/j.bodyim.2004.03.001

Keum, B. T., Wong, S. N., DeBlaere, C., & Brewster, M. E. (2015). Body image and Asian American men: Examination of the Drive for Muscularity Scale. *Psychology of Men & Masculinity, 16,* 284–293. http://dx.doi.org/10.1037/a0038180

Kimmel, S. B., & Mahalik, J. R. (2004). Measuring masculine body ideal distress: Development of a measure. *International Journal of Men's Health, 3,* 1–10. http://dx.doi.org/10.3149/jmh.0301.1

Kimmel, S. B., & Mahalik, J. R. (2005). Body image concerns of gay men: The roles of minority stress and conformity to masculine norms. *Journal of Consulting and Clinical Psychology, 73,* 1185–1190. http://dx.doi.org/10.1037/0022-006X.73.6.1185

Labre, M. P. (2005). Burn fat, build muscle: A content analysis of *Men's Health* and *Men's Fitness. International Journal of Men's Health, 4,* 187–200. http://dx.doi.org/10.3149/jmh.0402.187

Lanzieri, N., & Cook, B. J. (2013). Examination of muscularity and body fat depictions in magazines that target heterosexual and gay men. *Body Image, 10,* 251–254. http://dx.doi.org/10.1016/j.bodyim.2012.12.003

Leit, R. A., Pope, H. G., Jr., & Gray, J. J. (2001). Cultural expectations of muscularity in men: The evolution of playgirl centerfolds. *International Journal of Eating Disorders, 29,* 90–93. http://dx.doi.org/10.1002/1098-108X(200101)29:1<90::AID-EAT15>3.0.CO;2-F

Litt, D., & Dodge, T. (2008). A longitudinal investigation of the Drive for Muscularity Scale: Predicting use of performance enhancing substances and weightlifting among males. *Body Image, 5,* 346–351. http://dx.doi.org/10.1016/j.bodyim.2008.04.002

MacKinnon, D. P., Goldberg, L., Clarke, G. N., Elliot, D. L., Cheong, J., Lapin, A., . . . Krull, J. L. (2001). Mediating mechanisms in a program to reduce intentions to use anabolic steroids and improve exercise self-efficacy and dietary behavior. *Prevention Science, 2,* 15–28. http://dx.doi.org/10.1023/A:1010082828000

Mahalik, J. R., Locke, B. D., Ludlow, L. H., Diemer, M. A., Scott, R. P. J., Gottfried, M., & Freitas, G. (2003). Development of the Conformity to Masculine Norms Inventory. *Psychology of Men & Masculinity, 4,* 3–25. http://dx.doi.org/10.1037/1524-9220.4.1.3

Mahalik, J. R., Mooray, E. B., Coonerty-Femiano, A., Ludlow, L. H., Slattery, S. M., & Smiler, A. (2005). Development of the Conformity to Feminine Norms Inventory. *Sex Roles, 52,* 417–435. http://dx.doi.org/10.1007/s11199-005-3709-7

Martins, Y., Tiggemann, M., & Kirkbride, A. (2007). Those speedos become them: The role of self-objectification in gay and heterosexual men's body image. *Personality and Social Psychology Bulletin, 33,* 634–647. http://dx.doi.org/10.1177/0146167206297403

Mayville, S. B., Williamson, D. A., White, M. A., Netemeyer, R. G., & Drab, D. L. (2002). Development of the Muscle Appearance Satisfaction Scale: A self-report measure for the assessment of muscle dysmorphia symptoms. *Assessment, 9,* 351–360. http://dx.doi.org/10.1177/1073191102238156

McCabe, M. P., & Ricciardelli, L. A. (2003). A longitudinal study of body change strategies among adolescent males. *Journal of Youth and Adolescence, 32,* 105–113. http://dx.doi.org/10.1023/A:1021805717484

McCabe, M. P., & Ricciardelli, L. A. (2004). Body image dissatisfaction among males across the lifespan: A review of past literature. *Journal of Psychosomatic Research, 56,* 675–685. http://dx.doi.org/10.1016/S0022-3999(03)00129-6

McCabe, M. P., Ricciardelli, L. A., & Finemore, J. (2002). The role of puberty, media and popularity with peers on strategies to increase weight, decrease weight and increase muscle tone among adolescent boys and girls. *Journal of Psychosomatic Research, 52,* 145–153. http://dx.doi.org/10.1016/S0022-3999(01)00272-0

McCreary, D. R., Hildebrandt, T. B., Heinberg, L. J., Boroughs, M., & Thompson, J. K. (2007). A review of body image influences on men's fitness goals and supplement use. *American Journal of Men's Health, 1,* 307–316. http://dx.doi.org/10.1177/1557988306309408

McCreary, D. R., & Sasse, D. K. (2000). An exploration of the drive for muscularity in adolescent boys and girls. *Journal of American College Health, 48,* 297–304. http://dx.doi.org/10.1080/07448480009596271

McCreary, D. R., Sasse, D. K., Saucier, D. M., & Dorsch, K. D. (2004). Measuring the drive for muscularity: Factorial validity of the Drive for Muscularity Scale in men and women. *Psychology of Men & Masculinity, 5*, 49–58. http://dx.doi.org/10.1037/1524-9220.5.1.49

McCreary, D. R., Saucier, D. M., & Courtenay, W. H. (2005). The drive for muscularity and masculinity: Testing the associations among gender-role traits, behaviors, attitudes, and conflict. *Psychology of Men & Masculinity, 6*, 83–94. http://dx.doi.org/10.1037/1524-9220.6.2.83

McPherson, K. E., McCarthy, P., McCreary, D. R., & McMillan, S. (2010). Psychometric evaluation of the Drive for Muscularity Scale in a community-based sample of Scottish men participating in an organized sporting event. *Body Image, 7*, 368–371. http://dx.doi.org/10.1016/j.bodyim.2010.06.001

Mendle, J., Turkheimer, E., & Emery, R. E. (2007). Detrimental psychological outcomes associated with early pubertal timing in adolescent girls. *Developmental Review, 27*, 151–171.

Menzel, J. E., Schaefer, L. M., Burke, N. L., Mayhew, L. L., Brannick, M. T., & Thompson, J. K. (2010). Appearance-related teasing, body dissatisfaction, and disordered eating: A meta-analysis. *Body Image, 7*, 261–270. http://dx.doi.org/10.1016/j.bodyim.2010.05.004

Menzel, J. E., Sperry, S. L., Small, B., Thompson, J. K., Sarwer, D. B., & Cash, T. F. (2011). Internalization of appearance ideals and cosmetic surgery attitudes: A test of the tripartite influence model of body image. *Sex Roles, 65*, 469–477. http://dx.doi.org/10.1007/s11199-011-9983-7

Mills, J. S., & D'Alfonso, S. R. (2007). Competition and male body image: Increased drive for muscularity following failure to a female. *Journal of Social and Clinical Psychology, 26*, 505–518. http://dx.doi.org/10.1521/jscp.2007.26.4.505

Moradi, B., & Huang, Y. P. (2008). Objectification theory and psychology of women: A decade of advances and future directions. *Psychology of Women Quarterly, 32*, 377–398. http://dx.doi.org/10.1111/j.1471-6402.2008.00452.x

Morrison, M. A., Morrison, T. G., & Sager, C. L. (2004). Does body satisfaction differ between gay men and lesbian women and heterosexual men and women? A meta-analytic review. *Body Image, 1*, 127–138.

Morrison, T. G., & Harriman, R. L. (2005). Additional evidence for the psychometric soundness of the Drive for Muscularity Attitudes Questionnaire (DMAQ). *The Journal of Social Psychology, 145*, 618–620. http://dx.doi.org/10.3200/SOCP.145.5.618-620

Morrison, T. G., Morrison, M. A., Hopkins, C., & Rowan, E. T. (2004). "Muscle mania" Development of a new scale examining the drive for muscularity in Canadian men. *Psychology of Men & Masculinity, 5*, 30–39. http://dx.doi.org/10.1037/1524-9220.5.1.30

Mulgrew, K. E., Johnson, L. M., Lane, B. R., & Katsikitis, M. (2014). The effect of aesthetic versus process images on men's body satisfaction. *Psychology of Men & Masculinity, 15*, 452–459. http://dx.doi.org/10.1037/a0034684

Murnen, S. K. (2011). Gender and body images. In T. F. Cash & L. Smolak (Eds.), *Body image: A handbook of science, practice, and prevention* (2nd ed., pp. 173–179). New York, NY: Guilford Press.

Murnen, S. K., & Don, B. P. (2012). Body image and gender roles. In T. Cash (Ed.), *Encyclopedia of body image and human appearance* (Vol. 1, pp. 128–134). http://dx.doi.org/10.1016/B978-0-12-384925-0.00019-5

Neumark-Sztainer, D., Paxton, S. J., Hannan, P. J., Haines, J., & Story, M. (2006). Does body satisfaction matter? Five-year longitudinal associations between body satisfaction and health behaviors in adolescent females and males. *Journal of Adolescent Health, 39*, 244–251. http://dx.doi.org/10.1016/j.jadohealth.2005.12.001

Ogden, C. L., Carroll, M. D., Kit, B. K., & Flegal, K. M. (2014). Prevalence of childhood and adult obesity in the United States, 2011–2012. *JAMA, 311*, 806–814. http://dx.doi.org/10.1001/jama.2014.732

Orbach, S. (2009). *Bodies.* London, England: Profile.

Parent, M. C., & Moradi, B. (2011). His biceps become him: A test of objectification theory's application to drive for muscularity and propensity for steroid use in college men. *Journal of Counseling Psychology, 58*, 246–256. http://dx.doi.org/10.1037/a0021398

Pope, C. G., Pope, H. G., Jr., Menard, W., Fay, C., Olivardia, R., & Phillips, K. A. (2005). Clinical features of muscle dysmorphia among males with body dysmorphic disorder. *Body Image, 2*, 395–400. http://dx.doi.org/10.1016/j.bodyim.2005.09.001

Pope, H. G., Jr., Olivardia, R., Gruber, A., & Borowiecki, J. (1999). Evolving ideals of male body image as seen through action toys. *International Journal of Eating Disorders, 26*, 65–72. http://dx.doi.org/10.1002/(SICI)1098-108X(199907)26:1<65::AID-EAT8>3.0.CO;2-D

Ricciardelli, L. A., McCabe, M. P., Williams, R. J., & Thompson, J. K. (2007). The role of ethnicity and culture in body image and disordered eating among males. *Clinical Psychology Review, 27*, 582–606. http://dx.doi.org/10.1016/j.cpr.2007.01.016

Ridgeway, R. T., & Tylka, T. L. (2005). College men's perceptions of ideal body composition and shape. *Psychology of Men & Masculinity, 6*, 209–220. http://dx.doi.org/10.1037/1524-9220.6.3.209

Robert, C. A., Munroe-Chandler, K. J., & Gammage, K. L. (2009). The relationship between the drive for muscularity and muscle dysmorphia in male and female weight trainers. *Journal of Strength and Conditioning Research, 23*, 1656–1662. http://dx.doi.org/10.1519/JSC.0b013e3181b3dc2f

Rodgers, R. F., Ganchou, C., Franko, D. L., & Chabrol, H. (2012). Drive for muscularity and disordered eating among French adolescent boys: A sociocultural model. *Body Image, 9*, 318–323. http://dx.doi.org/10.1016/j.bodyim.2012.03.002

Rohlinger, D. A. (2002). Eroticizing men: Cultural influences on advertising and male objectification. *Sex Roles, 46*, 61–74. http://dx.doi.org/10.1023/A:1016575909173

Rubinstein, S., & Caballero, B. (2000). Is Miss America an undernourished role model? *JAMA, 283*, 1569–1569. http://dx.doi.org/10.1001/jama.283.12.1569-JLT0322-18-1

Russell, C. J., & Keel, P. K. (2002). Homosexuality as a specific risk factor for eating disorders in men. *International Journal of Eating Disorders, 31*, 300–306. http://dx.doi.org/10.1002/eat.10036

Sladek, M. R., Engeln, R., & Miller, S. A. (2014). Development and validation of the Male Body Talk Scale: A psychometric investigation. *Body Image, 11*, 233–244. http://dx.doi.org/10.1016/j.bodyim.2014.02.005

Smolak, L., & Murnen, S. K. (2008). Drive for leanness: Assessment and relationship to gender, gender role, and objectification. *Body Image, 5*, 251–260. http://dx.doi.org/10.1016/j.bodyim.2008.03.004

Smolak, L., Murnen, S. K., & Thompson, J. K. (2005). Sociocultural influences and muscle building in adolescent boys. *Psychology of Men & Masculinity, 6*, 227–239. http://dx.doi.org/10.1037/1524-9220.6.4.227

Smolak, L., & Stein, J. A. (2006). The relationship of drive for muscularity to sociocultural factors, self-esteem, physical attributes gender role, and social comparison in middle school boys. *Body Image, 3*, 121–129. http://dx.doi.org/10.1016/j.bodyim.2006.03.002

Steinfeldt, J. A., Gilchrist, G. A., Halterman, A. W., Gomory, A., & Steinfeldt, M. C. (2011). Drive for muscularity and conformity to masculine norms among college football players. *Psychology of Men & Masculinity, 12*, 324–338. http://dx.doi.org/10.1037/a0024839

Stice, E., Rohde, P., Gau, J., & Shaw, H. (2009). An effectiveness trial of a dissonance-based eating disorder prevention program for high-risk adolescent girls. *Journal of Consulting and Clinical Psychology, 77*, 825–834. http://dx.doi.org/10.1037/a0016132

Stice, E., & Shaw, H. E. (2002). Role of body dissatisfaction in the onset and maintenance of eating pathology: A synthesis of research findings. *Journal of Psychosomatic Research, 53*, 985–993. http://dx.doi.org/10.1016/S0022-3999(02)00488-9

Swami, V., Diwell, R., & McCreary, D. R. (2014). Sexuality and the drive for muscularity: Evidence of associations among British men. *Body Image, 11*, 543–546. http://dx.doi.org/10.1016/j.bodyim.2014.08.008

Swami, V., Neofytou, R. V., Jablonska, J., Thirlwell, H., Taylor, D., & McCreary, D. R. (2013). Social dominance orientation predicts drive for muscularity among British men. *Body Image, 10*, 653–656. http://dx.doi.org/10.1016/j.bodyim.2013.07.007

Swami, V., & Voracek, M. (2013). Associations among men's sexist attitudes, objectification of women, and their own drive for muscularity. *Psychology of Men & Masculinity, 14*, 168–174. http://dx.doi.org/10.1037/a0028437

Thompson, J. K., Heinberg, L. J., Altabe, M. N., & Tantleff-Dunn, S. (1999). *Exacting beauty: Theory, assessment, and treatment of body image disturbance.* http://dx.doi.org/10.1037/10312-000

Thompson, J. K., & Stice, E. (2001). Thin-ideal internalization: Mounting evidence for a new risk factor for body-image disturbance and eating pathology. *Current Directions in Psychological Science, 10,* 181–183. http://dx.doi.org/10.1111/1467-8721.00144

Tod, D., Morrison, T. G., & Edwards, C. (2012). Evaluating validity and test–retest reliability in four drive for muscularity questionnaires. *Body Image, 9,* 425–428. http://dx.doi.org/10.1016/j.bodyim.2012.02.001

Tylka, T. L. (2011). Refinement of the tripartite influence model for men: Dual body image pathways to body change behaviors. *Body Image, 8,* 199–207. http://dx.doi.org/10.1016/j.bodyim.2011.04.008

Tylka, T. L., & Andorka, M. J. (2012). Support for an expanded tripartite influence model with gay men. *Body Image, 9,* 57–67. http://dx.doi.org/10.1016/j.bodyim.2011.09.006

Tylka, T. L., Bergeron, D., & Schwartz, J. P. (2005). Development and psychometric evaluation of the Male Body Attitudes Scale (MBAS). *Body Image, 2,* 161–175. http://dx.doi.org/10.1016/j.bodyim.2005.03.001

Williams, P. A., & Cash, T. F. (2001). Effects of a circuit weight training program on the body images of college students. *International Journal of Eating Disorders, 30,* 75–82. http://dx.doi.org/10.1002/eat.1056

Wiseman, M. C., & Moradi, B. (2010). Body image and eating disorder symptoms in sexual minority men: A test and extension of objectification theory. *Journal of Counseling Psychology, 57,* 154–166. http://dx.doi.org/10.1037/a0018937

Wright, S. M., & Aronne, L. J. (2012). Causes of obesity. *Abdominal Imaging, 37,* 730–732. http://dx.doi.org/10.1007/s00261-012-9862-x

Yager, Z., & O'Dea, J. A. (2008). Prevention programs for body image and eating disorders on University campuses: A review of large, controlled interventions. *Health Promotion International, 23,* 173–189. http://dx.doi.org/10.1093/heapro/dan004

Yang, C. F., Gray, P., & Pope, H. G., Jr. (2005). Male body image in Taiwan versus the West: *Yanggang Zhiqi* meets the Adonis Complex. *The American Journal of Psychiatry, 162,* 263–269. http://dx.doi.org/10.1176/appi.ajp.162.2.263

Yelland, C., & Tiggemann, M. (2003). Muscularity and the gay ideal: Body dissatisfaction and disordered eating in homosexual men. *Eating Behaviors, 4,* 107–116. http://dx.doi.org/10.1016/S1471-0153(03)00014-X

# III
# ETHNIC, RACIAL, AND SEXUAL MINORITY MEN

# 9

# THE INTERSECTION OF RACE, ETHNICITY, AND MASCULINITIES: PROGRESS, PROBLEMS, AND PROSPECTS

Y. JOEL WONG, TAO LIU, AND ELYSSA M. KLANN

*Intersectionality* is a conceptual framework that addresses how multiple interlocking social identities reflect diverse systems of power, privilege, oppression, and inequity (Bowleg, 2012; Shields, 2008; Stewart & McDermott, 2004). In particular, this framework emphasizes the manner in which multiple social identities, such as race, gender, and social class, are dependent on each other for meaning (Cole, 2009). The concept of intersectionality was first coined by legal scholar and critical race theorist Kimberlé Crenshaw (1989) to describe the marginalization of Black women in antidiscrimination law, feminist theory (which equated women with White women), and antiracist politics (which equated Blacks with Black men). Intersectionality has since made substantial inroads into diverse fields, such as women's studies (McCall, 2005), sociology (Choo & Ferree, 2010), and psychology (Cole, 2009). In the same vein, a small but growing body of psychological studies have recently used intersectionality as a framework to understand the

http://dx.doi.org/10.1037/0000023-010
*The Psychology of Men and Masculinities*, R. F. Levant and Y. J. Wong (Editors)

experiences of men of color[1] (e.g., Rogers, Sperry, & Levant, 2015; Schwing, Wong, & Fann, 2013; Y. J. Wong, Owen, Tran, Collins, & Higgins, 2012).

As a conceptual framework, intersectionality is ideally suited for the study of men of color for several reasons. For one, intersectionality highlights the notion that men of color have relatively unique experiences that differ from those of men in general and from women of color; therefore, they deserve to be studied in their own right rather than simply as men or as people of color. For another, intersectionality reflects the reality and complexities of men of color's lives in that they simultaneously occupy multiple social identities (Shields, 2008). As is demonstrated in the following section, intersectionality can also turn the spotlight on health disparities within subpopulations that might go unnoticed if racial/ethnic minority men are simply studied as men or as people of color (Bowleg, 2012; Y. J. Wong, Maffini, & Shin, 2014).

Nonetheless, several scholars have observed challenges and ambiguity regarding how to study intersectionality (Bowleg, 2012; Goff & Kahn, 2013; McCall, 2005; Nash, 2008). Although few scholars dispute the intersectionality framework's basic tenet that people have multiple, interlocking social identities, translating this insight into research questions and testable hypotheses remains substantially more challenging. For example, Bowleg (2008) criticized the additive approach to intersectionality, which focuses on the independent and summative effects of multiple identities, as inadequate to capture the complexities of people's experiences; however, she noted that "it is virtually impossible, particularly in quantitative research, to ask questions about intersectionality that are not inherently additive" (p. 314).

Therefore, the goal of this chapter is to elucidate research paradigms for the application of intersectionality to the psychology of racial/ethnic minority men. Throughout this chapter, we provide examples of theoretical concepts, research questions, research design, and statistical methods that reflect each of these three paradigms. Our basic premise is that there are multiple approaches to studying intersectionality, which can be categorized into at least three research paradigms, each with a different focus. We label these paradigms (a) the *intergroup paradigm*, (b) the *interconstruct paradigm*, and (c) the *intersectional uniqueness paradigm*. Although we believe these three paradigms can be applied to almost all types of intersectionality social science research, in this chapter, we focus mainly on the intersection of race, ethnicity, and gender as applied to men of color.

Before continuing, we provide clarifications regarding our terminology, namely, intersectionality as a framework, as research paradigms, and as concepts. As a framework, intersectionality is a broad, overarching perspective that addresses *why* we should focus on the lives of certain populations (e.g.,

---

[1]In this chapter, the term *men of color* is used interchangeably with *racial/ethnic minority men*.

men of color; refer to the definition of intersectionality at the beginning of this chapter). Intersectionality concepts focus on the *what* of intersectionality—they specify the types of constructs (e.g., gendered racism; Liang, Rivera, Nathwani, Dang, & Douroux, 2010) and theories (e.g., gendered race theory; Schug, Alt, & Klauer, 2015) that intersectionality research should address. Finally, research paradigms focus on the *how* of intersectionality; that is, they explicate how researchers can approach intersectionality by indicating illustrative research questions and methods (see Table 9.1). This chapter is organized around three intersectionality research paradigms, although throughout the chapter we provide relevant examples of intersectionality constructs and theories. What follows is a discussion of studies that exemplify these paradigms, the strengths and limitations of these paradigms, and directions for future research.

## INTERGROUP PARADIGM

The intergroup paradigm, which involves quantitative group comparisons based on individuals' social identities, is the most commonly employed paradigm in psychological research on intersectionality. Given our focus on the intersection of gender and race/ethnicity, we break down studies on men of color into two categories: (a) those that compare multiple racial/ethnic groups of men and (b) those that compare women and men from the same race/ethnicity. This categorization reflects our relative focus for this chapter, but of course, there are some studies that compare groups across gender and race/ethnicity.

### Studies Comparing Racial/Ethnic Groups of Men

Several studies have examined how men from diverse racial backgrounds differ in their endorsement of masculinity-related constructs. One study on White, Latino, and Black men found that Black men showed the strongest endorsement of traditional masculinity ideology, White men showed the weakest endorsement, and Latino men fell in between (Levant et al., 2003). These differences may be explained by a number of factors, including the interplay of traditional masculinity ideology and privilege.

Decades of literature have also linked masculinity-related constructs to men's physical and mental health (O'Neil, 2012); more recent literature has disaggregated these data to explain which of these links may differ across racial/ethnic groups (e.g., Levant & Wong, 2013). One study that used latent class regression to investigate masculinity profiles of Latino, Asian American, and White men identified two latent classes of participants that exhibited

## TABLE 9.1
### Intersectionality Research Paradigms: Illustrative Research Questions and Methods

| Research paradigm | Focus | Illustrative research questions | Illustrative research methods |
|---|---|---|---|
| Intergroup paradigm | Quantitative group comparisons based on individuals' social identities | Do men and women from diverse racial groups differ in their levels of conformity to masculine norms? Does the link between men's conformity to masculine norms and psychological help-seeking attitudes differ across diverse racial groups? | ANOVA and MANOVA Multiple regression: test conformity to masculine norms × race interaction effects |
| Interconstruct paradigm | Relations among constructs associated with individuals' social identities | Are various dimensions of Black men's racial identity associated with their subjective masculinity stress? Do Latino men who are exposed to racist behavior (vs. neutral behavior) experience greater vigilance to masculinity threat cues? | Pearson correlation and multiple regression Experimental design: ANOVA |
| Intersectional uniqueness paradigm | Unique, nonadditive experiences arising from the intersection of social identities | How do Native American men subjectively define Native American manhood? What are the dimensions of Asian American men's experience of gendered racism? | Qualitative methods (e.g., interviews or open-ended survey questions) Scale development: factor analysis of newly developed scale items |

Note. ANOVA = analysis of variance; MANOVA = multivariate analysis of variance.

very different profiles in the relation between conformity to masculine norms and psychological distress (Y. J. Wong, Owen, & Shea, 2012). Compared with White and Latino men, Asian American men had greater odds of belonging to the latent class of participants in which conformity to several masculine norms was more strongly associated with psychological distress. On the basis of these findings, the authors argued that masculinity researchers should not simply be studying whether masculinity constructs are associated with men's psychological well-being but also how specific dimensions of masculinity are related to psychological well-being among diverse groups of men.

Levant, Wong, Karakis, and Welsh (2015) proposed the masculinity cultural incongruence hypothesis to explain cultural differences in the link between masculinity-related constructs and men's well-being. Specifically, the authors posited that men's endorsement of the masculinity ideology of restrictive emotionality would engender psychological distress when this ideology conflicts with the norms of the cultural group to which they belong. Consistent with the idea that Latino cultural norms encourage the expression of emotions, which conflicts with the White masculinity ideology of restrictive emotionality, the authors found that the positive association between endorsing restrictive emotionality and alexithymia was greater for Latino men than for Asian, Black, and White American men.

Men of color may also seek and receive mental health care at rates that differ along racial lines. For example, Beals et al. (2005) found that Native American men sought professional help for issues related to substance use at greater rates than the general population, whereas Woodward (2011) compared Black Caribbean, Black African, and non-Hispanic White men in the United States and found that Black Caribbean and Black African men were significant less likely to be receiving professional mental health treatment for mood or anxiety disorders. Using structural equation modeling to test a model of help-seeking in men, Vogel, Heimerdinger-Edwards, Hammer, and Hubbard (2011) found that although there was a strong relationship between conformity to masculine norms and help-seeking behaviors, this relationship differed significantly among White, Asian American, and Black men.

Similar studies have investigated physical health disparities as well. For example, a Centers for Disease Control and Prevention (CDC; 2013) report breaking down men's leading causes of death by race demonstrates that although homicide ranked as the fifth leading cause for Black men (ninth for Hispanic men, and 10th for American Indian men), it did not rank in the top 10 causes for racially aggregated data. This finding, only possible through data disaggregation, may help direct attention toward targeting the underlying causes of Black men's high rates of death by homicide. Understanding the rate at which men from different ethnic/racial backgrounds experience health issues and seek professional help, as well as the reasons why they do so, is essential to reducing health disparities due to oppression and privilege. By studying these differences, health professionals can begin to tackle the barriers that may keep men of color from receiving the care they need.

By studying men of color's educational outcomes, researchers can also begin to understand what forces of inequity and oppression may be at play in the resultant disparities we see between men of different ethnic/racial groups. Comparing Latino, Mexicano, White, Black, and Asian American men in community colleges, Harris, Wood, and Newman (2015) found that different factors related to masculinity were linked to academic focus and effort for diverse ethnic/racial groups. For example, healthy perceptions of men as breadwinners were correlated with academic effort for Mexicano and Latino men but not for Black, Asian American, or White men. Studies like these that investigate factors affecting educational outcomes may help prevention professionals identify risk and protective factors for men of color in higher education.

Additionally, a body of research has looked at perceptions and stereotypes of men of color. Y. J. Wong, Horn, and Chen (2013) had study participants picture the "typical" White, Black, or Asian American man and found that Black men were rated as the most masculine and Asian American men as least masculine among the three groups. A content analysis of magazine advertisements found similar results, in that Black and White models were more frequently portrayed as tough and "macho" than Asian models (Shaw & Tan, 2014). In a two-study analysis, one team of researchers investigated the idea that certain ethnic or racial groups are perceived as more masculine or feminine, which results in gendered race prototypes, or stereotypical racial representations that are gender specific. For example, because Black Americans are generally perceived as masculine and Asian Americans are generally perceived as feminine, a Black man is more prototypical than a Black woman and an Asian American woman is more prototypical than an Asian American man (Schug et al., 2015). This team found support for gendered race prototypes in that statements made by Asian American men were least likely to be remembered by undergraduate participants and that when asked to write a story about a person of a certain ethnicity, undergraduates were significantly less likely to write about a man when assigned to write about an Asian American individual and significantly less likely to write about a woman when assigned to write about a Black individual. Thus, it seems that gendered racial stereotypes affect individuals' implicit perceptions.

## Studies Comparing Men and Women
## From the Same Racial/Ethnic Group

Studies that compare men and women from the same ethnic group have found similar patterns as studies between groups of men and have also broadened our understanding of men of color in unique ways. For example, several studies have investigated one of two competing hypotheses: the cumulative discrimination hypothesis (Beal, 1979) and the subordinate male target hypothesis (Sidanius & Pratto, 1999). The cumulative discrimination hypothesis suggests that because women of color hold (at least) two marginalized identities, they experience greater inequity than men. In contrast, the subordinate male target hypothesis asserts that men from ethnic/racial minority groups may face greater oppression than their female counterparts. This is because, from an evolutionary perspective, racial discrimination is conceptualized as a form of intrasex competition in which men seek to prevent outgroup men from obtaining material and symbolic resources (Sidanius & Pratto, 1999).

Some gender-stratified studies have found support for the cumulative disadvantage hypothesis; for example, Asian American and Black women experience more stress or are more negatively affected by discrimination than Asian American and Black men (Hahm, Ozonoff, Gaumond, & Sue, 2010; Landers, Rollock, Rolfes, & Moore, 2011). But other studies have found that men of color experience more discrimination than women from their racial groups, which would support the subordinate male target hypothesis (Brondolo et al., 2015; Liang, Alvarez, Juang, & Liang, 2007; Yoshihama, Bybee, & Blazevski, 2012). In these studies, discrimination and racism were experienced and reported more by Asian American, Latino, Black, and Indian (Gujarati) men than women. Further investigation is needed to understand the contexts in which the cumulative disadvantage hypothesis and the subordinate male target hypothesis might hold true in intersectional studies of race and gender.

In investigations of attitudes toward help-seeking, studies of men of color have found that Asian American and Black men were less likely to seek professional help than were women of the same racial/ethnic groups (Liang et al., 2007; Ward, Wiltshire, Detry, & Brown, 2013). The findings of these two studies mirror those found in studies of men and women of all ethnicities, but other investigations show more complex patterns. For example, one study that compared Black and Latino men and women found that Black men had less favorable attitudes toward therapy than did Black women, but Latino men had more favorable attitudes toward therapy than did Latina women (Chiang, Hunter, & Yeh, 2004). It may be that the reason for the differences between men and women of color is not simply gender, but the impact of their culture on their gender attitudes. For example, in commenting on their surprising finding regarding Latino men and women, Chiang and colleagues (2004) suggested that perhaps Latina women have stronger cultural self-identification than Latino men and are therefore more inclined to seek support from sources more accepted by their culture (e.g., family) than from professionals. It is clear that the interplay between gender and race is multi-dimensional, multidirectional, and changes depending on cultural differences.

## Evaluation and Future Directions

A key contribution of the intergroup paradigm to intersectionality research is that it highlights subpopulations of men that deserve greater research or clinical attention (Bowleg, 2013). This is particularly important in health disparities research in which a particular subgroup's elevated risk (e.g., Black men's vulnerability to homicide) might not be as visible when that subgroup is classified within a broader racial (e.g., Black) or gender category (e.g., men). From a multicultural perspective, the identification of subpopulations of men that are at risk for adverse outcomes allows for a tai-lored approach to treatment and prevention that takes into account salient norms and customs within these subpopulations (Y. J. Wong, Vaughan, & Klann, in press). To illustrate, among gay and bisexual men from diverse racial groups, Black men accounted for the largest proportion of men diag-nosed with HIV infection in 2013 (39%; CDC, 2015). The identification of this at-risk group has enabled prevention professionals to develop interven-tions that address the customs and nomenclature salient to these Black men. For instance, many Black men who have sex with men do not identify as gay or bisexual at all; therefore, prevention professionals need to be familiar with the diversity of identity labels used by such men (e.g., *men on the down low*) in their outreach efforts to this population (e.g., Bowleg, 2013; Mays, Cochran, & Zamudio, 2004).

We also consider two serious conceptual limitations inherent in the inter-group paradigm. For one, this paradigm is premised on an additive approach to intersectionality that assumes people's multiple social identities are dis-tinct and summative (e.g., *I am Black, and I am also a man*) rather than inher-ently intertwined (e.g., *I am simply a Black man*). This additive approach has been criticized by some intersectionality scholars as incongruent with people's experiences of their social identities (Bowleg, 2008; Shields, 2008), a limitation we address in our subsequent discussion of the intersectional uniqueness paradigm.

Another serious limitation of the intergroup paradigm is that social categories such as race and gender are implicitly used as proxies for underlying constructs (e.g., racism-related stress), yet these constructs are not explicitly tested (Cole, 2009). Simply showing that White and Black men differ on several outcomes reveals nothing about why these differences exist. A focus on differences across social categories, rather than the underlying constructs associated with these social categories, might also produce the unintended consequence of reifying group differences, stereotyping underrepresented groups, and ignoring within-group diversity. To address these shortcomings, we turn to the interconstruct paradigm.

## INTERCONSTRUCT PARADIGM

The interconstruct paradigm addresses some of the aforementioned limitations in the intergroup paradigm by shifting the focus of intersectionality research from group comparisons to testing the relations among constructs associated with individuals' social identities. To the extent that multiple social identities are interdependent (Cole, 2009), individuals' experiences associated with their social identities (e.g., racism, acculturation, and ethnic identity) should also be interrelated. Given our focus on the intersection of race, ethnicity, and gender as applied to racial/ethnic minority men, our literature review focuses in particular on the associations among gender, race, ethnicity, and culture-related constructs.

Before proceeding, we define several constructs used in this section of the chapter. *Ethnic identity and racial identity* refer to one's sense of self or social identity as a member of an ethnic group (e.g., Korean Americans; Phinney, 2003) and racial group (e.g., Asian Americans), respectively (Helms & Parham, 1996). Both ethnic and racial identities are multidimensional constructs. For example, ethnic identity encompasses dimensions such as ethnic belonging as well as ethnic behaviors and customs, whereas racial identity includes diverse attitudes associated with racial identity statuses, such as preencounter (denigrating one's racial group) and internalization (a sense of pride in one's membership in a racial group; Helms & Parham, 1996). We use the term *cultural orientation* to refer to people of color's orientation toward their own ethnic culture as well as the dominant culture (Shin, Wong, & Maffini, 2016); these include *acculturation* (i.e., the degree of adherence to the dominant culture), *enculturation* (i.e., the extent of adherence to one's own ethnic culture), and *biculturalism* (i.e., high levels of acculturation and enculturation; Maffini & Wong, 2012).

### Interconstruct Studies

Drawing on the idea that social perceptions are influenced by intersecting identities, a few studies have examined the link between race- and gender-related perceptions. In one study, college students watched video clips of Black and White women and men engaged in various body movements (Wilkins, Chan, & Kaiser, 2011). The more stereotypically Black the target was perceived to be, the more the targets were rated as high on masculinity, thus underscoring the link between perceived Blackness and perceived masculinity. Similarly, Johnson, Freeman, and Pauker (2012) demonstrated that college students who held strong implicit associations between the categories of Black/male and Asian/female (as measured by the Implicit Association Test) exhibited greater sex categorization biases (e.g., slower response in categorizing Asian male faces as male). Collectively, these studies highlight the gendered nature of race and the idea that perceptions of race and gender are interdependent (Johnson et al., 2012).

To the extent that social perceptions of race and gender are correlated with each other, racism might also have an impact on men of color's masculinity-related experiences. There are several conceptual explanations for why racism might have gendered consequences for men of color. For one, aspects of dominant White American masculine norms (e.g., being assertive and controlling one's emotions) might be at odds with the masculine norms of cultural minority groups (e.g., emotional expression for Latino men and humility for Asian American men; Levant et al., 2015; Y. J. Wong, Nguyen, et al., 2012). Therefore, men of color might encounter racism expressed as social disapproval for their lack of conformity to White American masculine norms (Y. J. Wong, Tsai, Liu, Zhu, & Wei, 2014). For another, racism can be conceptualized as an impediment to men of color's ability to actualize goals relevant to traditional masculine roles, such as demonstrating power and control (Hammond, Fleming, & Villa-Torres, 2016). To illustrate, a Latino man who experiences career barriers as a result of racism at his workplace might feel that he cannot live up to the masculine gender role of being a breadwinner. Consequently, O'Neil (2008) argued that racism constitutes a form of psychological emasculation for men of color. In similar terms, racism might constitute a threat to men of color's self-efficacy, which threatens their masculine self-concept (Goff, Di Leone, & Kahn, 2012). In support of this hypothesis, Goff et al. (2012) demonstrated that Black men who were assigned to be exposed to racial discrimination became more attuned to masculinity threat cues, although racial discrimination did not affect White men's vigilance to masculinity threat cues. Similarly, Vinson (2010) found that ethnic discrimination was positively correlated with gender role conflict in a racially diverse sample of men.

Not only does racism have gendered consequences, it might also interact with masculinity-related constructs to affect negative psychosocial outcomes. In one study, perceived racism exacerbated the positive associations between Latino masculinity ideologies and various dimensions of gender role conflict among Latino men (Liang, Salcedo, & Miller, 2011). In another, Asian male international students' experience of racial discrimination was positively linked to subjective masculinity stress only when being a man was central to their self-concept (Y. J. Wong, Tsai, et al., 2014).

Beyond social perceptions and racism, a cluster of studies have examined the link between masculinity constructs and racial/ethnic identities and cultural orientation among men of color. Men of color's cultural orientation has been shown to be associated with gender role conflict, although findings on this association have not been consistent. Leka (1998) found that Mexican American men who were high on biculturalism scored lower on the restrictive emotionality dimension of gender role conflict than those from other acculturative typologies (e.g., low on biculturalism). Among Asian American men, enculturation to Asian values positively predicted several dimensions of gender role conflict (Liu & Iwamoto, 2006), whereas another study found that acculturation was negatively related to restrictive emotionality but positively associated with success, power, and competition (Kim, O'Neil, & Owen, 1996).

Studies on the link between racial and ethnic identities and masculinity-related constructs have also produced mixed findings. In a study of Black, Latino, and White men, Abreu, Goodyear, Campos, and Newcomb (2000) found that the ethnic belonging dimension of ethnic identity (defined as the degree of attachment to one's ethnic group) was the strongest, positive predictor of traditional masculinity ideology over and beyond participants' demographic ethnicities. This finding underscores the value of focusing on ethnicity-related constructs rather than on ethnicity as a social category in intersectionality research. In another study of racially diverse men, the overall construct of ethnic identity was not significantly correlated with gender role conflict and its dimensions, with the exception of a modest, positive association with the dimension of success, power, and competition (Vinson, 2010).

Beyond ethnic identity, several studies have identified links between dimensions of racial identity and gender role conflict (see O'Neil, 2015). Studies on Black men have generally found that racial identities that are externally defined, less mature, or that reflect internalized racism were related to greater gender role conflict (Carter, Williams, Juby, & Buckley, 2005; Wade, 1996; Wester, Vogel, Wei, & McLain, 2006). To the extent that gender role conflict reflects White American cultural norms, these findings make sense because Black men with less mature racial identity statuses may idealize White American culture and therefore experience greater gender role conflict (Carter et al., 2005). Nevertheless, researchers have found different patterns in the link between racial identity statuses and gender role conflict for Asian American and Latino men. For these men, the racial identity statuses of dissonance (conflicting attitudes toward White and minority groups), resistance (an active rejection of European American culture) and internalization (secure sense of one's racial identity) were positively associated with gender role conflict (Carter et al., 2005; Liu, 2002). Overall, these conflicting findings are difficult to reconcile and reflect the need for greater theoretical grounding in understanding the relations among masculinity constructs and racial, ethnic, and cultural identity–related constructs.

## Evaluation and Future Directions

Overall, the interconstruct paradigm contributes to intersectionality research in several important ways. Research in this paradigm addresses calls by intersectionality scholars to address within-group diversity rather than focus solely on group comparisons (Parent, DeBlaere, & Moradi, 2013). In so doing, interconstruct research underscores the notion that racial/ethnic minority men deserve to be studied in their own right without the need for group comparisons with other social groups (e.g., women and Whites; Stewart & McDermott, 2004). By turning the spotlight to the associations among racial, cultural, and gender constructs, the interconstruct paradigm also emphasizes that it is not social identity categories per se (e.g., Native American men) but experiences associated with these categories (e.g., racism) that shape individuals' lives (Cole, 2009). Importantly, these constructs draw direct attention to a central tenet of the intersectionality framework: the idea that multiple identities reflect systems of power, privilege, oppression, and inequity, such as racism and traditional masculinity ideology (Shields, 2008).

Despite these strengths, intersectionality research in this paradigm is still in its infancy compared with the intergroup paradigm, and several limitations warrant attention. Most research in this area has focused on the relations among race, ethnicity, and masculinity-related constructs rather than on how these constructs conjointly influence other outcomes (for exceptions, see Liang et al., 2011; Y. J. Wong, Tsai, et al., 2014). More research that examines interaction effects involving such constructs is needed. To illustrate, researchers can study whether racial identity buffers or accentuates the relation between men of color's adherence to traditional masculinity ideology and well-being. Such research has the potential to present a more nuanced analysis of how diverse constructs associated with power, privilege, and oppression interact to influence men of color's well-being.

Another limitation is that interconstruct research has focused mainly on individual-level variables rather than on macro-level racial or gender constructs, such as country-level masculinity (Hofstede, 2016) or the racial/ethnic density of a community (e.g., Hong, Zhang, & Walton, 2014). Given the focus of the intersectionality framework on multiple systems of oppression and power (Cole, 2009), it behooves researchers to study these constructs at the systemic level. To illustrate, researchers could use multilevel modeling to investigate whether the proportion of men in an organization (an organization-level construct) interacts with racial/ethnic minority men's experiences of racism (an individual-level construct) to impact their well-being in diverse organizations (Y. J. Wong & Horn, 2016).

A third limitation is that interconstruct research, particularly studies on the interface of masculinities and racial/ethnic identities and cultural constructs, tends to lack a strong theoretical grounding. The atheoretical nature of such research might in part explain the morass of conflicting findings on the links among racial identity, cultural orientation, and masculinity-related constructs described in the aforementioned literature review. What is needed are comprehensive intersectionality theories and theoretical models that clearly articulate why, how, when, and for whom race-related and masculinity-related constructs are linked. Several recent attempts have been made to develop new theoretical models that explain the relations among race- and masculinity-related constructs. Building on social self-preservation theory and challenge-threat appraisal theories, Hammond et al. (2016) proposed a theoretical model that conceptualizes everyday racism as a social evaluative threat to Black men's masculine self as well as the processes through which these constructs ultimately result in Black male health disparities. Additionally, O'Neil (2015) proposed a multicultural model of the psychology of men in which oppressive macro-level influences, such as racism, stereotypes, and institutional discrimination, influence micro-level multicultural variables (e.g., racial identities), which in turn influence gender role conflict and well-being. These efforts should be commended and expanded. To illustrate, scholars have posited that men of color who have experienced racial threats to their masculinity from immigration and acculturative stress might resort to sexism and patriarchal behaviors (e.g., domestic violence) to reassert their masculine self (Liu & Chang, 2007; Wester, 2008). This hypothesis could be tested empirically and also developed into a more comprehensive intersectionality theory that explains the relation between acculturative stress and sexism.

Finally, a key limitation of interconstruct research is that it lacks appropriate terminology to describe men of color's experience of gender-based discrimination (Bowleg, 2012). Although sexism is often viewed as an oppressive experience affecting women rather than men, men of color may experience unique forms of gender-based discrimination that are interlaced with racism (Liang et al., 2010). These experiences are not adequately captured by current research rooted the interconstruct paradigm. To address this limitation, we turn to the intersectional uniqueness paradigm.

## INTERSECTIONAL UNIQUENESS PARADIGM

The intersectional uniqueness paradigm focuses on how the intersection of social identities creates unique, nonadditive experiences. In her article that first proposed the concept of intersectionality, Crenshaw (1989) argued that although sometimes Black women experienced the combined effects of discrimination arising from race and sex, sometimes they also "experience discrimination as Black women—not the sum of race and sex discrimination, but as Black women" (p. 139). This emphasis on unique experiences is premised on the proposition that social identities are inherently intertwined; thus, experiences associated with multiple identities cannot be separated, nor can they be simply added together to account for individuals' overall experiences (Cole & Zucker, 2007). To illustrate, the experiences of a Native American man cannot be understood simply by adding the experiences of being a man to being Native American. Rather, each intersection of social identities creates distinctive experiences of social status, oppression, and privileges. Therefore, the experiences of men of color are qualitatively different from those of women of the same racial or ethnic groups and from men of other racial groups. Studies based on the intersectional uniqueness paradigm focus on either the salient experiences of one social group based on individuals' multiple social identities (e.g., Asian American men) or qualitative (rather than quantitative) differences between social groups. In this section, we review three areas of research in which scholars have used this paradigm to study men of color: men's construction of their social identities, masculine norms, and gendered racism.

## Studies on Intersectional Uniqueness and the Construction of Social Identities

The first area of intersectional uniqueness research that we present relates to how men of color conceptualize their own identities on the basis of the intersection of race, ethnicity, and gender. Researchers who are interested in this topic might address the question "What does it mean to be a Black/Asian/Latino/Native American man?" using qualitative methods. To illustrate, studies have shown that Black men construct masculinity with a stronger relational and ethical focus than White men (Hunter & Davis, 1992, 1994; Rogers et al., 2015). Analyzing open-ended answers to the question "What does manhood mean to you?" Hammond and Mattis (2005) found that mainstream masculinity expectations were rarely endorsed by Black men. Rather, responsibility and accountability were viewed as the most salient features of manhood, endorsed by almost half of the participants. In addition, consistent with other researchers (Hunter & Davis, 1992, 1994), they found that Black men defined their manhood with relational and spiritual emphases. They valued family centeredness, community involvement, and spirituality in their understanding of what it means to be a man. Building on Hammond and Mattis's (2005) study, Rogers et al. (2015) elicited responses to the core question "What characteristics should Black men have?" and found that "positive role model" was the most commonly endorsed theme. The authors interpreted this as indicating that Black men adopted this strategy to cope with the systemic barriers created by racism. That is, they constructed their culturally unique definition of masculinity in the context of racial oppression and institutional barriers.

In another qualitative study, Pompper (2010) found almost all Black, Latino, and Asian American male participants explained that their individual understanding of masculinity was steeped in their ethnic culture, whereas White men never mentioned culture. Pride, conflict, and responsibility were major themes addressed by these men of color in their definitions of masculinity, issues that White men rarely raised. In general, studies on the construction of meaning of manhood among men of color challenge the view that masculinity is a unitary entity that cuts across culture, race, and ethnicity. Rather, the meaning of manhood is unique at the intersection of race and gender.

## Studies on Intersectional Uniqueness and Masculine Norms

The second area of research that is based on the intersectional uniqueness paradigm is the investigation of masculinity norms in specific ethnic and racial groups. Masculine norms do not exist in a vacuum independent of race and culture. Rather, to the extent that intersecting social identities are associated with unique experiences, the content of masculine norms is also dependent on specific racial, ethnic, and cultural contexts. Hence, some masculine norms in cultural minority groups likely differ from those in White American culture. For example, Arciniega, Anderson, Tovar-Blank, and Tracey (2008) argued that machismo norms in Mexican culture comprise at least two dimensions: traditional machismo and *caballerismo*. Interestingly, caballerismo, which focuses on emotional connectedness, is diametrically different from the masculine norm of emotional control in White American culture (Mahalik et al., 2003). Arciniega et al. also developed a scale to assess these two dimensions of machismo in Mexican culture. Results on this new scale showed that traditional machismo was correlated with negative outcomes such as antisocial behavior, whereas caballerismo was related to positive outcomes such as problem-solving coping.

Research on Asians and Asian Americans also suggests that some Asian masculine norms may be qualitatively different from White American masculine norms (Chua & Fujino, 1999). In a cross-country study of masculinity in five Asian countries, participants reported that "having a good job" was the most important attribute of being a man. Asian men also valued family relationships and financial stability over sexual attributes, compared with Western men (Ng, Tan, & Low, 2008). Similarly, a study of university students' perceptions of the most important masculine norms in Singapore identified norms that were similar to those in Western cultures (e.g., emotional toughness) as well as those that differed from norms in Western cultures, such as nonaggression and fidelity in monogamous relationships (Y. J. Wong, Ho, Wang, & Fisher, 2016). In summary, the idea of intersectional uniqueness has inspired researchers to identify culture-specific masculine norms that may include dimensions that differ qualitatively from White American masculine norms.

## Studies on Intersectional Uniqueness and Gendered Racism and Stereotypes

Arguably, the most fertile area of research based on the intersectional uniqueness paradigm is the study of gendered racism and stereotypes. A cluster of studies have focused on identifying salient dimensions of stereotypes of racial minority men (Ghavami & Peplau, 2013; Schwing et al., 2013). These studies are premised on the notion that racial stereotypes are intrinsically gendered and gender stereotypes are inherently racialized (Liang et al., 2010).

Studies that apply the intersectional uniqueness paradigm to Asian American men have identified at least eight potential stereotypes that speak to Asian American men's experience of gendered racism in the United States. Results from interviews, media analysis, and survey studies have shown that Asian American men are stereotyped as martial art experts, asexual nerds, unattractive romantic partners, emasculated males, lacking in leadership skills, untrustworthy villains, excessively competitive, and overly patriarchal (Cheng, 1996a, 1996b; Chua & Fujino, 1999; Do, 2006; Ghavami & Peplau, 2013; Guo & Harlow, 2014; Ho, 2011; Liu, Iwamoto, & Chae, 2011; Mok, 1998; Niemann, Jennings, Rozelle, Baxter, & Sullivan, 1994; Phua, 2007; Wilkins et al., 2011; R. P. Wong, 2008; Y. J. Wong et al., 2013; Y. J. Wong, Owen, et al., 2012). These stereotypes are particularly striking because some of them differ dramatically from stereotypes about Asian American women. For instance, the unattractive, asexual stereotype of Asian American men is in direct contrast to the hypersexualized stereotype of Asian American women (Shimizu, 2007), thus underscoring the distinctiveness of gendered racist stereotypes.

In contrast to the hypomasculine stereotypes of Asian American men, stereotypes of Black men are diametrically different. They are viewed as dangerous criminals and aggressors and are portrayed as absent and irresponsible fathers (Schwing & Wong, 2014). In conflict with the intelligent but physically weak image of Asian American men, Black men are assumed to be gifted sports players with lower intellectual abilities (Schwing et al., 2013). They are also viewed as angry, poor, lazy, hypersexual, tall, and gangsters (Ghavami & Peplau, 2013).

Consistent with Black men, Latino men are also stereotyped as hypermasculine, but in different ways. Despite diverse conceptions of machismo, the stereotype of machismo as applied to Latino men only focuses on the exaggerated negative aspects of masculine roles. These distorted images of Latino men depict them as sexist machos, heavy drinkers, domineering, and sexually promiscuous (Ghavami & Peplau, 2013; Niemann, 2001). They are thus viewed as endorsing an extreme form of traditional masculine ideology.

Stereotypes of American Indian/Native American men reflect perceptions of rigid social roles. The most prominent images are "the doomed warrior"; the wild, passionate, exotic, sexual savage; or "the wise elder" who is highly knowledgeable (Bird, 1999). Although the warrior stereotype is highly sexualized, the wise elder is desexualized. These binary stereotypes were also noted by Rouse (2016), who observed that the polar opposite stereotypes of warrior chief and mystic shaman reflected an imposition of the traditional gender paradigm to Native American cultures. The warrior chief is brutal, while the mystic shaman is highly romanticized.

Our literature review also uncovered research that compared gender-by-race stereotypes of Asian, Black, Latino, and Middle Eastern Americans. Researchers identified several unique race-by-gender stereotypes for men and women of each race that were not simply the sum of gender and racial stereotypes (Ghavami & Peplau, 2013; Jackson, Lewandowski, Ingram, & Hodge, 1997). For example, the stereotypes of Asian American men as effeminate and having small penises were not shared with any other gender or racial groups (Ghavami & Peplau, 2013).

Another line of research on gendered stereotypes and racism relates to the development of scales to measure these constructs. For instance, Schwing et al. (2013) developed the African American Men's Gendered Racism Stress Inventory (AMGRaSI) with three subscales to assess Black men's perceived gendered racism based on stereotypes of Black men as physically and sexually violent, absent fathers, and gifted sportsmen. Schwing et al. demonstrated that Black men's experience of gendered racism stress, as measured by the AMGRaSI, uniquely predicted psychological distress above and beyond what could be explained by generic racism stress and masculine gender role stress (Schwing et al., 2013), thus lending support to the idea that gendered racism is a unique phenomenon.

In sum, our literature review demonstrates that some stereotypes about specific groups of men of color are qualitatively different from those of women from the same racial group as well as stereotypes of men from other racial groups. In general, stereotypes of men of color tend to portray men of color as exhibiting deviant forms of masculinities that are benchmarked against White standards of masculinities. Some racial groups (e.g., Black and Latino men) are stereotyped as exhibiting negative forms of hypermasculinity, while men of other races (e.g., Asian American men) are stereotyped as insufficiently masculine.

## Evaluation and Future Directions

Several strengths in the intersectional uniqueness paradigm are noteworthy. First, by emphasizing the interdependent nature of social identities and associated experiences, this paradigm enables researchers to examine the ways in which meanings of race, culture, and masculinities are intertwined. Such a conceptualization avoids the pitfall of assuming that the content of masculine norms, stereotypes, and racism is invariant across culture and gender.

Second, the intersectional uniqueness paradigm's emphasis on distinct experiences arising from the nexus of social identities addresses an important limitation in the intergroup paradigm's focus on the independent and summative effects of multiple identities (Shields, 2008). In contrast, research that captures the intersectional uniqueness of multiple identities best reflects the complex reality of men of color's lived experiences.

A third strength of this paradigm is the diversity of research methods that can address the intersectional uniqueness of men of color's experiences. Qualitative methods, such as interviews, can be used to explore men of color's conjoint experiences of race and gender (e.g., Rogers et al., 2015). Similarly, as illustrated by Schwing et al.'s (2013) scale development project on Black men's experiences of gendered racism stress, quantitative methods can also be used to measure constructs that reflect intersectional uniqueness.

Despite these strengths, there is a dearth of empirical research applying this paradigm to the study of men of color. For instance, scale development research focusing on constructs that reflect intersectional uniqueness is still in its infancy. Although researchers have developed two measures of internalization of stereotypes concerning Asian American men (Do, 2006; R. P. Wong, 2008), there are currently no scales that assess Latinos', Native Americans', and Asian Americans' experiences of gendered racism and stereotypes as exhibited by others.

Similarly, the promise of the intersectional uniqueness paradigm has not been fully realized in qualitative research. Although many qualitative studies have examined men of color's perceptions of manhood or masculinity, several of these studies (e.g., Hammond & Mattis, 2005; Hurtado & Sinha, 2008) did not explicitly invite participants to discuss their experiences as men from specific racial groups (e.g., Latino men). Thus, we encourage more qualitative and quantitative research on men of color's experiences of social identities, masculine norms, and gendered racism that is explicitly grounded in the intersectional uniqueness paradigm.

Finally, there is an overall lack of intersectional uniqueness research on Native American men. Linguistic scholars have documented that Native American worldviews and languages do not recognize the gender binary

(Rouse, 2016). Rather, they recognize three or four genders. Instead of assigning gender roles based on biological sex, traditional Native American cultures assign their role by one's purpose for an individual, community, or Nation. Thus, American Indian/Native American men may adopt a broader range of normative gender possibilities than men from other races, who follow prescribed and restricted gender norms. Their flexible definition of gender may allow American Indian/Native American men to assume roles or responsibilities that are traditionally considered to be for women (Rouse, 2016). Despite these postulations, empirical research on the unique masculine norms and subjective meanings of manhood among Native Americans is sorely lacking.

## OVERALL RECOMMENDATIONS AND CONCLUSIONS

We conclude this chapter with three overall recommendations for future intersectionality scholarship on the psychology of racial/ethnic minority men. First, we echo Cole's (2009) call for researchers to examine the diversity within social categories to address who is included and excluded in research. In the United States, intersectionality research on men of color tends to privilege racial diversity over ethnic diversity. Far more research has been conducted on Asian, Black, and Latino American men than on ethnic groups such as Asian Indian, Jamaican, and Cuban American men. Additionally, psychological research is lacking on Native American and Alaskan men (Rouse, 2016) and boys of color, as well as on racial minority men in countries beyond the United States. Clearly, more research is needed on these populations.

Second, it is worth emphasizing that as a conceptual framework, intersectionality does not merely emphasize the need to study individuals' multiple social identities but also how these identities reflect systems of power, privilege, oppression, and inequity (Bowleg, 2012; Shields, 2008). Hence, it is not sufficient for intersectionality researchers simply to identify differences between groups of individuals with diverse social identities; they must also explain how these differences relate to structural constructs such as sexism, White privilege, and internalized racism. In this regard, one fruitful area for the advancement of intersectionality scholarship is the development of theories that can adequately explain men of color's experiences of power, privilege, oppression, and inequity. Throughout this chapter, we have highlighted a few of these emerging theories and theoretical models (e.g., Hammond et al., 2016). Our hope is that scholars will build on and synthesize these theories to provide a comprehensive account of racial and ethnic minority men's lived experiences.

Third, we encourage psychologists to adopt an interdisciplinary perspective in their research on intersectionality. Psychology is not the only discipline to use the intersectionality framework in research on men of color. We therefore urge psychologists to be familiar with the theories, constructs, and research methods from other disciplines, such as women's studies (e.g., McCall, 2005) and sociology (e.g., Choo & Ferree, 2010) to foster the cross-fertilization of ideas. In so doing, psychologists can contribute to and learn from other disciplines. For instance, Christensen and Jensen (2014) argued that although the concept of hegemonic masculinity developed by sociologist Raewyn Connell acknowledges the hegemony of some masculinities over others, it does not sufficiently address the power relations between diverse groups of men based on their multiple identities. In this regard, psychological intersectionality research methods, theories (e.g., gendered race theory), and constructs (e.g., gendered racism) could be used to enrich the concept of hegemonic masculinity and the sociological study of men and masculinities.

In this chapter, we discussed three intersectionality research paradigms for the psychological study of racial/ethnic minority men. We examined the intergroup paradigm, which examines intersectionality through the use of quantitative comparisons between social groups (e.g., Black men vs. Black women). Next, we discussed the interconstruct paradigm, which focuses on the relations among constructs associated with individuals' social identities (e.g., the link between men of color's racial identity and gender role conflict). Finally, we reviewed the intersectionality uniqueness paradigm, which addresses unique nonadditive experiences arising from the intersection of multiple social identities. An overarching theme in this chapter is that there are diverse approaches to studying intersectionality. We therefore encourage researchers interested in intersectionality research to be aware of the strengths and limitations of the three research paradigms and to be explicit about which research paradigms they use in their research. Our hope is that these paradigms will draw attention to the benefits of applying the intersectionality framework to clinical practice and research on men of color as well as help researchers and clinicians think more critically and intentionally about how to conceptualize men of color's experiences from an intersectionality framework.

## REFERENCES

Abreu, J. M., Goodyear, R. K., Campos, A., & Newcomb, M. D. (2000). Ethnic belonging and traditional masculinity ideology among African Americans, European Americans, and Latinos. *Psychology of Men & Masculinity, 1,* 75–86. http://dx.doi.org/10.1037/1524-9220.1.2.75

Arciniega, G. M., Anderson, T. C., Tovar-Blank, Z. G., & Tracey, T. J. (2008). Toward a fuller conception of machismo: Development of a traditional machismo and caballerismo scale. *Journal of Counseling Psychology, 55*, 19–33. http://dx.doi.org/10.1037/0022-0167.55.1.19

Beal, F. (1979). Double jeopardy: To be Black and female. In T. Cade (Ed.), *The Black woman* (pp. 90–100). New York, NY: New American Library.

Beals, J., Novins, D. K., Whitesell, N. R., Spicer, P., Mitchell, C. M., & Manson, S. M. (2005). Prevalence of mental disorders and utilization of mental health services in two American Indian reservation populations: Mental health disparities in a national context. *The American Journal of Psychiatry, 162*, 1723–1732. http://dx.doi.org/10.1176/appi.ajp.162.9.1723

Bird, S. E. (1999). Gendered construction of the American Indian in popular media. *Journal of Communication, 49*, 61–83. http://dx.doi.org/10.1111/j.1460-2466.1999.tb02805.x

Bowleg, L. (2008). When Black + lesbian + woman ≠ Black lesbian woman: The methodological challenges of qualitative and quantitative intersectionality research. *Sex Roles, 59*, 312–325. http://dx.doi.org/10.1007/s11199-008-9400-z

Bowleg, L. (2012). The problem with the phrase *women and minorities*: Intersectionality—An important theoretical framework for public health. *American Journal of Public Health, 102*, 1267–1273. http://dx.doi.org/10.2105/AJPH.2012.300750

Bowleg, L. (2013). "Once you've blended the cake, you can't take the parts back to the main ingredients": Black gay and bisexual men's descriptions and experiences of intersectionality. *Sex Roles, 68*, 754–767. http://dx.doi.org/10.1007/s11199-012-0152-4

Brondolo, E., Monge, A., Agosta, J., Tobin, J. N., Cassells, A., Stanton, C., & Schwartz, J. (2015). Perceived ethnic discrimination and cigarette smoking: Examining the moderating effects of race/ethnicity and gender in a sample of Black and Latino urban adults. *Journal of Behavioral Medicine, 38*, 689–700. http://dx.doi.org/10.1007/s10865-015-9645-2

Carter, R. T., Williams, B., Juby, H. L., & Buckley, T. R. (2005). Racial identity as mediator of the relationship between gender role conflict and severity of psychological symptoms in Black, Latino, and Asian men. *Sex Roles, 53*, 473–486. http://dx.doi.org/10.1007/s11199-005-7135-7

Centers for Disease Control and Prevention. (2013). *Leading causes of death in males: All males by race/ethnicity.* Retrieved from http://www.cdc.gov/men/lcod/2013/race_ethnicitymen2013.pdf

Centers for Disease Control and Prevention. (2015). *HIV among African American gay and bisexual men.* Retrieved from http://www.cdc.gov/hiv/group/msm/bmsm.html

Cheng, C. (1996a). *"Nerds" need not apply: Masculinity and racial discrimination against Asian and Asian American men in an assessment center laboratory.* Unpublished manuscript, University of Southern California, Los Angeles.

Cheng, C. (1996b). "We choose not to compete": The "merit" discourse in the selection process, and Asian and Asian American men and their masculinity. In C. Cheng (Ed.), *Masculinities in organizations* (pp. 177–200). Thousand Oaks, CA: Sage.

Chiang, L., Hunter, C. D., & Yeh, C. J. (2004). Coping attitudes, sources, and practices among Black and Latino college students. *Adolescence, 39,* 793–815.

Choo, H. Y., & Ferree, M. M. (2010). Practicing intersectionality in sociological research: A critical analysis of inclusions, interactions, and institutions in the study of inequalities. *Sociological Theory, 28,* 129–149. http://dx.doi.org/10.1111/j.1467-9558.2010.01370.x

Christensen, A. D., & Jensen, S. Q. (2014). Combining hegemonic masculinity and intersectionality. *NORMA: International Journal for Masculinity Studies, 9,* 60–75.

Chua, P., & Fujino, D. (1999). Negotiating new Asian-American masculinities: Attitudes and gender expectations. *The Journal of Men's Studies, 7,* 391–413. http://dx.doi.org/10.3149/jms.0703.391

Cole, E. R. (2009). Intersectionality and research in psychology. *American Psychologist, 64,* 170–180. http://dx.doi.org/10.1037/a0014564

Cole, E. R., & Zucker, A. N. (2007). Black and White women's perspectives on femininity. *Cultural Diversity and Ethnic Minority Psychology, 13,* 1–9. http://dx.doi.org/10.1037/1099-9809.13.1.1

Crenshaw, K. (1989). Demarginalizing the intersection of race and sex: A Black feminist critique of antidiscrimination doctrine, feminist theory, and antiracist politics. *University of Chicago Legal Forum, 140,* 139–167.

Do, V. T. (2006). *Asian American men and the media: The relationship between ethnic identity, self-esteem, and the endorsement of stereotypes* [Doctoral dissertation]. Retrieved from ProQuest Dissertations & Theses. (UMI No. 3220826)

Ghavami, N., & Peplau, L. A. (2013). An intersectional analysis of gender and ethnic stereotypes: Testing three hypotheses. *Psychology of Women Quarterly, 37,* 113–127. http://dx.doi.org/10.1177/0361684312464203

Goff, P. A., Di Leone, B. A. L., & Kahn, K. B. (2012). Racism leads to pushups: How racial discrimination threatens subordinate men's masculinity. *Journal of Experimental Social Psychology, 48,* 1111–1116. http://dx.doi.org/10.1016/j.jesp.2012.03.015

Goff, P. A., & Kahn, K. B. (2013). How psychological science impedes intersectional thinking. *Du Bois Review: Social Science Research on Race, 10,* 365–384. http://dx.doi.org/10.1017/S1742058X13000313

Guo, L., & Harlow, S. (2014). User-generated racism: An analysis of stereotypes of African Americans, Latinos, and Asians in YouTube videos. *Howard Journal of Communication, 25,* 281–302.

Hahm, H. C., Ozonoff, A., Gaumond, J., & Sue, S. (2010). Perceived discrimination and health outcomes: A gender comparison among Asian-Americans nationwide. *Women's Health Issues, 20,* 350–358. http://dx.doi.org/10.1016/j.whi.2010.05.002

Hammond, W. P., Fleming, P. J., & Villa-Torres, L. (2016). Everyday racism as a threat to the masculine social self: Framing investigations of African American male health disparities. In Y. J. Wong & S. R. Wester (Eds.), *APA handbook of men and masculinities* (pp. 259–283). http://dx.doi.org/10.1037/14594-012

Hammond, W. P., & Mattis, J. S. (2005). Being a man about it: Manhood meaning among African American men. *Psychology of Men & Masculinity, 6,* 114–126. http://dx.doi.org/10.1037/1524-9220.6.2.114

Harris, F., III, Wood, J. L., & Newman, C. (2015). An exploratory investigation of the effect of racial and masculine identity on focus: An examination of White, Black, Mexicano, Latino, and Asian men in community colleges. *Culture, Society and Masculinities, 7,* 61–72.

Helms, J. E., & Parham, T. A. (1996). The development of the Racial Identity Attitude Scale. In R. L. Jones (Ed.), *Handbook of tests and measurements for Black populations.* Berkeley, CA: Cobb Henry.

Ho, H. K. (2011). *Negotiating the boundaries of (in)visibility: Asian American men and Asian/American masculinity on screen* [Doctoral dissertation]. Retrieved from ProQuest Dissertations & Theses. (UMI No. 3476446)

Hofstede, G. (2016). Masculinity at the national cultural level. In Y. J. Wong & S. R. Wester (Eds.), *APA handbook of men and masculinities* (pp. 173–186). http://dx.doi.org/10.1037/14594-008

Hong, S., Zhang, W., & Walton, E. (2014). Neighborhoods and mental health: Exploring ethnic density, poverty, and social cohesion among Asian Americans and Latinos. *Social Science & Medicine, 111,* 117–124. http://dx.doi.org/10.1016/j.socscimed.2014.04.014

Hunter, A. G., & Davis, J. E. (1992). Constructing gender: An exploration of Afro-American men's conceptualization of manhood. *Gender & Society, 6,* 464–479. http://dx.doi.org/10.1177/089124392006003007

Hunter, A. G., & Davis, J. E. (1994). Hidden voices of Black men: Meaning, structure, and complexity of manhood. *Journal of Black Studies, 25,* 20–40. http://dx.doi.org/10.1177/002193479402500102

Hurtado, A., & Sinha, M. (2008). More than men: Latino feminist masculinities and intersectionality. *Sex Roles, 59,* 337–349. http://dx.doi.org/10.1007/s11199-008-9405-7

Jackson, L. A., Lewandowski, D. A., Ingram, J. M., & Hodge, C. N. (1997). Group stereotypes: Content, gender specificity, and affect associated with typical group members. *Journal of Social Behavior & Personality, 12,* 381–396.

Johnson, K. L., Freeman, J. B., & Pauker, K. (2012). Race is gendered: How covarying phenotypes and stereotypes bias sex categorization. *Journal of Personality and Social Psychology, 102,* 116–131. http://dx.doi.org/10.1037/a0025335

Kim, E. J., O'Neil, J. M., & Owen, S. V. (1996). Asian-American men's acculturation and gender-role conflict. *Psychological Reports, 79,* 95–104. http://dx.doi.org/10.2466/pr0.1996.79.1.95

Landers, A. J., Rollock, D., Rolfes, C. B., & Moore, D. L. (2011). Police contacts and stress among African American college students. *American Journal of Orthopsychiatry, 81*, 72–81. http://dx.doi.org/10.1111/j.1939-0025.2010.01073.x

Leka, G. E. (1998). Acculturation of a Mexican American male population and gender role conflict [Master's thesis]. *Dissertation Abstracts International, 36*, 1178.

Levant, R. F., Richmond, K., Majors, R. G., Inclan, J. E., Rossello, J. M., Heesacker, M., . . . Sellers, A. (2003). A multicultural investigation of masculinity ideology and alexithymia. *Psychology of Men & Masculinity, 4*, 91–99. http://dx.doi.org/10.1037/1524-9220.4.2.91

Levant, R. F., & Wong, Y. J. (2013). Race and gender as moderators of the relationship between the endorsement of traditional masculinity ideology and alexithymia: An intersectional perspective. *Psychology of Men & Masculinity, 14*, 329–333. http://dx.doi.org/10.1037/a0029551

Levant, R. F., Wong, Y. J., Karakis, E. N., & Welsh, M. M. (2015). Mediated moderation of the relationship between restrictive emotionality and alexithymia among men from diverse racial groups. *Psychology of Men & Masculinity, 16*, 459–467. http://dx.doi.org/10.1037/a0039739

Liang, C. T. H., Alvarez, A. N., Juang, L. P., & Liang, M. X. (2007). The role of coping in the relationship between perceived racism and racism-related stress for Asian Americans: Gender differences. *Journal of Counseling Psychology, 54*, 132–141. http://dx.doi.org/10.1037/0022-0167.54.2.132

Liang, C. T. H., Rivera, A. L., Nathwani, A., Dang, P., & Douroux, A. N. (2010). Dealing with gendered racism and racial identity among Asian American men. In W. M. Liu, D. H. Iwamoto, & M. H. Chae (Eds.), *Culturally responsive counseling with Asian American men* (pp. 63–81). New York, NY: Routledge.

Liang, C. T. H., Salcedo, J., & Miller, H. A. (2011). Perceived racism, masculinity ideologies, and gender role conflict among Latino men. *Psychology of Men & Masculinity, 12*, 201–215. http://dx.doi.org/10.1037/a0020479

Liu, W. M. (2002). Exploring the lives of Asian American men: Racial identity, male role norms, gender role conflict, and prejudicial attitudes. *Psychology of Men & Masculinity, 3*, 107–118. http://dx.doi.org/10.1037/1524-9220.3.2.107

Liu, W. M., & Chang, T. (2007). Asian American masculinities. In F. T. L. Leong, A. Ebreo, L. Kinoshita, A. G. Inman, & L. H. Yang (Eds.), *Handbook of Asian American psychology* (pp. 197–211). Thousand Oaks, CA: Sage.

Liu, W. M., & Iwamoto, D. K. (2006). Asian American men's gender role conflict: The role of Asian values, self-esteem, and psychological distress. *Psychology of Men & Masculinity, 7*, 153–164. http://dx.doi.org/10.1037/1524-9220.7.3.153

Liu, W. M., Iwamoto, D. K., & Chae, M. H. (Eds.). (2011). *Culturally responsive counseling with Asian American men.* New York, NY: Routledge.

Maffini, C. S., & Wong, Y. J. (2012). Psychology of biculturalism. In G. R. Hayes & M. H. Bryant (Eds.), *Psychology of culture* (pp. 87–104). Hauppauge, NY: Nova Science.

Mahalik, J. R., Locke, B. D., Ludlow, L. H., Diemer, M. A., Scott, R. P. J., Gottfried, M., & Freitas, G. (2003). Development of the Conformity to Masculine Norms Inventory. *Psychology of Men & Masculinity, 4,* 3–25. http://dx.doi.org/10.1037/1524-9220.4.1.3

Mays, V. M., Cochran, S. D., & Zamudio, A. (2004). HIV prevention research: Are we meeting the needs of African American men who have sex with men? *Journal of Black Psychology, 30,* 78–105. http://dx.doi.org/10.1177/0095798403260265

McCall, L. (2005). The complexity of intersectionality. *Signs: Journal of Women in Culture and Society, 30,* 1771–1800. http://dx.doi.org/10.1086/426800

Mok, T. A. (1998). Getting the message: Media images and stereotypes and their effect on Asian Americans. *Cultural Diversity and Mental Health, 4,* 185–202. http://dx.doi.org/10.1037/1099-9809.4.3.185

Nash, J. (2008). Rethinking intersectionality. *Feminist Review, 89,* 1–15. http://dx.doi.org/10.1057/fr.2008.4

Ng, C. J., Tan, H. M., & Low, W. Y. (2008). What do Asian men consider as important masculinity attributes? Findings from the Asian Men's Attitudes to Life Events and Sexuality (MALES) study. *The Journal of Men's Health, 5,* 350–355. http://dx.doi.org/10.1016/j.jomh.2008.10.005

Niemann, Y. F. (2001). Stereotypes about Chicanas and Chicanos: Implications for counseling. *The Counseling Psychologist, 29,* 55–90. http://dx.doi.org/10.1177/0011000001291003

Niemann, Y. F., Jennings, L., Rozelle, R. M., Baxter, J. C., & Sullivan, E. (1994). Use of free response and cluster analysis to determine stereotypes of eight groups. *Personality and Social Psychology Bulletin, 20,* 379–390. http://dx.doi.org/10.1177/0146167294204005

O'Neil, J. M. (2008). Summarizing 25 years of research on men's gender role conflict using the Gender Role Conflict Scale. *The Counseling Psychologist, 36,* 358–445. http://dx.doi.org/10.1177/0011000008317057

O'Neil, J. M. (2012). The psychology of men. In E. M. Altmaier & J.-I. C. Hansen (Eds.), *The Oxford handbook of counseling psychology* (pp. 375–408). New York, NY: Oxford University Press.

O'Neil, J. M. (2015). *Men's gender role conflict: Psychological costs, consequences, and an agenda for change.* http://dx.doi.org/10.1037/14501-000

Parent, M. C., DeBlaere, C., & Moradi, B. (2013). Approaches to research on intersectionality: Perspectives on gender, LGBT, and racial/ethnic identities. *Sex Roles, 68,* 639–645. http://dx.doi.org/10.1007/s11199-013-0283-2

Phinney, J. S. (2003). Ethnic identity and acculturation. In K. M. Chun, P. Balls Organista, & G. Marin (Eds.), *Acculturation: Advances in theory, measurement, and applied research* (pp. 63–81). http://dx.doi.org/10.1037/10472-006

Phua, V. C. (2007). Contesting and maintaining hegemonic masculinities: Gay Asian American men in mate selection. *Sex Roles, 57,* 909–918. http://dx.doi.org/10.1007/s11199-007-9318-x

Pompper, D. (2010). Masculinities, the metrosexual, and media images: Across dimensions of age and ethnicity. *Sex Roles, 63*, 682–696. http://dx.doi.org/10.1007/s11199-010-9870-7

Rogers, B. K., Sperry, H. A., & Levant, R. F. (2015). Masculinities among African American men: An intersectional perspective. *Psychology of Men & Masculinity, 16*, 416–425. http://dx.doi.org/10.1037/a0039082

Rouse, L. M. (2016). American Indians, Alaska Natives, and the psychology of men and masculinity. In Y. J. Wong (Ed.), *APA handbook of men and masculinities* (pp. 319–337). http://dx.doi.org/10.1037/14594-015

Schug, J., Alt, N. P., & Klauer, K. C. (2015). Gendered race prototypes: Evidence for the non-prototypicality of Asian men and Black women. *Journal of Experimental Social Psychology, 56*, 121–125. http://dx.doi.org/10.1016/j.jesp.2014.09.012

Schwing, A. E., & Wong, Y. J. (2014). African American boys' and young men's experiences of racism-related stress. In W. Spielberg & K. Vaughans (Eds.), *The psychology of African American boys and young men* (pp. 107–119). Santa Barbara, CA: Praeger.

Schwing, A. E., Wong, Y. J., & Fann, M. D. (2013). Development and validation of the African American Men's Gendered Racism Stress Inventory. *Psychology of Men & Masculinity, 14*, 16–24. http://dx.doi.org/10.1037/a0028272

Shaw, P., & Tan, Y. (2014). Race and masculinity: A comparison of Asian and Western models in men's lifestyle magazine advertisements. *Journalism & Mass Communication Quarterly, 91*, 118–138. http://dx.doi.org/10.1177/1077699013514410

Shields, S. A. (2008). Gender: An intersectionality perspective. *Sex Roles, 59*, 301–311. http://dx.doi.org/10.1007/s11199-008-9501-8

Shimizu, C. P. (2007). *The hypersexuality of race: Performing Asian/American women on screen and scene.* http://dx.doi.org/10.1215/9780822389941

Shin, M., Wong, Y. J., & Maffini, C. S. (2016). Correlates of Asian American emerging adults' perceived parent–child cultural orientation: Testing a bilinear and bidimensional model. *Asian American Journal of Psychology, 7*, 31–40.

Sidanius, J., & Pratto, F. (1999). *Social dominance: An intergroup theory of social hierarchy and oppression.* http://dx.doi.org/10.1017/CBO9781139175043

Stewart, A. J., & McDermott, C. (2004). Gender in psychology. *Annual Review of Psychology, 55*, 519–544. http://dx.doi.org/10.1146/annurev.psych.55.090902.141537

Vinson, C. A. (2010). Influence of ethnic identity and perceived discrimination on male gender role conflict's impact on well-being. *Dissertation Abstracts International, 71–11.*

Vogel, D. L., Heimerdinger-Edwards, S. R., Hammer, J. H., & Hubbard, A. (2011). "Boys don't cry": Examination of the links between endorsement of masculine norms, self-stigma, and help-seeking attitudes for men from diverse backgrounds. *Journal of Counseling Psychology, 58*, 368–382. http://dx.doi.org/10.1037/a0023688

Wade, J. C. (1996). African American men's gender role conflict: The significance of racial identity. *Sex Roles, 34*, 17–33. http://dx.doi.org/10.1007/BF01544793

Ward, E. C., Wiltshire, J. C., Detry, M. A., & Brown, R. L. (2013). African American men and women's attitude toward mental illness, perceptions of stigma, and preferred coping behaviors. *Nursing Research, 62,* 185–194. http://dx.doi.org/10.1097/NNR.0b013e31827bf533

Wester, S. R. (2008). Male gender role conflict and multiculturalism: Implications for counseling psychology. *The Counseling Psychologist, 36,* 294–324. http://dx.doi.org/10.1177/0011000006286341

Wester, S. R., Vogel, D. L., Wei, M., & McLain, R. (2006). African American men, gender role conflict, and psychological distress: The role of racial identity. *Journal of Counseling & Development, 84,* 419–429. http://dx.doi.org/10.1002/j.1556-6678.2006.tb00426.x

Wilkins, C. L., Chan, J. F., & Kaiser, C. R. (2011). Racial stereotypes and interracial attraction: Phenotypic prototypicality and perceived attractiveness of Asians. *Cultural Diversity and Ethnic Minority Psychology, 17,* 427–431. http://dx.doi.org/10.1037/a0024733

Wong, R. P. (2008). Development and validation of the Stereotypes of Asian American Men Endorsement Scale (SAAMES). *Dissertation Abstracts International, 69*(4-B), 2669.

Wong, Y. J., Ho, R. M., Wang, S.-Y., & Fisher, A. (2016). Subjective masculine norms among university students in Singapore: A mixed-methods study. *Psychology of Men & Masculinity, 17,* 30–41.

Wong, Y. J., & Horn, A. J. (2016). Enhancing and diversifying research methods in the psychology of men and masculinities. In Y. J. Wong & S. R. Wester (Eds.), *APA handbook of men and masculinities* (pp. 231–255). http://dx.doi.org/10.1037/14594-011

Wong, Y. J., Horn, A. J., & Chen, S. (2013). Perceived masculinity: The potential influence of race, racial essentialist beliefs, and stereotypes. *Psychology of Men & Masculinity, 14,* 452–464. http://dx.doi.org/10.1037/a0030100

Wong, Y. J., Maffini, C. S., & Shin, M. (2014). The Racial-Cultural Framework: A framework for addressing suicide-related outcomes in communities of color. *The Counseling Psychologist, 42,* 13–54. http://dx.doi.org/10.1177/0011000012470568

Wong, Y. J., Nguyen, C. P., Wang, S.-Y., Chen, W., Steinfeldt, J. A., & Kim, B. S. K. (2012). A latent profile analysis of Asian American men's and women's adherence to cultural values. *Cultural Diversity and Ethnic Minority Psychology, 18,* 258–267. http://dx.doi.org/10.1037/a0028423

Wong, Y. J., Owen, J., & Shea, M. (2012). A latent class regression analysis of men's conformity to masculine norms and psychological distress. *Journal of Counseling Psychology, 59,* 176–183. http://dx.doi.org/10.1037/a0026206

Wong, Y. J., Owen, J., Tran, K. K., Collins, D. L., & Higgins, C. E. (2012). Asian American male college students' perceptions of people's stereotypes about Asian American men. *Psychology of Men & Masculinity, 13,* 75–88.

Wong, Y. J., Tsai, P.-C., Liu, T., Zhu, Q., & Wei, M. (2014). Male Asian international students' perceived racial discrimination, masculine identity, and subjective masculinity stress: A moderated mediation model. *Journal of Counseling Psychology, 61,* 560–569. http://dx.doi.org/10.1037/cou0000038

Wong, Y. J., Vaughan, E. L., & Klann, E. M. (in press). The science and practice of prevention from multicultural and social justice perspectives. In M. Israelashvili & J. L. Romano (Eds.), *Cambridge handbook of international prevention science.* Cambridge, England: Cambridge University Press.

Woodward, A. T. (2011). Discrimination and help-seeking: Use of professional services and informal support among African Americans, Black Caribbeans, and non-Hispanic Whites with a mental disorder. *Race and Social Problems, 3,* 146–159. http://dx.doi.org/10.1007/s12552-011-9049-z

Yoshihama, M., Bybee, D., & Blazevski, J. (2012). Day-to-day discrimination and health among Asian Indians: A population-based study of Gujarati men and women in metropolitan Detroit. *Journal of Behavioral Medicine, 35,* 471–483. http://dx.doi.org/10.1007/s10865-011-9375-z

# 10

# GAY, BISEXUAL, AND TRANSGENDER MASCULINITIES

MIKE C. PARENT AND TYLER C. BRADSTREET

As the study of masculinities has evolved, researchers have turned attention to various forms of diversity among men. Among these have been sexual orientation and gender diversity. Following the depathologization of homosexuality in the mid-20th century (culminating, among mental health professionals, with the removal of homosexuality as a formal diagnosis in the *Diagnostic and Statistical Manual of Mental Disorders*; Drescher, 2012; Silverstein, 2009), research on masculinities among gay, bisexual, and transgender (GBT) men has expanded and extended into research domains that include relationships, health, body image, and help-seeking, among other topics. The goal of the present chapter is to provide a critical overview of empirical, theory-driven research on GBT men's masculinities and to elucidate areas for growth of the field.

http://dx.doi.org/10.1037/0000023-011
*The Psychology of Men and Masculinities*, R. F. Levant and Y. J. Wong (Editors)

# THEORETICAL PARADIGMS

A variety of theoretical approaches to the study of masculinities have been used in qualitative and quantitative research. Because these approaches are reviewed in detail in other sections of this book, this brief introduction focuses solely on the approaches as they apply to research on GBT men.

Within qualitative work, the dominant theoretical perspective is Connell's (1995) hegemonic masculinity paradigm. In Connell's framework, GBT masculinities are viewed as subordinate or marginalized identities that frame other aspects of identity, and this marginalization and subordination persists even when individual men possess other privileged or high-status identities (e.g., being an athlete, being youthful and able-bodied, being physically attractive). Research in the framework of hegemonic masculinity generally seeks to understand the interrelationships of power that apply to (and thus marginalize or subordinate) GBT men.

Within quantitative inquiry, several paradigms have emerged. Often, these paradigms have reciprocal relationships with scale development; a construct is hypothesized to exist and a measure is developed to assess that construct, then the measure can be used for additional research within the paradigm. Operationalization of gender roles in this way generally takes the work of Bem (1974) as a paradigm shift in the analysis of gender in social sciences. Since the work of Bem, three major theoretical paradigms specific to understanding masculinity have emerged: gender role strain or conflict, gender role ideology, and gender role conformity.

## Gender Role Strain or Conflict, Ideology, and Conformity

As described in Chapter 1 of this volume, the *gender role strain paradigm* (GRSP), developed by Pleck (1981, 1995), posits that men may experience stress ("strain") as a result of violating prescribed gender roles. Similarly, as described in Chapter 3, the *gender role conflict* (GRC; O'Neil, 2008; O'Neil, Helm, Gable, David, & Wrightsman, 1986) paradigm posits that individuals experience conflict because of adherence to traditional gender roles (O'Neil, 2008). Specifically, O'Neil (2008) posited that nonheterosexual men may have lower scores on measures of GRC as a result of forming a nonheterosexual sexual identity within a heterosexist society, which he hypothesized may force nonheterosexual men to examine their own adherence to masculine norms. O'Neil further posited that resolving such conflicts might be reinforcing to nonheterosexual men. For example, resolution of conflicting feelings around affectionate behavior toward other men has different practical rewards for gay men than straight men (e.g., formation and maintenance of romantic and sexual relationships is predicated on affectionate behavior among men for gay men, but not for heterosexual men). Nonheterosexual men may also be more comfortable than heterosexual men in adopting more flexible or androgynous gender roles (Hooberman, 1979), which may allow for lowered restrictive emotionality, success–power–competition, and conflict between work and family among nonheterosexual men. However, as noted by O'Neil (2008), the developmental trajectory of GRC as it pertains to sexual orientation has not been explored, and although a fair number of studies have applied the GRC paradigm to gay men, bisexual men and transgender men have been largely absent from the literature base.

As defined in Chapter 2 of this volume, *gender role ideology* refers to acceptance or internalization of a perceived social message about definitions of masculinity. Nonheterosexual men are typically hypothesized as having lower endorsement of traditional masculinity ideology compared with heterosexual men (Wade & Donis, 2007). The reasons offered for this are similar to the reasons posited for GRC.

As described in Chapter 5, the *gender conformity paradigm* posits that individuals receive messages about how they, personally, should behave by virtue of their sex or gender. Sexuality is a core aspect of the conformity paradigm and is included in operationalization of the construct (e.g., the Heterosexual Self-Presentation subscale of the Conformity to Masculine Norms Inventory [CMNI]). Regardless of levels of endorsement relative to heterosexual men, aspects of conformity to masculine norms are posited to hold associations with variables found among other groups of men (Mahalik et al., 2003) and also have some unique relationships among nonheterosexual men (Hamilton & Mahalik, 2009; Parent, Torrey, & Michaels, 2012).

## Additional Paradigms

Other paradigms exist that have informed the study of GBT masculinities. For example, biological perspectives have examined the role of factors such as testosterone, primarily in work on the etiology of homosexuality. Kolodny, Masters, Hendryx, and Toro (1971) reported that, among a sample of gay men referred from a medical clinic, plasma testosterone levels were lower than among a comparison group of heterosexual men; this finding was not replicated by Barlow, Abel, Blanchard, and Mavissakalian (1974); subsequent investigations also failed to replicate this finding or found higher levels of testosterone among gay men compared with heterosexual men (e.g., Brodie, Gartrell, Doering, & Rhue, 1974).

# RESEARCH ON GBT MASCULINITIES

The present review of GBT masculinities focuses on qualitative and quantitative work with GBT men that has been conducted within the frameworks of the paradigms described in the preceding section. Incumbent with this focus on theory-driven research, some aspects of the body of literature on GBT men are not addressed; specifically, research using atheoretical approaches to understanding GBT men's masculinities are not given a great deal of attention. Atheoretical research presents a challenge across all branches of psychology; approaches to research not grounded in theory are not easily integrated into larger bodies of research and scholarship (Tracey & Glidden-Tracey, 1999). Related to this, throughout the present chapter, effect sizes are presented for research when they were either provided by study authors or were calculable from the data presented within published studies.

## Heterosexuals' Attitudes Toward GBT Masculinities

Perceived gender roles, and violations of those roles, are in part constructed by dominant social groups (Connell, 1992; Wilson et al., 2010). Because of this, the construction of GBT masculinities among heterosexual persons is important, and this topic in general has been the focus of a number of research programs. Numerous studies have found negative attitudes toward GBT men among the general population (Herek, 1988, 1994), although attitudes appear to be improving in general as well (Hicks & Lee, 2006; Loftus, 2001). In research that has included examinations of gender roles, research indicates that heterosexual men and women view gay men as less masculine, and more feminine, than heterosexual men, and that adherence to traditional masculinity ideology or gender role conformity is related to holding negative attitudes toward GBT men (Jellison, McConnell, & Gabriel, 2004; Keiller, 2010; Kerns & Fine, 1994; Lemelle & Battle, 2004; Mellinger & Levant, 2014; Parrott, Peterson, Vincent, & Bakeman, 2008). Less research has paid attention specifically to the perceived masculinity of bisexual men, and none has addressed perceptions of transgender men.

Several mechanisms have been posited for the finding that gay men are perceived to be less masculine. Glick, Gangl, Gibb, Klumpner, and Weinberg (2007) investigated undergraduate men's affect toward hypothetical gay targets that varied on masculinity (specifying that the hypothetical target liked either football/cars or dance/musicals, was in a fraternity/adventure club or choir/sewing club, and hoped to be a CEO/lawyer/surgeon or a dancer/fashion designer/hairdresser). Subjects were also exposed to an experimental manipulation in which they were told either that their personality was typically masculine (control condition) or typically feminine (masculinity threat condition). The results indicated that when the subjects' masculinity was threatened, participants responded with more negative affect toward effeminate gay men (but not masculine gay men; effect sizes not obtainable from published data). This further supports the notion of social construction of masculinity; a stable and nonexternally referent masculinity would have meant that participants would have responded to the effeminate targets in the same manner regardless of the masculinity threat condition. However, because the effect only appeared in the threat condition, it is possible that negative reactions to the effeminate gay men targets were made as a defensive reaction to that threat.

Kroeper, Sanchez, and Himmelstein (2014) explored the concept of precarious manhood as it applied to heterosexual men's attitudes toward gay men. With 88 heterosexual-identified men undergraduate students, Kroeper et al. told participants that they would be completing a study on technology in hiring decisions through use of an online chat system. Participants were told that they and a second participant (a confederate) would be evaluating job applicants. The applicant resume included involvement with an LGBT organization and interests that included fashion and baking. The participant was told that he and the confederate would be evaluating the applicant over an online chat system. After some scripted discussion of the candidate, in one condition, the confederate remarked that the applicant's involvement in an LGBT group might make some people uncomfortable; in the other condition, the confederate stated that the applicant doesn't have enough experience. Participants were asked after the experiment how much they disagreed with the remark. Participants also reported whether they perceived that the partner did anything inappropriate and whether the participant confronted the partner on the behavior. Higher scores on a measure of precarious manhood were associated with decreased likelihood to report having confronted the inappropriate behavior. Thus, the results suggested that the greater endorsement of beliefs related to precarious manhood was associated with less likelihood to act in a supportive manner toward a hypothetical gay man.

Although research also exists on general attitudes toward bisexual men and transgender men (Herek, 2002; Norton & Herek, 2013), much less work has been done on gender role ideology/conformity and attitudes toward these groups. Research does indicate that gender conformity may influence attitudes toward these groups; in one study of Portuguese adolescents, Costa and Davies (2012), gender role ideology (items were novel or taken from other measures and reflected support for rigidly defined traditional gender roles for men and women) and scores on the Genderism and Transphobia Scale (D. B. Hill & Willoughby, 2005) were correlated (transphobia correlated $r = .76$ with ideology about women's gender roles, and $r = .55$ with ideology about men's gender roles). However, more nuanced issues (e.g., heterosexual men's construction of masculinity for bisexual men who are in relationships with men versus women, or their construction of masculinity of transgender men at various points in the transitioning process) remain unclear, and more work is needed in this area.

## Relationships

In the past, research on gay men's romantic relationships was predominantly invalidating and pathologizing (and, for bisexual and transgender men, nonexistent), depicting these relationships as dysfunctional and deviant (Sonenschein, 1968), although research has moved toward less biased or even positive analyses of GBT men's relationships (Vaughan et al., 2014). Men's relationships are influenced by gender role norms (Levant, Hirsch, Celentano, & Cozza, 1992; Mahalik et al., 2003), especially emotional control and restricted affectionate expression among men. Indeed, fearing how society will react to expressions of affection, admiration, or love of other men, some avoid these behaviors and decide to present a more stoic persona (Wester, Pionke, & Vogel, 2005). Additionally, given that restriction of emotionality and affectionate behavior among men is associated with fear of femininity (O'Neil, 2013) and the fact that GBT men are typically assumed to be feminine (Boysen, Vogel, Madon, & Wester, 2006), GBT men, in an attempt to enact masculinity, may be more unwilling to disclose vulnerabilities to others, which may result in poorer interpersonal relationships and psychological adjustment, compared with heterosexual men (Addis & Mahalik, 2003).

Regarding GBT men's friendships with heterosexual men, heterosexual men report being able to relax and reduce rigid adherence of conformity to traditional masculine norms and engage in healthful friendship relationships with gay men (Barrett, 2013; Fee, 2000). Other research has indicated that, among college students, variables such as appreciation of diversity, shyness, and religiosity influence openness to friendships with gay men (Mohr & Sedlacek, 2000). In terms of friendships with women, extant work has focused on the friendships between heterosexual women and gay men, indicating positive interactions between women and gay men (Bartlett, Patterson, VanderLaan, & Vasey, 2009; Grigoriou, 2004; Tillmann-Healy, 2001), including findings that the benefits of gay men–heterosexual women relationships may arise from a functional perspective of human mating (Russell, DelPriore, Butterfield, & Hill, 2013); heterosexual women may allow greater emotional closeness to gay men and take gay men's advice on relationships more seriously, because they may perceive that gay men do not have deceptive mating motivations (i.e., that sexually interested men may give bad relationship advice in an effort to keep a woman available to themselves for mating).

However, research has generally not incorporated masculinities variables into these investigations, nor has friendship research examined bisexual men (perhaps because bisexual men are not allowed the same emotional closeness and trust from heterosexual women as gay men are afforded). Although work does exist on the friendships of transgender persons (Galupo, Bauerband, et al., 2014; Galupo, Krum, Hagen, Gonzalez, & Bauerband, 2014), focusing on issues such as coming out as transgender and the benefits of friendships, this work has generally not incorporated a masculinities perspective.

Some work has examined GBT men's romantic relationships, investigating topics such as relationship cohesion, relationship satisfaction, and distribution of labor (Frost & Meyer, 2009; Green, Bettinger, & Zacks, 1996; Kurdek, 2007), primarily among gay men. Little work has applied measures of masculinity to GBT men's romantic relationships. Wade and Donis (2007) sampled university students and snowballed acquaintances of the research team, and found that traditional masculinity ideology was correlated with lower romantic relationship quality for both gay ($r = -.36$) and heterosexual ($r = -.31$) men. In another study using data from gay men collected online, Wester and colleagues (2005) found that although gay men experienced conflict associated with emotional and affective restriction, that variable accounted for only 5% of the variance of relationship satisfaction scores. These results suggest that although greater GRC is associated with lower levels of relationship satisfaction, relationship satisfaction among gay men may not be heavily driven by GRC any more so than among heterosexual relationships, as previously suggested (Ossana, 2000). Sánchez, Bocklandt, and Vilain (2009) explored the relation among GRC, casual sex, and relationship satisfaction in single and partnered gay men because it has been suggested that interest in casual sex impedes gay men's ability to find and maintain long-term relationships. Sánchez et al. reported that single, compared with partnered, gay men scored higher on restrictive affectionate behavior between men ($r = .14$) and were more interested in casual sex ($r = .13$); partnered men, compared with single men, scored higher on drive for success ($r = .20$). Additionally, they found that GRC scores were positively correlated with interest in casual sex in both groups ($r = .32$ among partnered gay men, $r = .23$ among single gay men), suggesting that male socialization might influence GBT men's interest in casual sex and avoidance of committed relationships. Some work has explored bisexual men's romantic relationships, often addressing topics such as negotiation of monogamy or consensual nonmonogamy (McLean, 2004), and a nascent literature is exploring transgender persons' relationships (Iantaffi & Bockting, 2011), although concepts related to masculinities have not been applied in these bodies of work.

A small amount of research has explored fatherhood among gay men, investigating topics such as relationship satisfaction as a function of remaining in or leaving their other-sex relationship, parenting stress among gay fathers, or parent–child relationships among gay fathers (Golombok et al., 2014; Tornello, Farr, & Patterson, 2011; Tornello & Patterson, 2012); this work has not integrated concepts related to masculinities. Although some work has sampled bisexual fathers (and, typically, merged them into the same analysis group as gay fathers), no work has focused exclusively on bisexual fathers (indeed, even the case study literature and popular books focus almost exclusively on gay fathers; bisexual fathers are invisible within the literature). There is a small base of literature on transgender parenting issues, particularly related to custody issues (Chang, 2002); a large body of literature addressing psychological outcomes for children of gay or lesbian parents exists (Crowl, Ahn, & Baker, 2008) and has been useful in legal battles for gay and lesbian parenting rights (Patterson, 2009), but no parallel literature base exists for transgender persons.

## Mental Health

Many GBT men have and maintain good mental health despite research indicating GBT men are at greater risk for psychological distress and mental health issues, compared with heterosexual men (Cochran & Mays, 2000). Although early research on GBT men tended to pathologize sexual orientation and gender identity minority statuses through interpreting differing prevalence rates of disorders to indicate lower psychological health among GBT men, more recent work, such as that using the minority stress model, has contextualized these concerns and placed mental health concerns for GBT men within the contexts of prejudice and discrimination (I. H. Meyer, 1995, 2003). The minority stress model posits that GBT men are subject to chronic stress related to stigmatization and oppression from the dominant group in society, which in turn leads to higher rates of morbidity (I. H. Meyer, 1995). Population-based research has corroborated that GBT men experience mental health problems at a greater rate than heterosexual men (to varying degrees). One study indicated that GBT men were 3.6 times more likely to suffer from major depression, 5 times more likely to suffer from panic-related anxiety disorders, and 3.9 times more likely to experience comorbid mental health disorders (Cochran, Sullivan, & Mays, 2003). A meta-analysis of 3 decades worth of LGBT mental health research indicated that GBT men were 2.7 times more likely to experience a mood disorder and 2.4 times more likely to experience an anxiety disorder (I. H. Meyer, 2003). More recent research has indicated GBT men were 1.5 to 2 times more likely to experience some form of mood, anxiety, or substance use disorder during their lifetime, and 2 times more likely to attempt suicide, compared with heterosexual men (Bostwick, Boyd, Hughes, & McCabe, 2010; King et al., 2008).

Pachankis and Goldfried (2006) explored social anxiety among gay men by comparing the occurrence and correlates of social anxiety among gay and heterosexual men. Results indicated that gay men reported a greater fear of negative evaluation ($d = .66$) and social interaction anxiety ($d = .55$), as well as lower self-esteem ($d = .50$) and gender conformity ($d = 2.40$) than heterosexual men. Additionally, results indicated that among gay men, comfort about being gay was negatively associated with gender conformity ($r = -.35$), and gender conformity was negatively associated with anxiety related to concealment of homosexuality ($r = -.35$). Overall, these results suggest that hiding a core aspect of identity involves near constant self-monitoring, which has been found to impair interpersonal functioning among socially anxious individuals and increase feelings of shame and worthlessness (Pachankis & Goldfried, 2006). The majority of the gay population in this study reported changing behaviors due to fear of being identified as gay; this fear, and thus, concealment of homosexuality, has been indicated to be associated with lowered satisfaction with life and social support (Safren & Pantalone, 2006).

Safren, Reisner, Herrick, Mimiaga, and Stall (2010) explored the impact that psychosocial health problems had on the sexual health concerns of men who have sex with men. Specifically, their results indicated that endorsement of psychosocial health problems significantly increased the odds of unprotected anal intercourse, odds ratio (OR) = 1.42, 95% confidence interval (CI) [1.19, 1.68]; multiple sex partners, OR = 1.24, 95% CI [1.05, 1.47]; and HIV seroprevalence, OR = 1.42, 95% CI [1.12, 1.80]. This suggests that as individuals become exposed to additional psychosocial stressors, such as those stemming from violation of traditional masculine norms, their odds of engagement in HIV sexual risk behaviors increased, which may in fact be an important factor driving the HIV epidemic among GBT men.

Men experience difficulties with alexithymia (i.e., difficulty experiencing, fantasizing, thinking about, and expressing one's emotions; Taylor, Ryan, & Bagby, 1985) more often than women (Levant, Hall, Williams, & Hasan, 2009; Vorst & Bermond, 2001). Men who are socialized via traditional masculinity ideology or who experience higher levels of GRC experience greater levels of alexithymia (Fischer & Good, 1997; Levant, Rankin, Williams, Hasan, & Smalley, 2010; Levant & Wong, 2013). Levant (1998) indicated that alexithymia resulting from socialization to the traditional masculine norm of restricting emotionality manifests as deficits in expressing emotions that reflect a sense of vulnerability or that express attachment. Other research suggests alexithymia may be a secondary characteristic of HIV because it is associated with poor utilization and perception of social support, occurring as a reaction to stressful circumstances surrounding the diagnosis (Fukunishi, Hirabayashi, Matsumoto, Yamanaka, & Fukutake, 1999). However, other than assessing the relationship between HIV status and alexithymia, research is scant on alexithymia among GBT men, much less on masculinity's influence. Past research has not restricted GBT men from participating, but the number of GBT men participants has typically been small. Future research may use purposeful sampling of GBT men to allow for accurate comparisons and for greater understanding of the relationship between alexithymia and masculinity ideology in GBT men.

## Physical Health

Research on GBT men's health has been largely dominated by research on HIV/AIDS and risky sexual behaviors among gay men, although the health of bisexual and transgender populations has also been recently explored in more detail (Boehmer, 2002; Huang et al., 2010). The concept of masculinities has been applied to understanding health-related behaviors among GBT men and has been integrated into some of the theoretical models within this area.

Health, and especially unprotected sex, has been a major area of focus in qualitative research on GBT men. Research has consistently linked unprotected (or "bareback") sex with concepts of masculinity. This finding has been borne out in analyses of bisexual men's HIV risk behaviors (LaPollo, Bond, & Lauby, 2014), Black men's sexual risk behaviors (Malebranche, Fields, Bryant, & Harper, 2009), men's risk-reduction behaviors (Holmes, Gastaldo, O'Bryrne, & Lombardo, 2008), and in analysis of content of dating/sexual websites for GBT men (Dowsett, Williams, Ventuneac, & Carballo-Diéguez, 2008). This research has generally indicated that unsafe sex practices are associated with construction of masculinity related to sex; that is, that to have unsafe sex enacts masculinity and (either implicitly or explicitly) that safer sex practices are unmasculine.

Relatedly, in quantitative paradigms, Parent, Torrey, and Michaels (2012) investigated HIV testing practices among an online sample of 170 U.S. men who have sex with men. After controlling for the influence of number of sexual partners (which was positively related to being tested for HIV), Parent et al. assessed the relationships between being tested for HIV and masculine gender role conformity (measured with the CMNI–46). Heterosexual self-presentation alone was associated negatively with having been recently tested for HIV, $OR = 0.48$, 95% CI [0.24, 0.96], suggesting that gay men were less likely to be tested for HIV to the degree that they valued being perceived by others as heterosexual. Hamilton and Mahalik (2009) explored the relationships among minority stress and masculinity (assessed with the CMNI) in predicting health risk behaviors (alcohol use, tobacco use, illicit drug use, and risky sexual behavior) among a sample of 315 gay men recruited online. Masculinity was positively but weakly associated with health risks ($r = .17$). Pachankis, Westmaas, and Dougherty (2011) explored the relationships between masculinity (measured with a novel single-item measure) and tobacco smoking among 136 gay and 56 heterosexual university students. Gay men rated themselves as moderately less masculine than heterosexual participants ($d = .36$), and masculinity was associated with greater smoking among all participants, $I = 1.68$, 95% CI [1.18, 2.40].

Regarding other health risks, men engage in more health risk behaviors than women in nearly all domains (Courtenay, 2000), with GBT men, overall, engaging in more health risk behaviors than heterosexual men (Cochran, Ackerman, Mays, & Ross, 2004). GBT men may engage in health risk behaviors to conform to traditional masculine norms and promote heterosexual self-presentation, or they may choose not to conform to traditional masculine norms and avoid risky behaviors. Indeed, greater conflict with masculine ideals is associated with lowered self-esteem and greater depression and anxiety among GBT men (Simonsen, Blazina, & Watkins, 2000; Szymanski & Carr, 2008).

Research on the health of transgender persons has increased in the past decade, with attention being given to health issues such as HIV risk and drug use (Clements-Nolle, Marx, Guzman, & Katz, 2001; Herbst et al., 2008), although much of this work focuses on male-to-female transgender persons and persons who are homeless and/or sex workers. Although clearly important populations to examine (especially as rates of homelessness and sex work are high among transgender persons; Spicer, 2010), such samples may not be reflective of transgender persons who are employed and not involved in sex work; it is also important that research examine health among female-to-male transgender persons, transgender persons who are not homeless, and transgender persons who do not work in the sex trade.

### Body Image and Eating Disorders

In the past 2 decades, research on men's body image has expanded significantly, including work on GBT men's body image. Because early research on body image was largely adapted from research on women's body image, early work focused on thinness-related concerns. However, in the past 2 decades, research has increasingly focused on muscularity in relation to men's body image. In qualitative research, muscularity has often been conceptualized as an enactment of masculinity and an opportunity to enhance social status (Drummond, 2005; Duncan, 2010), as a remasculinizing reaction against the implicit demasculinization of one's same-sex desire (Ridge, Plummer, & Peasley, 2006), or used as a semiotic sign that one does not have HIV (Drummond, 2005; Klein, 1993).

Quantitative research has also examined GBT men's body image. Kimmel and Mahalik (2005) examined relations between scores on the CMNI and measures of body image among 357 gay men recruited from online sources. Their results indicated that total scores on the CMNI were not correlated with scores on the Body Image Ideals Questionnaire (a measure of perceived discrepancy between current and ideal physical attributes; $r = -.04$) and were correlated weakly with scores on the Masculine Body Ideal Distress Scale (a measure of distress for failing to have an ideal body; $r = .24$). Subsequent hierarchical regressions indicated that CMNI total scores contributed to explaining variance in Masculine Body Ideal Distress Scale scores, but not Body Image Ideals Questionnaire scores. Because the Body Image Ideals Questionnaire focuses on several physical attributes (e.g., face), while the Masculine Body Ideal Distress Scale focuses on muscularity, this may indicate that masculinity is linked primarily to muscular body composition and not to general, overall attractiveness, among gay men.

There has been some work on sexual orientation and eating disorder symptoms. In one investigation, C. Meyer, Blissett, and Oldfield (2001) studied the occurrence of eating disorder symptoms (measured with the Eating Attitudes Test) among heterosexual and gay/lesbian men and women university students, while also examining the role of masculinity and femininity (measured by scores on the Bem Sex Role Inventory). Among all groups, scores on the BSRI Masculinity subscale were associated negatively with eating pathology ($r = -.28$), whereas scores on the BSRI Femininity subscale were associated positively with eating pathology ($r = .27$). This work built on previous work that found high levels of disordered eating among gay men and focused on gay men's desire to be attractive to other men as the underlying cause (Heffernan, 1994; Silberstein, Mishkind, Striegel-Moore, Timko, & Rodin, 1989), and pointed toward gender role conformity as an important potential moderator of the relationship between sexual orientation and eating pathology.

Research on masculinity, body image, and eating disorders among bisexual and transgender persons is scant. Research generally indicates the presence of body image disturbance among transgender individuals before beginning the transition process and improvement in body image as transitioning proceeds (Fleming, MacGowan, Robinson, Spitz, & Salt, 1982; Kraemer, Delsignore, Schnyder, & Hepp, 2008), although some work has not replicated this finding (Vocks, Stahn, Loenser, & Legenbauer, 2009); research on bisexual persons, and on transgender persons and persons transitioning genders, has not been incorporated into a masculinities framework.

## Help-Seeking

In general, men engage in fewer health-promoting and preventive behaviors than women and seek medical and mental help at much lower rates than women (Bertakis, Azari, Helms, Callahan, & Robbins, 2000; Garfield, Isacco, & Rogers, 2008; Owens, 2008). This lack of health care utilization has led to personal, relational, physical, mental, and economic costs (World Health Organization, 2002). Conformity to and endorsement of traditional masculinity ideologies is one important predictor of men's help-seeking behavior (Addis & Mahalik, 2003; Levant, Stefanov, et al., 2013; Vogel, Heimerdinger-Edwards, Hammer, & Hubbard, 2011).

Help-seeking among sexual minority men, however, has not received great attention among researchers or incorporated the concept of masculinities. In regard to medical health help-seeking, many GBT men avoid coming out to their physicians (Brotman, Ryan, Jalbert, & Rowe, 2002; Kitts, 2010), view them as distrustful (Whetten, Reif, Whetten, & Murphy-McMillan, 2008), report discrimination and heterosexist assumptions from care providers (Dean et al., 2000; Keogh et al., 2004), and report that their health care needs are often not being met (Burgess, Lee, Tran, & van Ryn, 2007). Despite these findings, population-based research has indicated GBT men seek health care help more frequently than heterosexual men (Bakker, Sandfort, Vanwesenbeeck, van Lindert, & Westert, 2006; Tjepkema, 2008). It is possible that although GBT men may seek help more often for typical health concerns, they might not seek or receive help for GBT-specific health concerns because of perceptions of homophobia among health care professionals or their reluctance to come out (Cant, 2006; Parent et al., 2012). In regard to mental health help-seeking, research suggests that GBT men hold more favorable attitudes toward and are more likely to seek help than heterosexual men (Cochran, Sullivan, & Mays, 2003; Eisenberg, Downs, Golberstein, & Zivin, 2009; Grella, Greenwell, Mays, & Cochran, 2009). However, despite a large literature base on men's help-seeking (Addis & Mahalik, 2003), little work has extended this literature to gay men, and none has extended it to bisexual or transgender men.

Hegemonic masculinity may play an important role in GBT men's help-seeking because it can lead to avoidance of help-seeking, endurance of physical and mental pain, and high levels of risk-taking behavior (Courtenay, 2000). Adherence to hegemonic masculinity may lead GBT men to experience thoughts of not being "man" enough, which in turn influences how they negotiate conflicting societal and personal beliefs about the relationship between sexual orientation and masculinity (Wilson et al., 2010). Thus, if GBT men who are traditionally masculine experience higher levels of minority stress due to preservation of social status, they may have negative attitudes toward and be less likely to engage in help-seeking behaviors.

Sánchez, Bocklandt, and Vilain (2013) sampled 38 pairs of monozygotic male twins who were raised together and were discordant for sexual orientation; the authors assessed whether the twin pairs differed in mental health help-seeking attitudes and the effect of masculinity on help-seeking attitudes. Heterosexual twins held less favorable views of seeking mental health help ($r = -.25$), and heterosexual twins also indicated greater adherence to traditional masculine roles than their gay cotwins ($r = .26$). Specifically, results indicated that positive help-seeking attitudes were related to Gender Role Conflict Scale scores more strongly for gay men ($r = -.37$) than their heterosexual twins ($r = -.11$; Sánchez et al., 2013; Sánchez, Westefeld, Liu, & Vilain, 2010). Thus, differences emerged in endorsement of GRC and attitudes toward help-seeking, as well as the strength of association between those two constructs.

Despite this work, limited research has addressed help-seeking behaviors among bisexual men and transgender men. Future research is needed to build on the substantial literature base on masculinity and help-seeking through purposeful sampling from GBT men to gain a clearer understanding of how masculinity influences help-seeking decisions among these groups of men.

## AREAS FOR FUTURE RESEARCH

The present chapter aimed to review research and scholarship on gay, bisexual, and transgender masculinities. In doing so, it also aimed to elucidate areas where there is a dearth of knowledge and a need for greater empirical investigation. Although there has been significant work on the intersections of these constructs and identities, much work is yet needed.

Intimate partner violence (IPV) is an established area of research (McHugh & Frieze, 2006; Rennison & Welchans, 2000). Although the majority or work in this area has focused on violence against women in heterosexual relationships, attention has recently been focused on violence against men and violence in same-sex relationships (e.g., Finneran & Stephenson, 2013). Concepts of masculinity have been integrated into this research within mixed-gender couples, indicating that masculinity ideology and conformity to masculine norms are associated positively with IPV and related variables such as rape myth acceptance or sexual aggression (M. S. Hill & Fischer, 2001; Locke & Mahalik, 2005; Schwartz, Waldo, & Daniel, 2005). However, little work has quantitatively assessed the role of masculinity in GBT men's experiences of or perpetration of IPV. Indeed, masculinities may be integrated into existing models of IPV, such as Riggs and O'Leary's

(1989) model, which incorporates the belief that violence is appropriate in response to conflict (an aspect of masculine gender role conformity), and alcohol use (which has been reliably linked to endorsement of masculine role norms; Iwamoto, Cheng, Lee, Takamatsu, & Gordon, 2011; Iwamoto, Corbin, Lejuez, & MacPherson, 2014).

Substance use has also been understudied in GBT men within a masculinities framework. Previous research has demonstrated the utility of applying masculinities frameworks to understanding substance use within other minority populations (e.g., Liu & Iwamoto, 2007). Extension of this research to GBT populations may prove useful to prevention and intervention efforts. Substance use has also been demonstrated to be higher among GBT men than the general population for both legal substances (e.g., nicotine; Blosnich, Lee, & Horn, 2013) and illegal substances (Marshal et al., 2008). Further extension of this body of work to smoking and to illicit substances may have important public health implications.

Career-related research on GBT men and masculinities is also lacking, although masculinity has been integrated into vocational literature (Mahalik, 2006; Tokar & Jome, 1998). Because GBT men and heterosexual men tend to differ in scores on measures of masculinities, it is possible that those differences have effects on learning experiences, career decision-making self-efficacy, college major choice, satisfaction with education, and other variables. For example, longitudinal research on high school students, which has proven fruitful in investigating young women's career trajectories (Watt & Eccles, 2008), may be applied to GBT young men as well.

Precarious manhood (Vandello, Bosson, Cohen, Burnaford, & Weaver, 2008) has been underexplored in research on GBT men. Precarious manhood focuses on the construction of masculinity, especially on how masculinity can be seen as "easily lost"; that is, that actions are needed to "prove" manhood and that other actions can result in losing manhood. Endorsement of the concept of precarious manhood can be measured through assessment of beliefs about the unstable nature of masculinity (Kroeper et al., 2014). Pursuant to GBT men, precarious manhood may be especially important to understanding intergroup attitudes and relations. However, only one published study (Kroeper et al., 2014) has specifically examined this.

Finally, in general, across all areas, research has focused on cisgender gay men to the exclusion of bisexual and transgender men. Notably absent is research on the construction of masculinity for bisexual men (and, more complexly, constructions of masculinities in bisexual men varying by the gender of bisexual men's partner or partners) and the construction of masculinities in transgender men (and, more complexly, constructions of masculinities in transgender men varying by perceived "degree" of transition). Such research is important to extending work on the topics covered here and in other areas of work.

# REFERENCES

Addis, M. E., & Mahalik, J. R. (2003). Men, masculinity, and the contexts of help seeking. *American Psychologist, 58*, 5–14. http://dx.doi.org/10.1037/0003-066X.58.1.5

Bakker, F. C., Sandfort, T. G. M., Vanwesenbeeck, I., van Lindert, H., & Westert, G. P. (2006). Do homosexual persons use health care services more frequently than heterosexual persons: Findings from a Dutch population survey. *Social Science & Medicine, 63*, 2022–2030. http://dx.doi.org/10.1016/j.socscimed.2006.05.024

Barlow, D. H., Abel, G. G., Blanchard, E. B., & Mavissakalian, M. (1974). Plasma testosterone levels and male homosexuality: A failure to replicate. *Archives of Sexual Behavior, 3*, 571–575. http://dx.doi.org/10.1007/BF01541139

Barrett, T. (2013). Friendships between men across sexual orientation: The importance of (others) being intolerant. *The Journal of Men's Studies, 21*, 62–77. http://dx.doi.org/10.3149/jms.2101.62

Bartlett, N. H., Patterson, H. M., VanderLaan, D. P., & Vasey, P. L. (2009). The relation between women's body esteem and friendships with gay men. *Body Image, 6*, 235–241. http://dx.doi.org/10.1016/j.bodyim.2009.04.005

Bem, S. L. (1974). The measurement of psychological androgyny. *Journal of Consulting and Clinical Psychology, 42*, 155–162. http://dx.doi.org/10.1037/h0036215

Bertakis, K. D., Azari, R., Helms, L. J., Callahan, E. J., & Robbins, J. A. (2000). Gender differences in the utilization of health care services. *The Journal of Family Practice, 49*, 147–152.

Blosnich, J., Lee, J. G. L., & Horn, K. (2013). A systematic review of the aetiology of tobacco disparities for sexual minorities. *Tobacco Control, 22*, 66–73. http://dx.doi.org/10.1136/tobaccocontrol-2011-050181

Boehmer, U. (2002). Twenty years of public health research: Inclusion of lesbian, gay, bisexual, and transgender populations. *American Journal of Public Health, 92*, 1125–1130. http://dx.doi.org/10.2105/AJPH.92.7.1125

Bostwick, W. B., Boyd, C. J., Hughes, T. L., & McCabe, S. E. (2010). Dimensions of sexual orientation and the prevalence of mood and anxiety disorders in the United States. *American Journal of Public Health, 100*, 468–475. http://dx.doi.org/10.2105/AJPH.2008.152942

Boysen, G. A., Vogel, D. L., Madon, S., & Wester, S. R. (2006). Mental health stereotypes about gay men. *Sex Roles, 54*, 69–82. http://dx.doi.org/10.1007/s11199-006-8870-0

Brodie, H. K. H., Gartrell, N., Doering, C., & Rhue, T. (1974). Plasma testosterone levels in heterosexual and homosexual men. *The American Journal of Psychiatry, 131*, 82–83. http://dx.doi.org/10.1176/ajp.131.1.82

Brotman, S., Ryan, B., Jalbert, Y., & Rowe, B. (2002). The impact of coming out on health and health care access: The experiences of gay, lesbian, bisexual, and two-spirit people. *Journal of Health & Social Policy, 15,* 1–29. http://dx.doi.org/10.1300/J045v15n01_01

Burgess, D., Tran, A., Lee, R., & van Ryn, M. (2007). Effects of perceived discrimination on mental health and mental health services utilization among gay, lesbian, bisexual, and transgender persons. *Journal of LGBT Health Research, 3,* 1–14. http://dx.doi.org/10.1080/15574090802226626

Cant, B. (2006). Exploring the implications for health professionals of men coming out as gay in healthcare settings. *Health & Social Care in the Community, 14,* 9–16. http://dx.doi.org/10.1111/j.1365-2524.2005.00583.x

Chang, H. Y. (2002). My father is a woman, oh no: The failure of the courts to uphold individual substantive due process rights for transgender parents under the guise of the best interest of the child. *Santa Clara Law Review, 43,* 649–698.

Clements-Nolle, K., Marx, R., Guzman, R., & Katz, M. (2001). HIV prevalence, risk behaviors, health care use, and mental health status of transgender persons: Implications for public health intervention. *American Journal of Public Health, 91,* 915–921. http://dx.doi.org/10.2105/AJPH.91.6.915

Cochran, S. D., Ackerman, D., Mays, V. M., & Ross, M. W. (2004). Prevalence of nonmedical drug use and dependence among homosexually active men and women in the U.S. population. *Addiction, 99,* 989–998. http://dx.doi.org/10.1111/j.1360-0443.2004.00759.x

Cochran, S. D., & Mays, V. M. (2000). Lifetime prevalence of suicide symptoms and affective disorders among men reporting same-sex sexual partners: Results from NHANES III. *American Journal of Public Health, 90,* 573–578. http://dx.doi.org/10.2105/AJPH.90.4.573

Cochran, S. D., Sullivan, J. G., & Mays, V. M. (2003). Prevalence of mental disorders, psychological distress, and mental health services use among lesbian, gay, and bisexual adults in the United States. *Journal of Consulting and Clinical Psychology, 71,* 53–61. http://dx.doi.org/10.1037/0022-006X.71.1.53

Connell, R. W. (1992). A very straight gay: Masculinity, homosexual experience, and the dynamics of gender. *American Sociological Review, 57,* 735–751. http://dx.doi.org/10.2307/2096120

Connell, R. W. (1995). *Masculinities.* Berkeley: University of California Press.

Costa, P. A., & Davies, M. (2012). Portuguese adolescents' attitudes toward sexual minorities: Transphobia, homophobia, and gender role beliefs. *Journal of Homosexuality, 59,* 1424–1442. http://dx.doi.org/10.1080/00918369.2012.724944

Courtenay, W. H. (2000). Constructions of masculinity and their influence on men's well-being: A theory of gender and health. *Social Science & Medicine, 50,* 1385–1401. http://dx.doi.org/10.1016/S0277-9536(99)00390-1

Crowl, A., Ahn, S., & Baker, J. (2008). A meta-analysis of developmental outcomes for children of same-sex and heterosexual parents. *Journal of GLBT Family Studies, 4,* 385–407. http://dx.doi.org/10.1080/15504280802177615

Dean, L., Meyer, I. H., Robinson, K., Sell, R. L., Sember, R., Silenzio, V. M. B., . . . Xavier, J. (2000). Lesbian, gay, bisexual, and transgender health: Findings and concerns. *Journal of the Gay and Lesbian Medical Association, 4,* 102–151. http://dx.doi.org/10.1023/A:1009573800168

Dowsett, G. W., Williams, H., Ventuneac, A., & Carballo-Diéguez, A. (2008). "Taking it like a man": Masculinity and barebacking online. *Sexualities, 11,* 121–141. http://dx.doi.org/10.1177/1363460707085467

Drescher, J. (2012). The removal of homosexuality from the *DSM*: Its impact on today's marriage equality debate. *Journal of Gay & Lesbian Mental Health, 16,* 124–135. http://dx.doi.org/10.1080/19359705.2012.653255

Drummond, M. J. (2005). Men's bodies: Listening to the voices of young gay men. *Men and Masculinities, 7,* 270–290. http://dx.doi.org/10.1177/1097184X04271357

Duncan, D. (2010). Embodying the gay self: Body image, reflexivity, and embodied identity. *Health Sociology Review, 19,* 437–450. http://dx.doi.org/10.5172/hesr.2010.19.4.437

Eisenberg, D., Downs, M. F., Golberstein, E., & Zivin, K. (2009). Stigma and help seeking for mental health among college students. *Medical Care Research and Review, 66,* 522–541. http://dx.doi.org/10.1177/1077558709335173

Fee, D. (2000). "One of the guys": Instrumentality and intimacy in gay men's friendships with straight men. In P. Nardi (Ed.), *Gay masculinities* (pp. 44–65). http://dx.doi.org/10.4135/9781452233987.n3

Finneran, C., & Stephenson, R. (2013). Intimate partner violence among men who have sex with men: A systematic review. *Trauma, Violence, & Abuse, 14,* 168–185. http://dx.doi.org/10.1177/1524838012470034

Fischer, A. R., & Good, G. E. (1997). Men and psychotherapy: An investigation of alexithymia, intimacy, and masculine gender roles. *Psychotherapy: Theory, Research, Practice, Training, 34,* 160–170. http://dx.doi.org/10.1037/h0087646

Fleming, M. Z., MacGowan, B. R., Robinson, L., Spitz, J., & Salt, P. (1982). The body image of the postoperative female-to-male transsexual. *Journal of Consulting and Clinical Psychology, 50,* 461–462. http://dx.doi.org/10.1037/0022-006X.50.3.461

Frost, D. M., & Meyer, I. H. (2009). Internalized homophobia and relationship quality among lesbians, gay men, and bisexuals. *Journal of Counseling Psychology, 56,* 97–109. http://dx.doi.org/10.1037/a0012844

Fukunishi, I., Hirabayashi, N., Matsumoto, T., Yamanaka, K., & Fukutake, K. (1999). Alexithymic characteristics of HIV-positive patients. *Psychological Reports, 85,* 963–970.

Galupo, M. P., Bauerband, L. A., Gonzalez, K. A., Hagen, D. B., Hether, S. D., & Krum, T. E. (2014). Transgender friendship experiences: Benefits and barriers of friendships across gender identity and sexual orientation. *Feminism & Psychology, 24,* 193–215. http://dx.doi.org/10.1177/0959353514526218

Galupo, M. P., Krum, T. E., Hagen, D. B., Gonzalez, K. A., & Bauerband, L. A. (2014). Disclosure of transgender identity and status in the context of friendship. *Journal of LGBT Issues in Counseling, 8,* 25–42. http://dx.doi.org/10.1080/15538605.2014.853638

Garfield, C. F., Isacco, A., & Rogers, T. E. (2008). A review of men's health and masculinity. *American Journal of Lifestyle Medicine, 2*, 474–487. http://dx.doi.org/10.1177/1559827608323213

Glick, P., Gangl, C., Gibb, S., Klumpner, S., & Weinberg, E. (2007). Defensive reactions to masculinity threat: More negative affect toward effeminate (but not masculine) gay men. *Sex Roles, 57*, 55–59. http://dx.doi.org/10.1007/s11199-007-9195-3

Golombok, S., Mellish, L., Jennings, S., Casey, P., Tasker, F., & Lamb, M. E. (2014). Adoptive gay father families: Parent–child relationships and children's psychological adjustment. *Child Development, 85*, 456–468. http://dx.doi.org/10.1111/cdev.12155

Green, R.-J., Bettinger, M., & Zacks, E. (1996). Are lesbian couples fused and gay male couples disengaged? Questioning gender straightjackets. In J. Laird & R.-J. Green (Eds.), *Lesbians and gays in couples and families: A handbook for therapists* (pp. 185–230). San Francisco, CA: Jossey-Bass.

Grella, C. E., Greenwell, L., Mays, V. M., & Cochran, S. D. (2009). Influence of gender, sexual orientation, and need on treatment utilization for substance use and mental disorders: Findings from the California Quality of Life Survey. *BMC Psychiatry, 9*, 52–62. http://dx.doi.org/10.1186/1471-244X-9-52

Grigoriou, T. (2004). *Friendship between gay men and heterosexual women: An interpretative phenomenological analysis: Families & Social Capital ESRC Research Group.* London, England: South Bank University.

Hamilton, C. J., & Mahalik, J. R. (2009). Minority stress, masculinity, and social norms predicting gay men's health risk behaviors. *Journal of Counseling Psychology, 56*(1), 132–141. http://dx.doi.org/10.1037/a0014440

Heffernan, K. (1994). Sexual orientation as a factor in risk for binge eating and bulimia nervosa: A review. *International Journal of Eating Disorders, 16*, 335–347. http://dx.doi.org/10.1002/1098-108X(199412)16:4<335::AID-EAT2260160403>3.0.CO;2-C

Herbst, J. H., Jacobs, E. D., Finlayson, T. J., McKleroy, V. S., Neumann, M. S., Crepaz, N., & the HIV/AIDS Prevention Research Synthesis Team. (2008). Estimating HIV prevalence and risk behaviors of transgender persons in the United States: A systematic review. *AIDS and Behavior, 12*, 1–17. http://dx.doi.org/10.1007/s10461-007-9299-3

Herek, G. M. (1988). Heterosexuals' attitudes toward lesbians and gay men: Correlates and gender differences. *Journal of Sex Research, 25*, 451–477. http://dx.doi.org/10.1080/00224498809551476

Herek, G. M. (1994). Assessing heterosexuals' attitudes toward lesbians and gay men: A review of empirical research with the ATLG scale. In B. Greene & G. M. Herek (Eds.), *Lesbian and gay psychology: Theory, research, and clinical applications* (pp. 206–228). http://dx.doi.org/10.4135/9781483326757.n11

Herek, G. M. (2002). Heterosexuals' attitudes toward bisexual men and women in the United States. *Journal of Sex Research, 39*, 264–274. http://dx.doi.org/10.1080/00224490209552150

Hicks, G. R., & Lee, T.-T. (2006). Public attitudes toward gays and lesbians: Trends and predictors. *Journal of Homosexuality, 51*, 57–77. http://dx.doi.org/10.1300/J082v51n02_04

Hill, D. B., & Willoughby, B. L. B. (2005). The development and validation of the Genderism and Transphobia Scale. *Sex Roles, 53*, 531–544. http://dx.doi.org/10.1007/s11199-005-7140-x

Hill, M. S., & Fischer, A. R. (2001). Does entitlement mediate the link between masculinity and rape-related variables? *Journal of Counseling Psychology, 48*, 39–50. http://dx.doi.org/10.1037/0022-0167.48.1.39

Holmes, D., Gastaldo, D., O'Bryrne, P., & Lombardo, A. (2008). Bareback sex: A conflation of risk and masculinity. *International Journal of Men's Health, 7*, 171–191. http://dx.doi.org/10.3149/jmh.0702.171

Hooberman, R. E. (1979). Psychological androgyny, feminine gender identity, and self-esteem in homosexual and heterosexual males. *Journal of Sex Research, 15*, 306–315. http://dx.doi.org/10.1080/00224497909551054

Huang, Y.-P., Brewster, M. E., Moradi, B., Goodman, M. B., Wiseman, M. C., & Martin, A. (2010). Content analysis of literature about LGB people of color: 1998–2007. *The Counseling Psychologist, 38*, 363–396. http://dx.doi.org/10.1177/0011000009335255

Iantaffi, A., & Bockting, W. O. (2011). Views from both sides of the bridge? Gender, sexual legitimacy, and transgender people's experiences of relationships. *Culture, Health & Sexuality, 13*, 355–370. http://dx.doi.org/10.1080/13691058.2010.537770

Iwamoto, D. K., Cheng, A., Lee, C. S., Takamatsu, S., & Gordon, D. (2011). "Man-ing" up and getting drunk: The role of masculine norms, alcohol intoxication, and alcohol-related problems among college men. *Addictive Behaviors, 36*, 906–911. http://dx.doi.org/10.1016/j.addbeh.2011.04.005

Iwamoto, D. K., Corbin, W., Lejuez, C., & MacPherson, L. (2014). College men and alcohol use: Positive alcohol expectancies as a mediator between distinct masculine norms and alcohol use. *Psychology of Men & Masculinity, 15*, 29–39. http://dx.doi.org/10.1037/a0031594

Jellison, W. A., McConnell, A. R., & Gabriel, S. (2004). Implicit and explicit measures of sexual orientation attitudes: In group preferences and related behaviors and beliefs among gay and straight men. *Personality and Social Psychology Bulletin, 30*, 629–642. http://dx.doi.org/10.1177/0146167203262076

Keiller, S. W. (2010). Masculine norms as correlates of heterosexual men's attitudes toward gay men and lesbian women. *Psychology of Men & Masculinity, 11*, 38–52. http://dx.doi.org/10.1037/a0017540

Keogh, P., Weatherburn, P., Henderson, L., Reid, D., Dodds, C., & Hickson, F. (2004). *Doctoring gay men: Exploring the contribution of general practice.* London, England: Sigma Research.

Kerns, J. G., & Fine, M. A. (1994). The relation between gender and negative attitudes toward gay men and lesbians: Do gender role attitudes mediate this relation? *Sex Roles, 31*, 297–307. http://dx.doi.org/10.1007/BF01544590

Kimmel, S. B., & Mahalik, J. R. (2005). Body image concerns of gay men: The roles of minority stress and conformity to masculine norms. *Journal of Consulting and Clinical Psychology, 73*, 1185–1190. http://dx.doi.org/10.1037/0022-006X.73.6.1185

King, M., Semlyen, J., Tai, S. S., Killaspy, H., Osborn, D., Popelyuk, D., & Nazareth, I. (2008). A systematic review of mental disorder, suicide, and deliberate self-harm in lesbian, gay, and bisexual people. *BMC Psychiatry, 8*, 70–87.

Kitts, R. L. (2010). Barriers to optimal care between physicians and lesbian, gay, bisexual, transgender, and questioning adolescent patients. *Journal of Homosexuality, 57*, 730–747. http://dx.doi.org/10.1080/00918369.2010.485872

Klein, A. (1993). *Little big men: Bodybuilding subculture and gender construction.* Albany: University of New York Press.

Kolodny, R. C., Masters, W. H., Hendryx, J., & Toro, G. (1971). Plasma testosterone and semen analysis in male homosexuals. *The New England Journal of Medicine, 285*, 1170–1174. http://dx.doi.org/10.1056/NEJM197111182852104

Kraemer, B., Delsignore, A., Schnyder, U., & Hepp, U. (2008). Body image and transsexualism. *Psychopathology, 41*, 96–100. http://dx.doi.org/10.1159/000111554

Kroeper, K. M., Sanchez, D. T., & Himmelstein, M. S. (2014). Heterosexual men's confrontation of sexual prejudice: The role of precarious manhood. *Sex Roles, 70*, 1–13. http://dx.doi.org/10.1007/s11199-013-0306-z

Kurdek, L. A. (2007). The allocation of household labor by partners in gay and lesbian couples. *Journal of Family Issues, 28*, 132–148. http://dx.doi.org/10.1177/0192513X06292019

LaPollo, A. B., Bond, L., & Lauby, J. L. (2014). Hypermasculinity and sexual risk among Black and White men who have sex with men and women. *American Journal of Men's Health, 8*, 362–372. http://dx.doi.org/10.1177/1557988313512861

Lemelle, A. J., Jr., & Battle, J. (2004). Black masculinity matters in attitudes toward gay males. *Journal of Homosexuality, 47*, 39–51. http://dx.doi.org/10.1300/J082v47n01_03

Levant, R. F. (1998). *Desperately seeking language: Understanding, assessing, and treating normative male alexithymia.* Hoboken, NJ: Wiley.

Levant, R. F., Hall, R. J., Williams, C., & Hasan, N. T. (2009). Gender differences in alexithymia: A meta-analysis. *Psychology of Men & Masculinity, 10*, 190–203. http://dx.doi.org/10.1037/a0015652

Levant, R. F., Hirsch, L. S., Celentano, E., & Cozza, T. M. (1992). The male role: An investigation of contemporary norms. *Journal of Mental Health Counseling, 14*, 325–337.

Levant, R. F., Rankin, T. J., Williams, C. M., Hasan, N. T., & Smalley, K. B. (2010). Evaluation of the factor structure and construct validity of scores on the Male Role Norms Inventory—Revised (MRNI–R). *Psychology of Men & Masculinity, 11*, 25–37. http://dx.doi.org/10.1037/a0017637

Levant, R. F., Stefanov, D. G., Rankin, T. J., Halter, M. J., Mellinger, C., & Williams, C. M. (2013). Moderated path analysis of the relationships between masculinity and men's attitudes toward seeking psychological help. *Journal of Counseling Psychology, 60*, 392–406. http://dx.doi.org/10.1037/a0033014

Levant, R. F., & Wong, Y. J. (2013). Race and gender as moderators of the relationship between the endorsement of traditional masculinity ideology and alexithymia: An intersectional perspective. *Psychology of Men & Masculinity, 14*, 329–333. http://dx.doi.org/10.1037/a0029551

Liu, W. M., & Iwamoto, D. K. (2007). Conformity to masculine norms, Asian values, coping strategies, peer group influences, and substance use among Asian American men. *Psychology of Men & Masculinity, 8*, 25–39. http://dx.doi.org/10.1037/1524-9220.8.1.25

Locke, B. D., & Mahalik, J. R. (2005). Examining masculinity norms, problem drinking, and athletic involvement as predictors of sexual aggression in college men. *Journal of Counseling Psychology, 52*, 279–283. http://dx.doi.org/10.1037/0022-0167.52.3.279

Loftus, J. (2001). America's liberalization in attitudes toward homosexuality, 1973 to 1998. *American Sociological Review, 66*, 762–782. http://dx.doi.org/10.2307/3088957

Mahalik, J. R. (2006). Examining conformity to masculinity norms as a function of RIASEC vocational interests. *Journal of Career Assessment, 14*, 203–213. http://dx.doi.org/10.1177/1069072705283761

Mahalik, J. R., Locke, B. D., Ludlow, L. H., Diemer, M. A., Scott, R. P. J., Gottfried, M., & Freitas, G. (2003). Development of the Conformity to Masculine Norms Inventory. *Psychology of Men & Masculinity, 4*, 3–25. http://dx.doi.org/10.1037/1524-9220.4.1.3

Malebranche, D. J., Fields, E. L., Bryant, L. O., & Harper, S. R. (2009). Masculine socialization and sexual risk behaviors among Black men who have sex with men: A qualitative exploration. *Men and Masculinities, 12*, 90–112. http://dx.doi.org/10.1177/1097184X07309504

Marshal, M. P., Friedman, M. S., Stall, R., King, K. M., Miles, J., Gold, M. A., . . . Morse, J. Q. (2008). Sexual orientation and adolescent substance use: A meta-analysis and methodological review. *Addiction, 103*, 546–556. http://dx.doi.org/10.1111/j.1360-0443.2008.02149.x

McHugh, M. C., & Frieze, I. H. (2006). Intimate partner violence: New directions. *Annals of the New York Academy of Sciences, 1087*, 121–141. http://dx.doi.org/10.1196/annals.1385.011

McLean, K. (2004). Negotiating (non)monogamy. *Journal of Bisexuality, 4*, 83–97. http://dx.doi.org/10.1300/J159v04n01_07

Mellinger, C., & Levant, R. F. (2014). Moderators of the relationship between masculinity and sexual prejudice in men: Friendship, gender self-esteem, same-sex attraction, and religious fundamentalism. *Archives of Sexual Behavior, 43*, 519–530. http://dx.doi.org/10.1007/s10508-013-0220-z

Meyer, C., Blissett, J., & Oldfield, C. (2001). Sexual orientation and eating psychopathology: The role of masculinity and femininity. *International Journal of Eating Disorders, 29*, 314–318. http://dx.doi.org/10.1002/eat.1024

Meyer, I. H. (1995). Minority stress and mental health in gay men. *Journal of Health and Social Behavior, 36,* 38–56. http://dx.doi.org/10.2307/2137286

Meyer, I. H. (2003). Prejudice, social stress, and mental health in lesbian, gay, and bisexual populations: Conceptual issues and research evidence. *Psychological Bulletin, 129,* 674–697. http://dx.doi.org/10.1037/0033-2909.129.5.674

Mohr, J. J., & Sedlacek, W. E. (2000). Perceived barriers to friendship with lesbians and gay men among university students. *Journal of College Student Development, 41,* 70–80.

Norton, A. T., & Herek, G. M. (2013). Heterosexuals' attitudes toward transgender people: Findings from a national probability sample of U.S. adults. *Sex Roles, 68,* 738–753. http://dx.doi.org/10.1007/s11199-011-0110-6

O'Neil, J. M. (2008). Summarizing 25 years of research on men's gender role conflict using the Gender Role Conflict Scale: New research paradigms and clinical implications. *The Counseling Psychologist, 36,* 358–445. http://dx.doi.org/10.1177/0011000008317057

O'Neil, J. M. (2013). Gender role conflict research 30 years later: An evidence-based diagnostic schema to assess boys and men in counseling. *Journal of Counseling & Development, 91,* 490–498. http://dx.doi.org/10.1002/j.1556-6676.2013.00122.x

O'Neil, J. M., Helm, B., Gable, R., David, L., & Wrightsman, L. (1986). Gender Role Conflict Scale (GRCS): College men's fears of femininity. *Sex Roles, 14,* 335–350.

Ossana, S. M. (2000). Relationship and couples counseling. In R. M. Perez, K. A. DeBord, & K. J. Bieschke (Eds.), *Handbook of counseling and psychotherapy with lesbian, gay, and bisexual clients* (pp. 275–302). http://dx.doi.org/10.1037/10339-012

Owens, G. M. (2008). Gender differences in health care expenditures, resource utilization, and quality of care. *Journal of Managed Care Pharmacy, 14*(Suppl.), 2–6. http://dx.doi.org/10.18553/jmcp.2008.14.S3-A.2

Pachankis, J. E., & Goldfried, M. R. (2006). Social anxiety in young gay men. *Journal of Anxiety Disorders, 20,* 996–1015. http://dx.doi.org/10.1016/j.janxdis.2006.01.001

Pachankis, J. E., Westmaas, J. L., & Dougherty, L. R. (2011). The influence of sexual orientation and masculinity on young men's tobacco smoking. *Journal of Consulting and Clinical Psychology, 79,* 142–152. http://dx.doi.org/10.1037/a0022917

Parent, M. C., Torrey, C., & Michaels, M. S. (2012). "HIV testing is so gay": The role of masculine gender role conformity in HIV testing among men who have sex with men. *Journal of Counseling Psychology, 59,* 465–470. http://dx.doi.org/10.1037/a0028067

Parrott, D. J., Peterson, J. L., Vincent, W., & Bakeman, R. (2008). Correlates of anger in response to gay men: Effects of male gender role beliefs, sexual prejudice, and masculine gender role stress. *Psychology of Men & Masculinity, 9,* 167–178. http://dx.doi.org/10.1037/1524-9220.9.3.167

Patterson, C. J. (2009). Children of lesbian and gay parents: Psychology, law, and policy. *American Psychologist, 64*, 727–736. http://dx.doi.org/10.1037/0003-066X.64.8.727

Pleck, J. H. (1981). *The myth of masculinity.* Cambridge, MA: MIT Press.

Pleck, J. H. (1995). The gender role strain paradigm: An update. In R. F. Levant & W. S. Pollack (Eds.), *A new psychology of men* (pp. 11–32). New York, NY: Basic Books.

Rennison, C. M., & Welchans, S. (2000). *Bureau of Justice Statistics Special Report: Intimate partner violence.* Washington, DC: U.S. Department of Justice.

Ridge, D., Plummer, D., & Peasley, D. (2006). Remaking the masculine self and coping in the liminal world of the gay "scene." *Culture, Health & Sexuality, 8*, 501–514. http://dx.doi.org/10.1080/13691050600879524

Riggs, D., & O'Leary, K. (1989). A theoretical model of courtship aggression. In M. A. Pirog-Good & J. E. Stets (Eds.), *Violence in dating relationships* (pp. 53–71). New York, NY: Praeger.

Russell, E. M., DelPriore, D. J., Butterfield, M. E., & Hill, S. E. (2013). Friends with benefits, but without the sex: Straight women and gay men exchange trustworthy mating advice. *Evolutionary Psychology, 11*, 132–147. http://dx.doi.org/10.1177/147470491301100113

Safren, S. A., & Pantalone, D. W. (2006). Social anxiety and barriers to resilience among lesbian, gay, and bisexual adolescents. In A. M. Omoto & H. S. Kurtzman (Eds.), *Sexual orientation and mental health: Examining identity and development in lesbian, gay, and bisexual people* (pp. 55–71). http://dx.doi.org/10.1037/11261-003

Safren, S. A., Reisner, S. L., Herrick, A., Mimiaga, M. J., & Stall, R. D. (2010). Mental health and HIV risk in men who have sex with men. *Journal of Acquired Immune Deficiency Syndromes, 55*(Suppl. 2), S74–S77. http://dx.doi.org/10.1097/QAI.0b013e3181fbc939

Sánchez, F. J., Bocklandt, S., & Vilain, E. (2009). Gender role conflict, interest in casual sex, and relationship satisfaction among gay men. *Psychology of Men & Masculinity, 10*, 237–243. http://dx.doi.org/10.1037/a0016325

Sánchez, F. J., Bocklandt, S., & Vilain, E. (2013). The relationship between help-seeking attitudes and masculine norms among monozygotic male twins discordant for sexual orientation. *Health Psychology, 32*, 52–56. http://dx.doi.org/10.1037/a0029529

Sánchez, F. J., Westefeld, J. S., Liu, W. M., & Vilain, E. (2010). Masculine gender role conflict and negative feelings about being gay. *Professional Psychology: Research and Practice, 41*, 104–111. http://dx.doi.org/10.1037/a0015805

Schwartz, J. P., Waldo, M., & Daniel, D. (2005). Gender-role conflict and self-esteem: Factors associated with partner abuse in court-referred men. *Psychology of Men & Masculinity, 6*, 109–113. http://dx.doi.org/10.1037/1524-9220.6.2.109

Silberstein, L. R., Mishkind, M. E., Striegel-Moore, R. H., Timko, C., & Rodin, J. (1989). Men and their bodies: A comparison of homosexual and heterosexual men. *Psychosomatic Medicine, 51*, 337–346. http://dx.doi.org/10.1097/00006842-198905000-00008

Silverstein, C. (2009). The implications of removing homosexuality from the *DSM* as a mental disorder. *Archives of Sexual Behavior, 38*, 161–163. http://dx.doi.org/10.1007/s10508-008-9442-x

Simonsen, G., Blazina, C., & Watkins, C. E., Jr. (2000). Gender role conflict and psychological well-being among gay men. *Journal of Counseling Psychology, 47*, 85–89. http://dx.doi.org/10.1037/0022-0167.47.1.85

Sonenschein, D. (1968). The ethnography of male homosexual relationships. *Journal of Sex Research, 4*, 69–83. http://dx.doi.org/10.1080/00224496809550559

Spicer, S. S. (2010). Healthcare needs of the transgender homeless population. *Journal of Gay & Lesbian Mental Health, 14*, 320–339. http://dx.doi.org/10.1080/19359705.2010.505844

Szymanski, D. M., & Carr, E. R. (2008). The roles of gender role conflict and internalized heterosexism in gay and bisexual men's psychological distress: Testing two mediation models. *Psychology of Men & Masculinity, 9*, 40–54. http://dx.doi.org/10.1037/1524-9220.9.1.40

Taylor, G. J., Ryan, D., & Bagby, R. M. (1985). Toward the development of a new self-report alexithymia scale. *Psychotherapy and Psychosomatics, 44*, 191–199. http://dx.doi.org/10.1159/000287912

Tillmann-Healy, L. M. (2001). *Between gay and straight: Understanding friendship across sexual orientation.* Lanham, MD: Rowman AltaMira.

Tjepkema, M. (2008). *Health care use among gay, lesbian and bisexual Canadians* (Catalogue No. 82-003-X Health Reports). Toronto, Ontario, Canada: Statistics Canada.

Tokar, D. M., & Jome, L. M. (1998). Masculinity, vocational interests, and career choice traditionality: Evidence for a fully mediated model. *Journal of Counseling Psychology, 45*, 424–435. http://dx.doi.org/10.1037/0022-0167.45.4.424

Tornello, S. L., Farr, R. H., & Patterson, C. J. (2011). Predictors of parenting stress among gay adoptive fathers in the United States. *Journal of Family Psychology, 25*, 591–600. http://dx.doi.org/10.1037/a0024480

Tornello, S. L., & Patterson, C. J. (2012). Gay fathers in mixed-orientation relationships: Experiences of those who stay in their marriages and of those who leave. *Journal of GLBT Family Studies, 8*, 85–98. http://dx.doi.org/10.1080/1550428X.2012.641373

Tracey, T. J. G., & Glidden-Tracey, C. E. (1999). Integration of theory, research design, measurement, and analysis: Toward a reasoned argument. *The Counseling Psychologist, 27*, 299–324. http://dx.doi.org/10.1177/0011000099273002

Vandello, J. A., Bosson, J. K., Cohen, D., Burnaford, R. M., & Weaver, J. R. (2008). Precarious manhood. *Journal of Personality and Social Psychology, 95*, 1325–1339. http://dx.doi.org/10.1037/a0012453

Vaughan, M. D., Miles, J., Parent, M. C., Lee, H. S., Tilghman, J. D., & Prokhorets, S. (2014). A content analysis of LGBT-themed positive psychology articles. *Psychology of Sexual Orientation and Gender Diversity, 1*, 313–324. http://dx.doi.org/10.1037/sgd0000060

Vocks, S., Stahn, C., Loenser, K., & Legenbauer, T. (2009). Eating and body image disturbances in male-to-female and female-to-male transsexuals. *Archives of Sexual Behavior, 38*, 364–377. http://dx.doi.org/10.1007/s10508-008-9424-z

Vogel, D. L., Heimerdinger-Edwards, S. R., Hammer, J. H., & Hubbard, A. (2011). "Boys don't cry": Examination of the links between endorsement of masculine norms, self-stigma, and help-seeking attitudes for men from diverse backgrounds. *Journal of Counseling Psychology, 58*, 368–382. http://dx.doi.org/10.1037/a0023688

Vorst, H. C. M., & Bermond, B. (2001). Validity and reliability of the Bermond–Vorst alexithymia questionnaire. *Personality and Individual Differences, 30*, 413–434. http://dx.doi.org/10.1016/S0191-8869(00)00033-7

Wade, J. C., & Donis, E. (2007). Masculinity ideology, male identity, and romantic relationship quality among heterosexual and gay men. *Sex Roles, 57*, 775–786. http://dx.doi.org/10.1007/s11199-007-9303-4

Watt, H. M. G., & Eccles, J. S. (Eds.). (2008). *Gender and occupational outcomes: Longitudinal assessments of individual, social, and cultural influences.* http://dx.doi.org/10.1037/11706-000

Wester, S. R., Pionke, D. R., & Vogel, D. L. (2005). Male gender role conflict, gay men, and same-sex romantic relationships. *Psychology of Men & Masculinity, 6*, 195–208. http://dx.doi.org/10.1037/1524-9220.6.3.195

Whetten, K., Reif, S., Whetten, R., & Murphy-McMillan, L. K. (2008). Trauma, mental health, distrust, and stigma among HIV-positive persons: Implications for effective care. *Psychosomatic Medicine, 70*, 531–538. http://dx.doi.org/10.1097/PSY.0b013e31817749dc

Wilson, B. D. M., Harper, G. W., Hidalgo, M. A., Jamil, O. B., Torres, R. S., Fernandez, M. I., & the Adolescent Medicine Trials Network for HIV/AIDS Interventions. (2010). Negotiating dominant masculinity ideology: Strategies used by gay, bisexual and questioning male adolescents. *American Journal of Community Psychology, 45*, 169–185. http://dx.doi.org/10.1007/s10464-009-9291-3

World Health Organization. (2002). *Prevention and promotion in mental health.* Geneva, Switzerland: Author.

# IV

## IMPLICATIONS
## FOR PRACTICE

# 11

# COUNSELING, PSYCHOTHERAPY, AND PSYCHOLOGICAL INTERVENTIONS FOR BOYS AND MEN

GARY R. BROOKS

At the core of the new psychology of men has been the emergence of a new way of thinking about people. For many decades, theorists and practitioners made efforts to understand only the universal commonalities among all people. Although this approach may have been well intentioned, it was vehemently attacked by the feminist corrective in mental health. The 1975 American Psychological Association (APA) Task Force on Sex Bias and Sex Role Stereotyping in Mental Health charged that by treating stereotypical masculine attributes as universal (i.e., applicable to both men and women), the mental health field was profoundly patriarchal, ignoring female experiences and silencing women's voices. Since the appearance of the feminist critique of psychotherapy and the subsequent 2007 APA *Guidelines for Psychological Practice With Girls and Women*, mental health practitioners are far more likely to be aware of the ways that women can be mistreated in the therapy situation. Ironically, however, awareness has been slower in coming

http://dx.doi.org/10.1037/0000023-012
*The Psychology of Men and Masculinities*, R. F. Levant and Y. J. Wong (Editors)

in terms of recognizing the ways that "gender-blind psychotherapy" (i.e., therapy that ignores gender differences) has poorly served males.[1]

This chapter contends that although conventional therapy practices have sometimes been harmful to women who have actually been in therapy, they have been less visibly harmful to men by discouraging men from entering therapy at all. It is pointed out that recent economic and political trends have created dramatic sociocultural shifts in gender status and gender relations. These upheavals have created a crisis of masculinity that has not only produced distress among men but has been poorly addressed by the fields of counseling and therapy. Despite the recognition that these fields have been male-dominated, it has only recently been recognized that in many ways, men have also been harmed by gender-blind psychotherapy practices. Furthermore, only recently have theorists and practitioners drawn on the advances in understanding of male socialization and masculinity ideologies (see earlier chapters) and begun to challenge the limitations of conventional therapy practices and offered new types of interventions that are more congruent with men's ways of being.

## THE CONTEMPORARY CRISIS OF MASCULINITY

More than 2 decades ago, Betcher and Pollack (1993) wrote, "We live in a time of fallen heroes. . . . Men have been brought to earth, their strengths put in perspective by their flaws. . . . The empire seems to be crumbling" (p. 1). Similarly, Levant and Kopecky (1995) wrote, "American manhood is in crisis . . . the social changes wrought by the feminist movement have left our traditional code of masculinity in a state of collapse" (p. 1). In her 1999 book *Stiffed: The Betrayal of the American Man*, Faludi described current thinking on the matter as follows: "A domestic apocalypse was underway: American manhood was under siege" (p. 6). To many, such alarm may now seem overstated in light of the continued dominance of men in corporate boardrooms, political offices, and higher echelons of academic administration. Yet there are many signs of escalating problems for most men.

In her provocative book *The End of Men and the Rise of Women*, Rosin (2012) cited data from multiple sources, including the Bureau of Labor Statistics and the American Council on Education, documenting seismic changes in the balance of power in the lives of women and men. The massive recession in the U.S. economy of 2009 affected all Americans, but three quarters of jobs lost were lost by men, with "male" occupations of construction,

---

[1]Throughout this chapter, the term *males* is used to avoid the need to continually repeat *men and boys*.

manufacturing, and finance the hardest hit (Rosin, 2012). Rosin further noted that

> women worldwide dominate colleges and professional schools . . . in the United States, for every two men who will receive a BA this year, for example, three women will do the same . . . of the fifteen job categories to grow the most in the United States over the next decade, twelve are occupied primarily by women. (pp. 3–4)

Within the profession of psychology, some concerns have been raised about what has been referred to as the "feminization" of psychology (Goodheart & Markham, 1992), that is, the declining rates of males within the field.

## THE PROBLEMS WITH MALES AND PSYCHOTHERAPY

One of the most pernicious realities of the crisis of masculinity has been that despite the level of distress, there has been long-standing antagonism between men and help-seeking in general, and psychotherapy in particular. Addis and Mahalik (2003) observed that an extensive body of empirical research has documented that men are less likely than women to seek help for a diversity of physical, emotional, and situation problems. Others (Tucker et al., 2013; Vessey & Howard, 1993) have narrowed this observation to the recognition that men are especially likely to avoid psychotherapy. Multiple factors have been implicated in this discordance, including stigma (Tucker et al., 2013), precarious manhood (Vandello & Bosson, 2013), social network factors (Angermeyer, Matschinger, & Riedel-Heller, 2001), and institutional restrictions in many male-dominated settings such as the military and police settings (Brooks, 2012; Vogel, Wester, Hammer, & Downing-Matibag, 2014). In his characterization of men's aversion to psychotherapy, Brooks (1998, 2010) criticized the fields of counseling and psychotherapy for their failure to develop creative variations in conventional therapy techniques and delivery modalities that are more harmonious with male coping and help-seeking styles.

## OVERCOMING THE IMPASSE— MODIFYING THERAPIES FOR MALES

In discussing the "culture clash" between men and therapy, Rochlen (2014) stated: "Counseling men needs to be more consistent with the way men relate, connect and open up. The process needs to feel less threatening, more problem-focused, and, ultimately, more 'male-friendly'" (p. 4). Fortunately, the past decade has witnessed a burgeoning of new publications devoted to new models and ideas for approaching men within the psycho-therapy hour. For example, in early 2015, the Resources section of the website of the Society for the Psychological Study of Men and Masculinity (SPSMM; http://www.apa.org/about/division/div51.aspx) identified 67 books authored by SPSMM members, addressing a multitude of issues, populations, and treatment approaches. The books have taken a variety of forms. Some of the books (Englar-Carlson, Evans, & Duffey, 2014; Good & Brooks, 2005; Rochlen & Rabinowitz, 2014) have been edited, with coverage of a broad array of topics. Some (Brooks, 2010; Donaldson & Flood, 2014; Glicken, 2005; Rabinowitz & Cochran, 2002; Wexler, 2009) have been one- or two-author books address-ing process and technique issues with men in general. Some have considered specific therapy modalities (Andronico, 1996; Shepard & Harway, 2012). Many (Courtenay, 2011; Kiselica, Englar-Carlson, & Horne, 2008; Lynch & Kilmartin, 2013; Oren & Oren, 2009; Robertson, 2012; Vacha-Haase, Wester, & Christianson, 2010) have described therapy interventions with specific problems or common male populations, while and others (Ellis & Carlson, 2016; Liu, Iwamoto, & Chae, 2010; Silverstein, 2011; Sweet, 2012) have con-sidered specific issues with diverse populations (diversity of age, ethnicity, and sexual identity).

Especially beneficial from this new literature have been ideas about how established therapy approaches, psychodynamic, cognitive behavioral, interpersonal, client-centered, and existential therapies can be adapted to fit more harmoniously with the needs and styles of male populations. Space permits only a brief overview of the more fully developed applications of these approaches to male clients.

## Psychodynamic Approaches for Male Clients

Psychodynamic approaches to therapy with men were thoroughly described by William Pollack (2005). Pollack posited that a required devel-opmental process of separation and disidentification from mothers is deeply wounding of the character development of young boys. He noted that "this premature push for separation [causes] a traumatic disruption of the early holding environment . . . a life cycle loss in boys that may show itself later in adulthood in symptomatic behavior and characterological disturbance" (p. 205). Pollack's emphasis on the shattering of a boy's holding environ-ment is congruent with the early-life wounding experiences described by Rabinowitz and Cochran (2002). These therapists contend that the ultimate problems with trust and intimate relationships can only be addressed by uncovering their roots in childhood. Pollack emphasizes the need for therapy to symbolically re-create the early holding environment as a path to healing the deep levels of psychic damage.

## Cognitive and Cognitive-Behavioral Approaches for Male Clients

Perhaps the therapeutic modalities with most "face validity" for many men are those of cognitive and cognitive-behavioral therapies (CBT). Mahalik (2005a) stated, "Although emotions are a central part of the work that goes on in cognitive therapy, its focus on the importance of thoughts is likely to feel more congruent for men who conform to traditional gender roles regarding emotional expression" (p. 217). In conducting cognitive therapy with men, the first step is to discover basic cognitive schemas and self-talk underlying distortions and maladaptive ideas about manhood. In this regard, Mahalik (2005a) identified "nine injunctions of traditional masculinity" and gender-related cognitive distortions. Therapy in this modality consists of disconfirming a man's masculinity-related cognitive distortions, pointing out inconsistencies and illogical thinking, and creating personal experiments to test the accuracy of cognitive distortions. More recently, Spendelow (2015) extended Mahalik's ideas to describe the application of CBT for treatment of depression in men.

## Interpersonal Approaches for Male Clients

Developed first in the 1970s and 1980s by Klerman and colleagues (Klerman, Weissman, Rounsaville, & Chevron, 1984), the interpersonal therapy (IPT) approach combines the concepts of attachment theory and the object relations approach with a cognitive-behavioral emphasis on reinforcing interpersonal patterns in the here and now. For males, the childhood failures in acquisition of sufficient emotional nurturance and associated behavioral skills produce poor-quality relations and ultimately produce despair, loneliness, and depression. There is some empirical evidence that men, in general, are more likely to display the damaging effects of this process with relationships characterized by hostile, detached, cold, distant, and mistrusting qualities (Tracey & Schneider, 1995).

Because the IPT approach has been described as "a short-term, present-oriented psychotherapy focused mainly on the patient's current interpersonal relationships and life situations" (Prochaska & Norcross, 2007, p. 178), it may have significant advantages in initial engagement of therapy reticent males. Mahalik (2005b) contended that IPT has unique benefits for men for unlearning some of the most basic messages they have received about relating with others. According to Mahalik (2005b),

> Whereas the masculine socialization process encourages developing a sense of self through renouncing "femininity," interpersonal psychotherapists can help traditionally socialized men integrate parts of themselves that have been underdeveloped . . . [and] move toward relationships with others and integrate an emotional life. (p. 244)

## Humanistic, Existential, and Experiential Therapies for Male Clients

Although an extremely small number of therapists identify themselves as exclusively Rogerian, gestalt, or humanistic/existential in their theoretical orientation (Bechtoldt, Norcross, Wyckoff, Pokrywa, & Campbell, 2001), the cumulative impact of these approaches has been substantial. Kilmartin and Smiler (2015) applied the Rogerian principle of *conditional worth* to male development by noting that the gender role strain paradigm illustrates how traditional male socialization calls for rejecting essential parts of oneself and makes authentic living impossible. They stated,

> If the vigorous experience of the self provides the data upon which to base existential decisions, then many men are basing their decisions on limited information. The socialization of boys to avoid emotion leaves a large gap in their experience of the self. (p. 241)

The most elaborated incorporation of humanistic and existential perspectives into therapy work with men has been provided by Rabinowitz and Cochran (2002). They contended that carefully conducted experiential activities allow for active expression of feelings and access to the deeper reaches of a man's psyche. From an existential perspective, they have suggested techniques such as "confronting internal discrepancies" and "asking existential questions" to allow a man to "move beyond his empty storytelling and intellectualizing toward more authentic engagement with his psychological dilemmas" (p. 66). Further, they describe the value of "acknowledging death and mortality, confronting freedom of choice, and facing aloneness" (p. 67) to help a client move beyond the surface of therapy concerns and face the basic complexities of life.

## Group Therapy for Males

With the appearance of the new literature on psychotherapy with men, all-male groups have become identified as particularly useful to help men cope with the demands of the male gender role and gender role strain (Andronico, 1996; Brooks, 2010; Rabinowitz, 2014). These authors have described several unique advantages of all-male groups, for men in general, whereas Franklin, Chen, Hammad, Capawana, and Hoogasian (2015) focused on the benefits of this modality for African American men. First, such groups help men overcome the shameful uniqueness they may experience in being in the situation of needing help. This situation allows males to realize the relative universality of problems that all men face. Second, groups call for lower levels of communication demand by substituting side-by-side interactions for the intensity of face-to-face interactions. Therapy groups also provide an opportunity for "participative self-disclosure" (Brooks, 2010, p. 106), whereby group members' alternating revelations are supported and members are encouraged to expose vulnerabilities. Also, men's groups are the only venue to help men learn something impossible in other therapy formats—that men can provide emotional support and comforting for each other without the usual reliance on women for that function. Finally, the all-male group can be an especially valuable source of encouragement through the "instillation of hope" curative factor (Yalom & Leszcz, 2005). By witnessing the progress of men further along in the gender-role journey, men can be empowered to undertake the needed changes in their lives.

Resolving the problematic impasse between men and psychotherapy has no doubt been helped by these thoughtful ideas for making men more comfortable within the conventional therapy hour—that is, finding better ways to conduct more male-syntonic psychotherapy interventions. Yet these valuable contributions may not go far enough because they all share a common limitation: They require a man to enter the therapist's office and to take on the client role. In light of the aforementioned issues of stigma and men's resistance, these improved modalities may nevertheless go unutilized. To call on a sadly overused metaphor, it seems that some significant "outside-the-box" thinking may be needed. Fortunately, there are many resources with the psychological literature than can be drawn from and applied to this dilemma. Brooks (2010), in his exposition of "outside-the-office" interventions, identified several of them based in well-recognized psychological practices and processes—primary prevention, consultation, psychoeducation, stage of change, and consciousness raising—all of which suggest alternative ways to help men and boys receive the help they need.

## NOT RESTRICTED BY CONVENTIONAL BOUNDARIES— EXPANDING POSSIBILITIES FOR INTERVENTIONS WITH BOYS AND MEN

Although primary prevention, stages of change, consciousness raising, psychoeducation, and consultation differ in terms of their bodies of literature and their adherents, they share a common element: They do not require that a recipient of these psychological change practices ever enter a therapist's office. In essence, they are consistent with the notion of "bringing the mountain to Muhammad": If men won't come to therapists' offices, we may want to take our therapeutic efforts to them—that is, go where they already are.

As one of the earliest proponents of primary prevention, George Albee noted, "you can't stop an epidemic by treating one person at a time . . . taking preventative actions before the epidemic occurs is the only way" (as cited in Bloom, 2008, p. 107). Conyne (1987) described primary prevention as a series of intentional programs that target groups to promote functioning in healthy ways. The primary prevention model, as articulated by Bloom (2008), comprises three essential elements: prevention of predictable and interrelated problems, protection of existing states of health, and promotion of psychosocial wellness for identified populations of people (p. 110).

With specific reference to the application of primary prevention to male populations, Kiselica and Look (1993) presented forceful arguments for greater attention to preventive mental health. That critique was echoed by others within counseling psychology who expressed concern that a trend toward tertiary prevention would cost counseling psychology its distinctiveness as advocate for primary prevention in mental health (Sprinthall, 1990). Years later, Kiselica and colleagues presented an approach to enhance the "developmental trajectory" of young men and build strengths of emotional competence and positive masculinity (Kiselica, Englar-Carlson, & Horne, 2008).

Although not overtly couching his ideas under a primary prevention rubric, Zur (2008) presented a compelling argument that interventions taking place "beyond the office walls" or "outside the office" may be most helpful in a variety of situations, especially those by culture-sensitive therapists wishing to "emphasize flexibility and respect for clients' tradition, culture" (p. 8). Brooks (2010) contended that out-of-the-office interventions allow therapists to address the dysfunctional aspects of men's everyday lives early and preventively, before the malaise of gender role strain produces more maladaptive coping mechanisms, such as violence, substance abuse, or sexual misconduct.

Perhaps one of the more intriguing arguments for the utility of primary prevention for males can be found in a seemingly unrelated, yet nevertheless especially valuable line of parallel paradigm development. The "process of change" and "stage of change" model (Prochaska & DiClemente, 1982; Prochaska & Norcross, 2007) has been exceptionally valuable across all therapies because it calls attention to the reality that intervention will succeed or fail according to whether the client's readiness to consider change is taken into account. At the earliest point of readiness—precontemplation—clients are not only unaware of a need to make changes but are likely to resist and, when relenting to coercion, will only make superficial changes until the pressure dissipates (Prochaska & Norcross, 2007).

An enormous appeal of the stage of change model is what seems to be its special relevance to male populations. In light of the foregoing observations of the antipathy of most males to psychotherapy, it is not a stretch to consider many males to be precontemplators. That is, many men are unaware of the need to change some aspects of their traditional male ideas and behaviors.

By moving outside their offices and adopting primary prevention activities for precontemplative males, therapists may be taking the vital first step to generate positive contacts between men and therapists. This process could bridge gaps and shatter negative therapist stereotypes and further the process of empathic connection. In addition to the benefits of consciousness raising, these out-of-office activities may facilitate a segue into further therapy in office settings by allowing men to realize that other men have similar struggles and problems.

### Consultation—Setting-Specific Interventions for Males

The mental health consultation model, as described by Zins and Erchul (2002), provides

> a method of providing preventively oriented psychological and educational services in which consultants and consultees form cooperative partnerships and engage in reciprocal, systemic, problem-solving partnerships . . . to enhance and empower consultee systems, thereby promoting clients well-being. (p. 625)

Carney and Jefferson (2014) identified mental health consultation as an underutilized opportunity for enhancement of practice opportunities and professional growth.

This mental health consultation model has already had considerable success in developing intervention strategies for a wide variety of male populations and presents promising potential for even greater expansion Among these setting-specific models, Courtenay's ideas for interventions in health care settings have been among the best articulated. His HEALTH model (Courtenay, 2011) offers guidance for health professionals seeking to recognize men's unique health problems and the barriers to accessing their needed care. In his work within the health care system, Courtenay exemplifies the possibilities of consultation and proactive outreach in which knowledge of men and masculinity enriches physical health and sometimes opens doors for entry in more formal psychotherapy.

Another focus of intervention for men has been that of using executive coaching to help them become more adaptive to changing environments within the world of business (Hills, Carlstrom, & Evanow, 2005). Because business and corporate communities are now more likely to emphasize interpersonal insight and skills over anachronistic authoritarian styles of leadership, there have been opportunities for coaches to reach many therapy-averse men and promote psychological growth. Hills et al. (2005) contended that the "inner-journey" emphasis of executive coaching is quite similar to the emphasis of counseling and therapy in their contention that "if a man becomes more interpersonally effective, he will probably become a better leader and a better friend, father and partner" (p. 55).

Despite the observation of Richards and Bergin (2000) that religion and the mental health professions have historically been alienated, there nevertheless are many opportunities for outreach to men through church and religious settings (Robertson, 2013). Men's groups are a common activity within many churches. Although most men's groups within churches have focused primarily on spiritual issues and have had a socially conservative agenda (e.g., Promise Keepers), there have been others (e.g., the Unitarian Universalist Men's Network) that are far more embracing of new ideas about manhood and intergender relations. Davidson (2000) contended that the efforts of many members of gay, lesbian, bisexual, and transgender communities to function within established religions or establish their own churches illustrates the potential of maintaining ties with religiously oriented persons and promoting psychological growth.

The U.S. military and the Veterans Affairs Health Care system have a long history of providing mental health care to soldiers and veterans, the majority of whom have been men. Sadly, it is only recently that interventions for male veterans have taken gender into account to understand many of these veterans' mental health problems. Brooks (1990) highlighted the need to consider masculinity and male gender norms in treatments for male veterans. Significant evidence for the value of this position has recently emerged with the work of Jakupcak and his colleagues at the Washington Puget Sound VA. These psychologists have completed numerous studies of the relationship between male gender role norms and distress among male (and female) veterans (Jakupcak & Varra, 2011) and have subsequently called for programmatic outreach efforts and clinical interventions that take these gender role norms into account (Jakupcak, Blais, Grossbard, Garcia, & Okiishi, 2014).

Because prison and forensic populations are more than 90% male, they represent settings with extraordinary access to troubled men (Kupers, 2001). Kupers (2001) described the prison setting as one of the most extreme for exacerbation of "toxic masculinity," which he considered to be the "constellation of traits in men that serve to foster domination, the devaluation of women, homophobia, and wanton violence" (p. 171). When it is recognized that ethnic minority men comprise more than 80% of the U.S. prison population (Wagner, 2012), it becomes evident that this setting has enormous potential for masculinity-informed interventions with African American, Latino, and Native American men.

Finally, physical and alcohol rehabilitation programs offer additional sites for enhancement of therapeutic efforts with gender-informed perspectives. Marini (2005) recommended that therapists working with men in physical rehabilitation settings become fully aware of the interaction between masculine identity and rehabilitation outcome to develop interventions that circumvent the dysfunctional aspects of traditional men's most common coping styles. Isenhart (2005) urged alcohol treatment programs to include components specifically addressing the interaction of the male role with alcohol abuse.

### Primary Prevention—Psychoeducational and Consciousness Raising Activities

Interventions that provide information to men (and loved ones) about masculinity, gender roles, and gender role strain can take place in a variety of settings, from formal classroom activities to community-based programs with a primary prevention focus. In a fashion similar to the way that many women first became part of the women's movement, many men are being given opportunities for greater awareness through formal men's studies courses. Urschel (2000) noted that such courses have displayed a steady rate of acceptance in academia. Further documentation of this trend has been provided by O'Neil and Renzulli (2013), who noted that "teaching the psychology of men is a new discipline that has been developing over the past 10 years . . . the [survey] results indicate that teaching the psychology of men is becoming established" (p. 230).

The best illustration of a carefully articulated psychoeducational activity for men has been that of the gender role journey workshops first described by O'Neil and Carroll (1988). Those workshops featured a mixture of lectures and experiential activities to increase participants' awareness of gender role restrictions, intergender conflicts, and sexist behaviors. The workshops were conducted annually with male and female students between 1984 and 2006 in a psychology graduate school program. In their review of many years of evaluations from workshop participants, O'Neil and Renzulli (2013) reported that a high percentage of them found the experiences emotionally impactful and enhancing of their understanding of the effects of gender role restrictions. Although these workshops are distinct from formal psychotherapy interventions, they can easily be recognized as consciousness raising in that they can facilitate many men's transition from precontemplation to a stage more welcoming of eventual therapy participation.

Two other psychoeducational programs merit attention here. One, the Boy's Forum (O'Neil, Challenger, Renzulli, Crapser, & Webster, 2013), was a 2-day program for middle school boys conducted in an urban setting. O'Neil described the approach as a simple and straightforward method that empowers middle school–age boys to understand their masculinity issues, psychosocial development, and gender role transitions (O'Neil et al., 2013). A second psychoeducational program was one to combat "normative male alexithymia," conducted by Levant and Kelly (1989) for fathers and later developed into a manualized treatment program for a broader population of men. This proactive outreach program, alexithymia reduction treatment (Levant, Halter, Hayden, & Williams, 2009), demonstrated success in helping men become more aware of their emotional lives and better able to interact with others on an affective level.

### Weekend Retreats, Adventure Therapy, and Men's Centers

Since the late 1980s, there have been multiple variants of the weekend retreats most known to the general public through the mythopoetic movement of Robert Bly. Those retreats are similar to those of the "Modern Men's Weekend" described by Wissocki and Andronico (1996). The intent of these weekends, they contend, is not to focus on political goals but to use "mythological, psychological, and spiritual information to help men find internal congruence and the strength to access empowering images of masculine energy" (p. 114). Another group, the Men Mentoring Men organization, holds bimonthly meetings to "provide a safe and shameless experience for men to discuss, share, explore, and live inside the best of masculinity" (http://www.mthree.org/what-is-m3).

Recently, Englar-Carlson and Stevens (2014), in describing their experiential weekend retreats for men, suggested that the retreats allow participants to "deeply connect with each other and experience the risks, fears, and thrills of living authentically in the moment with other men" (p. 88). They consider their objective as that of creating a humanistic gathering spot that is "outside of the masculinity box."

Another variant of outside the office therapeutic experiences is that of the adventure therapy (Scheinfeld & Buser, 2014). The critical characteristic of the adventure therapy approach is engaging men though shared physical activities in natural settings (e.g., mountains, wilderness, and rivers). Proponents have noted that "guys feel a greater sense of confidence and motivation when they come together to accomplish tasks . . . the gestalt of [adventure therapy] provides an invigorating and adventurous experience, while creating space for intrapersonal and interpersonal insights" (Scheinfeld & Buser, 2014, p. 78).

The men's center approach on college campuses (Davies, Shen-Miller, & Isacco, 2010) shares common components with other outside-the-office interventions for men. It is consultative in that it introduces men and masculinity perspectives into programs originally targeting only men's physical health, and it is psychoeducational in that it teaches relational and emotional skills. It is, importantly, innovative in terms of "locating interventions in existing academic and social structures of campus life . . . creating therapeutic environments in nontherapy settings allows us to reach men who would not normally seek help" (Davies, Shen-Miller, & Isacco, 2010, p. 348). Two representative programs described by these authors are Madskills and Fraternity Leadership Class. The first is an intervention for men who violate the campus conduct code and the second is designed to promote positive leadership skills and help fraternity leaders be more informed about high-risk behaviors of men.

### Public Service Announcements and Digital Media

In the Internet era, there may be no avenue of broader access to public awareness than Public Service Announcements (PSAs). These activities can reach men who might otherwise never be exposed to critical information about mental health issues and who are likely to be susceptible to stigma against any type of mental health intervention. Of the many of these PSAs relevant to men's mental health, the National Institute of Mental Health's "Real Men. Real Depression" campaign (http://www.nimh.nih.gov/health/topics/men-and-mental-health/nimhs-real-men-real-depression-campaign.shtml) has probably had the greatest penetration, having been viewed by more than 345 million people (Kersting, 2005). Of special interest here has been the research of Rochlen and colleagues related to that campaign. Rochlen, McKelley, and Pituch (2006) reported that "it's clearly tailored to the specific audience that research has shown needs some direct, targeted and specific attention" (p. 2). Another example of this type of activity would be the efforts of Bring Change to Mind, a self-described stigma-fighting nonprofit focusing on men and mental illness (http://www.BringChange2Mind.org). "A Call to Men: The Next Generation of Manhood" is a production of the TIDES Organization addressing men's violence against women (http://www.acalltomen.org). Stomp Out Bullying is an organization committed to "reducing and preventing bullying, cyberbullying, sexting, and other digital abuse" (http://www.stompoutbullying.org).

In the area of digital media, the *Tough Guise* videos of Jackson Katz and Sut Jhali are especially impactful and poignant in examining the destructive impact of violence and tough posturing among boys and men (http://www.mediaed.org). In his documentary video *Dreamworlds*, Sut Jhali "takes a clarifying look at the warped world of music videos" (http://www.mediaed.org). In *Hip-Hop: Beyond Beats and Rhymes*, Byron Hurt analyzes the effects of hip hop culture on (primarily) young African American males (http://www.pbs.org/independentlens/hiphop/film.htm).

## Primary Prevention for Vulnerable Boys and Young Men

A plethora of books have appeared over the past 2 decades related to the problematic issues of modern boyhood. William Pollack's (1998) *Real Boys* raised alarms about the sociocultural climate for young men, and others echoed his concerns (Kindlon & Thompson, 2000; Sax, 2007). A welcome outgrowth of these treatises has been the development of many primary prevention activities designed to insulate young males from the hazards inherent in traditional male socialization. Again, only a few representative programs can be noted here.

A central component of these primary prevention programs has been that of developing positive coping behaviors, as illustrated by the growing area of resilience research (Arbona & Coleman, 2008). In this vein, Danish and Forneris (2008) described a developmental approach to promote "competency across the life span" (p. 500). One of their specific programs, Going for the Goal, is designed to help children of both genders gain a sense of personal control and confidence about their futures. From this resilience model, an encouraging trend has appeared in terms of programs targeting especially vulnerable young men. For example, in the cover story of the October 2014 *Monitor on Psychology*, DeAngelis (2014) described a range of programs designed for "Building resilience among black boys" (p. 50). A similar resilience program addressing the needs of Mexican American young men has been described by Chapin (2015). Marzalek and Logan (2014) described a program developed to "protect sexual minority youth from the risks associated with minority stress" (p. 319). Supportive programs for special needs children are being offered by the Education-A-Must Organization (http://www.education-a-must.com).

## THE NEXT STEP—WELCOMING AND TREATING RELUCTANT MALES

As was noted earlier in this chapter, the shifting cultural landscape has profoundly altered the lives of most men. Some men have responded adaptively and creatively, but many have not. The greater empowerment of previously disadvantaged groups has undercut hegemonic masculinity and challenged defensive fallbacks of sexism, racism, and heterosexism. O'Neil (2014) noted that "a paradigm shift is occurring with conceptions of masculinity in America, and this transition is hopeful and significant" (p. ix). The signs of positive change are not overwhelming, but they are present. Some men are performing more domestic labor (Blair, 2012). The "reconstructed fathering role" (Silverstein, Auerbach, & Levant, 2002) has been illustrated by fathers in delivery rooms, as well as the recent appearance of the "stay-at-home dads" phenomenon (Rochlen, McKelley, & Whittaker, 2010). In recent years, there are signs of shifts in endorsement of some traditional male values. Levant, Hall, and Rankin (2013) found that some young men, when completing measures tapping their adherence to traditional male norms, do not endorse the expectations that males should be dominant, emotionally restricted, and negative toward sexual minorities.

However, regardless of the degree to which males have adapted to the changing culture, it has been apparent that there has not yet been a stampede of boys and men arriving at the offices of psychotherapists and counselors. Nevertheless, there are reasons to hope that the greater attention to the factors inhibiting men's therapy participation is being better addressed by the psychotherapy professions. Also, there is hope that the previously discussed out-of-office activities will raise men's consciousness about their lives, lessen stigma about revealing personal distress, disrupt precontemplative thinking, and, in some cases, lead to entry in formal psychotherapy. If this optimistic scenario is to produce the best possible outcome, then there will need to be continued reconceptualizing and reshaping of many aspects of typical practices.

This chapter has thus far discussed some of the creative alterations of standard therapy models. In the remainder of the chapter, attention is paid to some of the more general changes that can maximize chances for success. These include contextualizing the stage of change model, incorporating insights from research on the working alliance and multicultural competence, and offering an overall framework for male-friendly therapy.

## Expanding the Stage of Change Model

Most therapists quickly realize that it is a major error to assume that all males seeking appointments are fully motivated to launch a therapy experience. More often than not, their motivation is far more complex. Fisch, Weakland, and Segal (1982) identified the importance of determining the "true customer of therapy"—that is, determining whether the impetus is coming from the client or from forces in his social environment. It is in terms of the "customer of therapy" that the intrapsychic focus of the Prochaska and Norcross (2007) stage of change model can benefit by paying greater attention to social environment and contextual factors in the life of a wavering male client. Given the therapy resistance common to most men, the change process will be greatly affected by the environment in which the potential client functions. A male client may be at the precontemplative stage, or he may be further along and in the "action" stage (i.e., he is aware of his problems and ready to work to make needed changes). Likewise, the people and forces in his life may be supportive of therapy, or they may be hostile or indifferent. Brooks (2010) discussed the four extreme circumstances: (a) precontemplative man/precontemplative context, (b) precontemplative man/action stage context, (c) action stage man/precontemplative context, and (d) action stage man/action stage context. He contends that each of these circumstances calls for a differing approach by the therapist.

Of the four possible situations, the first is the least likely to produce successful therapy and the last is likely to be most successful. The third will be the least common, and the second will be the most common and most difficult to manage. This second circumstance (precontemplative man/action stage context) is best exemplified by Scher's (1990, p. 323) characterization that men enter therapy only when desperate or when something external has driven them to it. Brooks (2010) offered an expanded stage of change model, with alternative strategies for each of these four circumstances. Only the strategies for the most common situation—resistant man in a coercive situation—will be highlighted here.

The first feature of this strategy is the recognition of the vital importance of the first therapy contact. Brooks (1998) noted that when encountering a new male client the therapist must "take full advantage of this first chance to engage a reluctant man in therapy. They must turn the tide and shift the momentum, doing whatever is reasonable to demonstrate . . . that therapy has something to offer" (p. 71). Similarly, Good and Robertson (2010) wrote,

> Getting boys and men to avail themselves of psychological services is the first challenge. But when men do present, the second challenge is to get them to trust therapists sufficiently to share their issues and to form an effective working alliance. (p. 306)

Men's therapy experts have offered a number of suggestions for a successful first contact with a male client. Prominent among these has been the "strengths" aspect of the positive psychology/positive masculinity perspective (Englar-Carlson & Kiselica, 2013; Kiselica & Englar-Carlson, 2010). That orientation calls for initial contacts to focus on more than the client's failings and also highlight the more admirable aspects of his behavior (including the willingness to enter the alien therapy environment). In fact, the man's skepticism and hesitance can be recognized as understandable and respectable. This stance is consistent with the motivational interviewing ideas of Miller and Rollnick (2002), with emphasis on "expressing empathy . . . rolling with resistance and supporting self-efficacy" (p. 32). Related to this attitude, Kilmartin (2014) described the value of sensitive humor to facilitate a "foot-in the door" with men (p. 29). Wexler (2014) articulated the appropriate use of therapist self-disclosure: "Therapist self-disclosure, carefully calibrated, can be extremely effective in fostering the therapeutic alliance and helping bring men out of their shell" (p. 30).

To these creative suggestions, Brooks (2010) added another strategy: triangulation. According to Brooks, "In the common situation in which a male client has been more or less coerced into therapy, a therapist is prudent to maximize the strategic benefits of a *triangulated position*" (p. 78). In essence, the therapist positions himself or herself as the go-between in a struggle between the male client and the therapy-pressuring person or agency. The therapist might ask, "What is it that is causing folks to be so much on your case?" From a go-between position, the therapist can mediate benevolently between the troubled factions without losing credibility with either. Because this strategic position can be maintained only when the external parties are resolute in their pressure, it is often useful for the therapist to (privately and within ethical guidelines) be in contact with them to reinforce their insistence for change. Also, the benefits of this position will be lost if the therapist is seen as too closely allied with others and is just another person who doesn't appreciate the male client's distress.

### Critical Beginnings—The Working Alliance and Multicultural Competence

Successful therapy with male clients only begins when a male client understands (or discovers) that therapy has something positive to offer him. Proponents of three perspectives have much to offer in this area. These are researchers on the working alliance, proponents of multicultural competence, and advocates of user-friendly therapy for males.

Psychotherapy research over the past 15 years has demonstrated persuasively that the key components in successful therapy outcome are not tied to any specific therapy modality but are best represented by relationship process variables. These variables have been described as the *working alliance* (Bordin, 1994) or the *therapeutic alliance* (Norcross & Lambert, 2011). As described by Bordin, the working alliance comprises three components: agreement on therapy goals, consensus about the tasks and activities within the therapy sessions, and the relationship between the client and the therapist. This third component, the broadest and most encompassing, is that of the sense of a "bond" between the client and therapist. Horvath and Bedi (2002) considered this to include "mutual trust, liking, respect, and caring" (p. 41).

Sue and Sue (2015) have been the leading proponents of the view that all therapists working with cultural groups differing from their own should work assiduously to develop multicultural competence. They contend that ethical practice requires deep appreciation of the worldviews of differing groups to avoid imposing therapists' own values and beliefs on clients. This multicultural competence consists of *knowledge*—knowing a cultural group's central values and beliefs; *skills*—the ability to adapt interventions to the group's preferred help-seeking style; and *awareness*—recognition of one's own culture, values, beliefs, and biases. Although this perspective has most commonly been proposed for work with marginalized groups, an argument can be made that when it comes to the realm of psychotherapy, male clients have not been a dominant group. As has been elaborated earlier, the worlds of therapy and manhood have been mutually distinct and in need of efforts to promote greater harmony. In that vein, therapy contacts with male clients can be considered a form of cross-cultural counseling (Brooks, 2010, p. 44), thereby making the precepts of multicultural competence applicable.

### Synthesis—Male-Friendly Therapy

Drawing from the working alliance and the multicultural competence paradigms, and from reviewing the writing of many therapy-with-men authors (Brooks, 2010; Englar-Carlson, 2014; Robertson, 2012; Rochlen & Rabinowitz, 2014), a model of user-friendly therapy for men that integrates the perspectives can be constructed. First, the *agreement on goals* aspect of the working alliance researchers is an important component of any male-friendly approach. Many men avoid therapy for fear that therapists will be hypercritical and judgmental of them and their lifestyle and that therapy will attempt to undercut central aspects of their masculinity (i.e., make them less manly). Therefore, a primary element of a male-friendly approach is to correct that misconception and convey that the therapy mission is constructive and positive. The reluctant man needs to realize that the goal is to cooperatively explore his lifestyle and beliefs, consider the interaction between them and his current difficulties, and, when appropriate, to jointly decide on which change objectives would make the most sense.

The *knowledge* component of cross-cultural consoling is central to all male-friendly approaches. The essence of men's studies, of course, has been to augment the decades of writing on the life experiences of women with higher level of appreciation of "the male experience" (Doyle, 1994) and "the masculine self" (Kilmartin & Smiler, 2015). The foremost trend in writing about therapy with men has been the movement from a gender-blind perspective to recognition that the most effective therapy with men is "gender sensitive" (Philpot, Brooks, Lusterman, & Nutt, 1997) and "gender aware" (Good, Gilbert, & Scher, 1990). The implication of Sue and Sue's (2015) model of cultural competence for user-friendly therapy with men is quite apparent: Culturally competent therapy with men must be conducted with considerable knowledge of men's socialization and coping styles, as well as an appreciation of the "hazards of being male" (Goldberg, 1976).

When it comes to the subject of conducting psychotherapy, there is considerable overlap between Bordin's working alliance ideas and the multicultural competence ideas of Sue and Sue. Both emphasizes the need for therapy to be carried out in a manner congruent with the style and needs of the clientele. Bordin emphasizes agreement on tasks and activities, whereas Sue and Sue focus on requisite skills for work with the specific populations. These principles are quite consistent with user-friendly therapy for males because most of the writing in this area has emphasized alterations in typical practices within the therapy hour. Kilmartin (2014) stated,

> A key to effectively working with men is changing the way counseling is conducted . . . how counseling is framed . . . using less jargon in interactions, being more active and direct in order to address presenting concerns first, and modify one's relational style to the match the client's. The appropriate use of humor and small talk in male-friendly ways has been cited as sometimes helpful. (p. 21)

Because many male clients feel greater trust when they experience their therapist as a real and authentic person, therapist self-disclosure can have major benefits. Wexler (2014) observed that self-disclosure lessens the shame many male clients experience. Brooks (2010) contended that carefully considered self-disclosure lessens the potentially harmful perceptions of an all-knowing expert therapist, thereby allowing for greater connection between client and therapist. Jooma (2014) found that when presented with video examples of therapist self-disclosure and non–self-disclosure, men with high gender role conflict rated self-disclosing therapists as more expert and more attractive. Finally, the suggestions of Sue and Sue (2015) regarding *proxemics* (use of space) and *kinesics* (body movements, posture, facial expressions) also merit attention in work with male clients.

The third component critical to the working alliance—the *therapeutic bond*—seems to have considerable overlap with Sue and Sue's ideas about *awareness* in multicultural competence. For a therapeutic bond to exist, the therapist, of course, must transmit a sense of caring, respect, and empathy for the client. Additionally, however, the therapist must be in tune with any personal factors interfering with positive regard for the client. These factors, sometimes referred to as *countertransference* and sometimes simply as *emotional reactivity*, must be recognized and dealt with effectively for therapy to succeed. In the matter of multicultural competence, the concept of awareness is akin to the thinking about the therapeutic bond, but it also seems to place even greater emphasis on bias and negativity inherent in ethnocentric worldviews. That is, unless a therapist acknowledges the likelihood of seeing "difference" (rooted in cultural values) as "pathology" (rooted in intrapsychic function), ethical and effective therapy will not be possible.

These ideas about the therapeutic bond and multicultural awareness have major implications for developing male-friendly psychotherapy. As noted earlier, avid proponents of the positive masculinity model of psychotherapy with boys and men (Englar-Carlson & Kiselica, 2013; Kiselica & Englar-Carlson, 2010) have contended that a "deficit" model and remedial approach to therapy needs to be augmented with an approach that accentuates positive aspects of masculinity. Although there has been considerable controversy about the widest implications of this model (Richmond, 2014), there is no significant disagreement among theorists and clinicians that the individual male client needs to be approached with compassion, empathy, and positive regard (Brooks, 2010; Kiselica et al., 2008; Rabinowitz & Cochran, 2002; Robertson, 2012). Good and Robertson (2010) suggested that "therapists need to start therapy by seeking to join men 'where they are'" (p. 311). Brooks (2010) stated that monitoring one's emotional reactivity is essential for successful therapy with men. Because so many men cope with their psychic distress with destructive (and self-destructive) behaviors such as violence, substance abuse, sexual misconduct, or emotional withdrawal, Brooks and Silverstein (1995) contended that therapists must be able to recognize the pain behind the dark-side behavior and find ways to see positives and join with the troubled male (without condoning or enabling any behavior harmful to self or others).

## Masculinities and Diversity Among Men

One of the most demanding challenges of men's studies has been the need to make the shift from a single idea of hegemonic masculinity (Connell, 1995) to conceptualizations recognizing and accounting for variations among men based in race, ethnicity, social class, sexual identity, and physical capability. Levant and Wong (2013) called for greater attention to research and scholarship perspectives incorporating an "intersectional perspective" (p. 329), particularly as it relates to the interface of race, ethnicity, and masculinities. Furthermore, they called for the study of masculine norms within specific cultures, the experience of incongruence between dominant Western masculine norms and minority masculine norms, and the connection between racism and performance of masculinities.

A thorough review of the evolving literature on diversity among men is beyond the scope of this chapter (and is less critical because of the focus of other chapters in this volume), but several points need to be made. First, although there are sizable differences in the experiences of non-White, non-heterosexual, and less physically abled males, they share a common experience of marginalization and oppression that will inevitably affect their entry into therapy relationships. First and foremost, African American, Latino, Native American, and Asian American men have for centuries been subject to the pernicious effects of racism and multiple forms of oppression. The intersectional perspective adds further enlightenment in terms recognition of the experiences of gay, bisexual, and transgender men of who are of dominant White culture or, more problematically, subject to additional disadvantage from membership in racial minority groups. Closely related to the experiences of racism, heterosexism, and cultural oppression, men of color and sexual minority men are likely to share a broad distrust of most mental health professionals, whether this distrust is characterized as "healthy cultural paranoia" (Paniagua, 1998, p. 23) or as a more generalized minority distrust of the majority society (Ridley, 1995). A regrettable irony about the relationship between the psychotherapy and gay and bisexual men is that these men are more likely to seek psychotherapy, yet the therapists they see are much less likely to be prepared to treat them (Haldeman, 2005).

## CONCLUSION

The primary emphasis of this chapter has been on the past failure of the professions of counseling and psychotherapy to recognize the roots of the impasse between men and psychotherapy and to continue expecting all accommodations to come exclusively from males themselves, rather than develop interventions more congruent with men's common methods of coping with pain and ultimate help-seeking (and help-rejecting) style. Fortunately, in the 2 decades since the publication of A New Psychology of Men (Levant & Pollack, 1995), there have been exciting developments that promise far greater capacity to heal the divide between males and psychotherapy. As noted earlier in this chapter, many thoughtful volumes have appeared related to the general problematic issues. Additionally, several creative thinkers have offered male-friendly customizations of traditional therapy modalities. Perhaps the most exciting development has been the appearance of many ideas to shift from the strictures of in-office psychotherapy to consider augmenting therapies with out-of-office therapeutic interventions. Through consultation, psychoeducation, experiential retreats, public awareness campaigns, and men's collectives, general awareness of the stresses of boyhood and manhood can be better recognized. In many cases, these activities alone will produce salutary effects. In other cases, these activities will facilitate entry of formerly skeptical men into the actual therapy office (quite possibly to a therapist with a reputation of understanding men's issues and practicing in a male-friendly manner). To ensure continued progress with male clients, therapists and counselors must commit themselves to learn all they can about the male experience(s), develop skills harmonious with male interpersonal and help-seeking styles, and access their personal problem areas and assets in work with men in need. As this process occurs, therapists will be far more effective, and major benefits will accrue to men, their loved ones, and the culture at large.

# REFERENCES

Addis, M. E., & Mahalik, J. R. (2003). Men, masculinity, and the contexts of help seeking. *American Psychologist, 58,* 5–14. http://dx.doi.org/10.1037/0003-066X.58.1.5

American Psychological Association. (1975). Report of the Task Force on Sex Bias and Sex-Role Stereotyping in Psychotherapeutic Practice. *American Psychologist, 30,* 1169–1175. http://dx.doi.org/10.1037/0003-066X.30.12.1169

American Psychological Association. (2007). *Guidelines for psychological practice with girls and women.* Retrieved from http://www.apa.org/practice/guidelines/girls-and-women.aspx

Andronico, M. (Ed.). (1996). *Men in groups: Insights, interventions, and psychoeducational work.* http://dx.doi.org/10.1037/10284-000

Angermeyer, M. C., Matschinger, H., & Riedel-Heller, S. G. (2001). What to do about mental disorder—Help-seeking recommendations of the lay public. *Acta Psychiatrica Scandinavica, 103,* 220–225. http://dx.doi.org/10.1034/j.1600-0447.2001.103003220.x

Arbona, C., & Coleman, N. (2008). Risk and resilience. In S. D. Brown & R. W. Lent (Eds.), *Handbook of counseling psychology* (4th ed., pp. 483–499). New York, NY: Wiley.

Bechtoldt, H., Norcross, J., Wyckoff, L. A., Pokrywa, M. L., & Campbell, L. F. (2001). Theoretical orientations and employment settings of clinical and counseling psychologists: A comparative study. *Clinical Psychologist, 54,* 3–6.

Betcher, R. W., & Pollack, W. S. (1993). *In a time of fallen heroes: The re-creation of masculinity.* New York, NY: Atheneum.

Blair, S. L. (2012). The division of household labor. In G. W. Peterson & K. R. Bush (Eds.), *Handbook of marriage and the family* (3rd ed., pp. 613–635). New York, NY: Springer Science.

Bloom, M. (2008). Principles and approaches to primary prevention. In T. P. Gullotta & G. M. Blau (Eds.), *Handbook of childhood behavioral issues: Evidence-based approaches to prevention and treatment* (pp. 107–122). New York, NY: Routledge.

Bordin, E. S. (1994). Theory and research on the therapeutic working alliance: New directions. In A. O. Horvath & L. S. Greenberg (Eds.), *The working alliance: Theory, research, and practice* (pp. 13–37). New York, NY: Wiley.

Brooks, G. R. (1990). Post-Vietnam gender-role strain: A needed concept? *Professional Psychology: Research and Practice, 21,* 18–25. http://dx.doi.org/10.1037/0735-7028.21.1.18

Brooks, G. R. (1998). *A new psychotherapy for traditional men*. San Francisco, CA: Jossey-Bass.

Brooks, G. R. (2010). *Beyond the crisis of masculinity: A transtheoretical model for male-friendly therapy*. http://dx.doi.org/10.1037/12073-000

Brooks, G. R. (2012). Male-sensitive therapy for the returning veteran and his partner. In D. S. Shepard & M. Harway (Eds.), *Engaging men in couples therapy* (pp. 279–299). New York, NY: Routledge.

Brooks, G. R., & Silverstein, L. B. (1995). Understanding the dark side of masculinity: An integrative systems model. In R. H. Levant & W. S. Pollack (Eds.), *A new psychology of men* (pp. 280–336). New York, NY: Basic.

Carney, J. M., & Jefferson, J. F. (2014). Consultation for mental health counselors: Opportunities and guidelines for private practice. *Journal of Mental Health Counseling, 36*, 302–314. http://dx.doi.org/10.17744/mehc.36.4.821133r0414u37v7

Chapin, L. A. (2015). Mexican-American boys and positive outcomes and resilience. *Journal of Child and Family Studies, 24*, 1791–1799. http://dx.doi.org/10.1007/s10826-014-9982-8

Connell, R. W. (1995). *Masculinities*. Berkeley: University of California Press.

Conyne, R. (1987). *Primary preventive counseling: Empowering people and systems*. http://dx.doi.org/10.4324/9780203336052

Courtenay, W. H. (2011). *Dying to be men*. New York, NY: Routledge.

Danish, S. J., & Forneris, T. (2008). Promoting positive development and competence across the life span. In S. D. Brown & R. W. Lent (Eds.), *Handbook of counseling psychology* (4th ed., pp. 500–516). New York, NY: Wiley.

Davidson, M. G. (2000). Religion and spirituality. In P. S. Richards & A. E. Bergin (Eds.), *Handbook of psychotherapy and religious diversity* (pp. 409–433). Washington, DC: American Psychological Association.

Davies, J. A., Shen-Miller, D. S., & Isacco, A. (2010). The Men's Center approach to addressing the health crisis of college men. *Professional Psychology: Research and Practice, 41*, 347–354. http://dx.doi.org/10.1037/a0020308

DeAngelis, T. (2014). Building resilience among Black boys. *Monitor on Psychology, 45*(9), 50.

Donaldson, C., & Flood, R. (2014). *Mascupathy: Understanding and healing the malaise of American manhood*. Grand Rapids, MI: The Institute for the Prevention and Treatment of Mascupathy.

Doyle, J. A. (1994). *The male experience* (3rd ed.). Dubuque, IA: Brown.

Ellis, C. M., & Carlson, J. (Eds.). (2016). *Cross cultural awareness and social justice in counseling*. New York, NY: Routledge.

Englar-Carlson, M. (2014). Introduction: A primer on counseling men. In M. Englar-Carlson, M. P. Evans, & M. Duffey, M. (Eds.), *A counselor's guide to working with men* (pp. 1–31). Alexandria, VA: American Counseling Association.

Englar-Carlson, M., Evans, M. P., & Duffey, M. (Eds.). (2014). *A counselor's guide to working with men*. Alexandria, VA: American Counseling Association.

Englar-Carlson, M., & Kiselica, M. S. (2013). Affirming the strengths in men: A positive masculinity approach to assisting male clients. *Journal of Counseling and Development, 91*, 399–409.

Englar-Carlson, M., & Stevens, M. A. (2014). Creating experiential weekend retreats for men. In A. B. Rochlen & F. E. Rabinowitz (Eds.), *Breaking barriers in counseling men: Insights and innovations* (pp. 88–98). New York, NY: Routledge.

Faludi, S. (1999). *Stiffed: The betrayal of the American man*. New York, NY: Morrow.

Fisch, R., Weakland, J., & Segal, L. (1982). *The tactics of change: Doing therapy briefly*. San Francisco, CA: Jossey-Bass.

Franklin, A. J., Chen, M., Hammad, S., Capawana, M. R., & Hoogasian, R. O. (2015). Consensual qualitative research analysis of a therapeutic support group session for African American men. *Psychology of Men and Masculinity, 16*, 264–273.

Glicken, M. D. (2005). *Working with troubled men: A contemporary practitioner's guide*. Mahwah, NJ: Erlbaum.

Goldberg, H. (1976). *The hazards of being male*. New York, NY: New American Library.

Good, G. E., & Brooks, G. R. (Eds.). (2005). *The new handbook of psychotherapy and counseling with men: A comprehensive guide to settings, problems, and treatment approaches* (Rev. ed.). San Francisco, CA: Jossey-Bass.

Good, G. E., Gilbert, L. A., & Scher, M. (1990). Gender aware therapy: A synthesis of feminist therapy and knowledge about gender. *Journal of Counseling & Development, 68*, 376–380. http://dx.doi.org/10.1002/j.1556-6676.1990.tb02514.x

Good, G. E., & Robertson, J. M. (2010). To accept a pilot? Addressing men's ambivalence and altering their expectancies about therapy. *Psychotherapy: Theory, Research, Practice, Training, 47*, 306–315. http://dx.doi.org/10.1037/a0021162

Goodheart, C. D., & Markham, B. (1992). The feminization of psychology: Implications for psychotherapy. *Psychotherapy: Theory, Research, Practice, Training, 29*, 130–138. http://dx.doi.org/10.1037/0033-3204.29.1.130

Haldeman, D. C. (2005). Psychotherapy with gay and bisexual men. In G. E. Good & G. R. Brooks (Eds.), *The new handbook of psychotherapy and counseling with men: A comprehensive guide to settings, problems, and treatment approaches* (Rev. ed., pp. 369–383). San Francisco, CA: Jossey-Bass.

Hills, H. I., Carlstrom, A., & Evanow, M. (2005). Consulting with men in business and industry. In G. E. Good & G. R. Brooks (Eds.), *The new handbook of psychotherapy and counseling with men: A comprehensive guide to settings, problems, and treatment approaches* (Rev. ed., pp. 54–69). San Francisco, CA: Jossey-Bass.

Horvath, A. O., & Bedi, R. P. (2002). The alliance. In J. C. Norcross (Ed.), *Psychotherapy relationships that work* (pp. 37–70). New York, NY: Oxford University Press.

Isenhart, C. (2005). Treating substance abuse in men. In G. E. Good & G. R. Brooks (Eds.), *The new handbook of psychotherapy and counseling with men: A comprehen-*

*sive guide to settings, problems, and treatment approaches* (Rev. ed., pp. 134–146). San Francisco, CA: Jossey-Bass.

Jakupcak, M., Blais, R., Grossbard, J., Garcia, H., & Okiishi, J. (2014). "Toughness" in association with mental health symptoms among Iraq and Afghanistan war veterans seeking Veterans Affairs health care. *Psychology of Men & Masculinity*, *15*, 100–104. http://dx.doi.org/10.1037/a0031508

Jakupcak, M., & Varra, E. M. (2011). Treating Iraq and Afghanistan war veterans with PTSD who are a high risk for suicide. *Cognitive and Behavioral Practice*, *18*, 85–97. http://dx.doi.org/10.1016/j.cbpra.2009.08.007

Jooma, S. (2014). Men's reactions to variants of self-disclosure in male psychotherapists. *Dissertation Abstracts International: Section B. Sciences and Engineering*, *74*.

Kersting, K. (2005, June). Men and depression: Battling depression through public education. *Monitor on Psychology*, *36*, 66–68.

Kilmartin, C. (2014). Using humor and storytelling in men's work. In A. B. Rochlen & F. E. Rabinowitz (Eds.), *Breaking barriers in counseling men: Insights and innovations* (pp. 20–29). New York, NY: Routledge/Taylor & Francis.

Kilmartin, C. T., & Smiler, A. P. (2015). *The masculine self* (5th ed.). Cornwell-on-the-Hudson, NY: Sloan.

Kindlon, D., & Thompson, M. (2000). *Raising Cain: Protecting the emotional life of boys*. New York, NY: Ballantine.

Kiselica, M. S., & Englar-Carlson, M. (2010). Identifying, affirming, and building upon male strengths: The positive psychology/positive masculinity model of psychotherapy with boys and men. *Psychotherapy: Theory, Research, Practice, Training*, *47*, 276–287.

Kiselica, M. S., Englar-Carlson, M., & Horne, A. M. (Eds.). (2008). *Counseling troubled boys: A guidebook for professionals*. New York, NY: Routledge.

Kiselica, M. S., & Look, C. T. (1993). Mental health counseling and prevention: Disparity between philosophy and practice? *Journal of Mental Health Counseling*, *15*, 3–14.

Klerman, G. L., Weissman, M. M., Rounsaville, B. J., & Chevron, E. S. (1984). *Interpersonal psychotherapy of depression*. New York, NY: Basic.

Kupers, T. A. (2001). Psychotherapy with men in prison. In G. R. Brooks & G. E. Good (Eds.), *The new handbook of psychotherapy and counseling with men: Vol. 1. A comprehensive guide to settings, problems, and treatment approaches* (pp. 170–184). San Francisco, CA: Jossey-Bass.

Levant, R. F., Hall, R. J., & Rankin, T. J. (2013). Male Role Norms Inventory—Short Form (MRNI–SF): Development, confirmatory factor analytic investigation of structure, and measurement invariance across gender. *Journal of Counseling Psychology*, *60*, 228–238. http://dx.doi.org/10.1037/a0031545

Levant, R. F., Halter, M. J., Hayden, E., & Williams, C. (2009). The efficacy of Alexithymia Reduction Treatment: A pilot study. *The Journal of Men's Studies*, *17*, 75–84. http://dx.doi.org/10.3149/jms.1701.75

Levant, R. F., & Kelly, J. (1989). *Between father and child.* New York, NY: Viking.

Levant, R. F., & Kopecky, G. (1995). *Masculinity reconstructed: Changing the rules of manhood—At work, in relationships, and in family life.* New York, NY: Dutton.

Levant, R. F., & Pollack, W. S. (Eds.). (1995). *A new psychology of men.* New York, NY: Basic Books.

Levant, R. F., & Wong, Y. J. (2013). Race and gender as moderators of the relationship between the endorsement of traditional masculinity ideology and alexithymia: An intersectional perspective. *Psychology of Men & Masculinity, 14,* 329–333. http://dx.doi.org/10.1037/a0029551

Liu, W. M., Iwamoto, D. K., & Chae, M. H. (2010). *Culturally responsive counseling with Asian American men.* New York, NY: Routledge.

Lynch, J. R., & Kilmartin, C. (2013). *Overcoming masculine depression: The pain behind the mask* (2nd ed.). New York, NY: Routledge.

Mahalik, J. R. (2005a). Cognitive therapy for men. In G. E. Good & G. R. Brooks (Eds.), *The new handbook of psychotherapy and counseling with men: A comprehensive guide to settings, problems, and treatment approaches* (Rev. ed., pp. 217–233). San Francisco, CA: Jossey-Bass.

Mahalik, J. R. (2005b). Interpersonal therapy for men. In G. E. Good & G. R. Brooks (Eds.), *The new handbook of psychotherapy and counseling with men: A comprehensive guide to settings, problems, and treatment approaches* (Rev. ed., pp. 234–247). San Francisco, CA: Jossey-Bass.

Marini, I. D. (2005). Issues of males with physical disabilities in rehabilitation settings. In G. R. Brooks & G. E. Good (Eds.), *The new handbook of psychotherapy and counseling with men: A comprehensive guide to settings, problems, and treatment approaches* (Rev. ed., pp. 88–103). San Francisco, CA: Jossey-Bass.

Marzalek, J. F., & Logan, C. R. (2014). It takes a village: Advocating for sexual minority youth. In D. Capuzzi & D. R. Gross (Eds.), *Youth at risk: A prevention resource for counselors, teachers, and parents* (6th ed., pp. 319–336). Alexandria, VA: American Counseling Association.

Miller, W. R., & Rollnick, S. (2002). *Motivational interviewing: Preparing people to change* (2nd ed.). New York, NY: Guilford Press.

Norcross, J. C., & Lambert, M. J. (2011). Psychotherapy relationships that work II. *Psychotherapy: Theory, Research, Practice, Training, 48,* 4–8. http://dx.doi.org/10.1037/a0022180

O'Neil, J. M. (2014). Foreword. In M. Englar-Carlson, M. P. Evans, & M. Duffey (Eds.), *A counselor's guide to working with men* (p. ix). Alexandria, VA: American Counseling Association.

O'Neil, J. M., & Carroll, M. R. (1988). A gender role workshop focused on sexism, gender role conflict, and the gender role journey. *Journal of Counseling & Development, 67,* 193–197. http://dx.doi.org/10.1002/j.1556-6676.1988.tb02091.x

O'Neil, J. M., Challenger, C., Renzulli, S., Crapser, B., & Webster, E. (2013). The Boy's Forum: An evaluation of a brief intervention to empower middle-school urban boys. *The Journal of Men's Studies, 21,* 191–205. http://dx.doi.org/10.3149/jms.2102.191

O'Neil, J. M., & Renzulli, S. (2013). Introduction to the special section: Teaching the psychology of men—A call to action. *Psychology of Men & Masculinity, 14,* 221–229. http://dx.doi.org/10.1037/a0033258

Oren, C. Z., & Oren, D. C. (Eds.). (2009). *Counseling fathers.* New York, NY: Routledge.

Paniagua, F. A. (1998). *Assessing and treating culturally diverse clients: A practical guide.* Thousand Oaks, CA: Sage.

Philpot, C. L., Brooks, G. R., Lusterman, D.-D., & Nutt, R. L. (1997). *Bridging separate gender worlds: Why men and women clash and how therapists can bring them together.* Washington, DC: American Psychological Association.

Pollack, W. S. (1998). *Real boys: Rescuing our sons from the myths of boyhood.* New York, NY: Random House.

Pollack, W. S. (2005). "Masked men": New psychoanalytically oriented treatment models for adult and young adult men. In G. E. Good & G. R. Brooks (Eds.), *The new handbook of psychotherapy and counseling with men: A comprehensive guide to settings, problems, and treatment approaches* (Rev. ed., pp. 203–216). San Francisco, CA: Jossey-Bass.

Prochaska, J. O., & DiClemente, C. C. (1982). Transtheoretical therapy: Toward a more integrative model of change. *Psychotherapy: Theory, Research & Practice, 19,* 276–288. http://dx.doi.org/10.1037/h0088437

Prochaska, J. O., & Norcross, J. C. (2007). *Systems of psychotherapy: A transtheoretical analysis.* Belmont, CA: Thomson.

Rabinowitz, F. E. (2014). Counseling men in groups. In M. Englar-Carlson, M. P. Evans, & T. Duffey (Eds.), *A counselor's guide to working with men* (pp. 55–70). Alexandria, VA: American Counseling Association.

Rabinowitz, F. E., & Cochran, S. V. (2002). *Deepening psychotherapy with men.* http://dx.doi.org/10.1037/10418-000

Richards, P. S., & Bergin, A. E. (Eds.). (2000). *Handbook of psychotherapy and religious diversity.* http://dx.doi.org/10.1037/10347-000

Richmond, K. (2014, August). *Engaging in difficult dialogue regarding positive masculinity.* Symposium presented at the American Psychological Association Convention, Washington, DC.

Ridley, C. R. (1995). *Overcoming unintentional racism in counseling and therapy: A practitioner's guide to intentional intervention.* Thousand Oaks, CA: Sage.

Robertson, J. M. (2012). *Tough guys and true believers.* New York, NY: Routledge.

Robertson, J. M. (2013). Perceiving religious men through counselor eyes: Risks and tips. *Journal of Counseling & Development, 91,* 410–418. http://dx.doi.org/10.1002/j.1556-6676.2013.00112.x

Rochlen, A. B. (2014). Introduction: Jack, the Sun, and the Wind. In A. B. Rochlen & F. E. Rabinowitz (Eds.), *Breaking barriers in counseling men: Insights and innovations* (pp. 1–6). New York, NY: Routledge.

Rochlen, A. B., McKelley, R. A., & Pituch, K. A. (2006). A preliminary examination of the "Real Men. Real Depression" campaign. *Psychology of Men & Masculinity, 7,* 1–13. http://dx.doi.org/10.1037/1524-9220.7.1.1

Rochlen, A. B., McKelley, R. A., & Whittaker, T. A. (2010). Stay-at-home fathers' reasons for entering the role and stigma experiences: A preliminary report. *Psychology of Men & Masculinity, 11,* 279–285. http://dx.doi.org/10.1037/a0017774

Rochlen, A. B., & Rabinowitz, F. E. (Eds.). (2014). *Breaking barriers in counseling men: Insights and innovations.* New York, NY: Routledge.

Rosin, H. (2012). *The end of men: And the rise of women.* New York, NY: Riverhead Books.

Sax, L. (2007). *Boys adrift: The five factors driving the growing epidemic of unmotivated boys and underachieving young men.* New York, NY: Basic.

Scheinfeld, D. E., & Buser, S. J. (2014). Adventure therapy with men. In A. B. Rochlen & F. E. Rabinowitz (Eds.), *Breaking barriers in counseling men: Insights and innovations* (pp. 77–98). New York, NY: Routledge.

Scher, M. (1990). Effect of gender-role incongruities on men's experience as clients in psychotherapy. *Psychotherapy: Theory, Research, Practice, Training, 27,* 322–326. http://dx.doi.org/10.1037/0033-3204.27.3.322

Shepard, D. S., & Harway, M. (2012). *Engaging men in couples therapy.* New York, NY: Routledge.

Silverstein, C. (2011). *The initial psychotherapy interview: A gay man seeks treatment.* http://dx.doi.org/10.1016/B978-0-12-385146-8.00003-1

Silverstein, L. B., Auerbach, C. F., & Levant, R. F. (2002). Contemporary fathers reconstructing masculinity: Clinical implications of gender role strain. *Professional Psychology: Research and Practice, 33,* 361–369.

Spendelow, J. S. (2015). Cognitive–behavioral treatment of depression: Tailoring treatment and directions for future research. *American Journal of Men's Health, 9,* 94–102. http://dx.doi.org/10.1177/1557988314529790

Sprinthall, N. A. (1990). Counseling psychology from Greystone to Atlanta: On the road to Armageddon? *The Counseling Psychologist, 18,* 455–463. http://dx.doi.org/10.1177/0011000090183007

Sue, D. W., & Sue, D. (2015). *Counseling the culturally diverse: Theory and practice* (7th ed.). New York, NY: Wiley.

Sweet, H. B. (Ed.). (2012). *Gender in the therapy hour.* New York, NY: Routledge.

Tracey, T. J. G., & Schneider, P. L. (1995). An evaluation of the circular structure of the checklist of interpersonal transactions and the checklist of psychotherapy interactions. *Journal of Counseling Psychology, 42,* 496–507. http://dx.doi.org/10.1037/0022-0167.42.4.496

Tucker, J. R., Hammer, J. H., Vogel, D. L., Bitman, R. L., Wade, N. G., & Maier, E. J. (2013). Disentangling self-stigma: Are mental illness and help-seeking self-stigmas different? *Journal of Counseling Psychology, 60,* 520–531. http://dx.doi.org/10.1037/a0033555

Urschel, J. K. (2000). Men's studies and women's studies: Commonalities, dependence, and independence. *The Journal of Men's Studies, 8,* 407–411.

Vacha-Haase, T., Wester, S. R., & Christianson, H. F. (2010). *Psychotherapy with older men.* New York, NY: Routledge.

Vandello, J. A., & Bosson, J. K. (2013). Hard won and easily lost: A review and synthesis of theory and research on precarious manhood. *Psychology of Men & Masculinity, 14,* 101–113. http://dx.doi.org/10.1037/a0029826

Vessey, J. T., & Howard, K. I. (1993). Who seeks psychotherapy? *Psychotherapy: Theory, Research, Practice, Training, 30,* 546–553. http://dx.doi.org/10.1037/0033-3204.30.4.546

Vogel, D. L., Wester, S. R., Hammer, J. H., & Downing-Matibag, T. M. (2014). Referring men to seek help: The influence of gender role conflict and stigma. *Psychology of Men & Masculinity, 15,* 60–67. http://dx.doi.org/10.1037/a0031761

Wagner, P. (2012). *Incarceration is not an equal opportunity punishment.* Northampton, MA: Prison Policy Initiative. Retrieved from http://prisonpolicy.org/articles/notequal.html

Wexler, D. B. (2009). *Men in therapy: New approaches for effective treatment.* New York, NY: Norton.

Wexler, D. B. (2014). Approaching the unapproachable: Therapist self-disclosure to de-shame clients. In A. B. Rochlen & F. E. Rabinowitz (Eds.), *Breaking barriers in counseling men: Insights and innovations* (pp. 30–40). New York, NY: Routledge.

Wissocki, G. W., & Andronico, M. P. (1996). The Somerset Institute's modern men's weekend. In M. Andronico (Ed.), *Men in groups: Insights, interventions, and psychoeducational work* (pp. 113–126). Washington, DC: American Psychological Association.

Yalom, I. D., & Leszcz, M. (2005). *The theory and practice of group psychotherapy.* New York, NY: Basic Books.

Zins, J. E., & Erchul, W. P. (2002). Best practices in school consultation. In A. Thomas & J. Grimes (Eds.), *Best practices in school psychology* (pp. 625–643). Washington, DC: National Association of School Psychologists.

Zur, O. (2008). *Beyond the office walls: Home visits, celebrations, adventure therapy, incidental encounters, and other encounters outside the office walls.* Retrieved from http://www.zurinstitute.com/outofofficeexperiences.html

# 12

## DYSFUNCTION STRAIN AND INTERVENTION PROGRAMS AIMED AT MEN'S VIOLENCE, SUBSTANCE USE, AND HELP-SEEKING BEHAVIORS

CHRISTOPHER T. H. LIANG, CARIN MOLENAAR, CHRISTINA HERMANN, AND LOUIS A. RIVERA

The U.S. Department of Justice, Federal Bureau of Investigation (2012) reported that men are more likely to be offenders in cases involving sexual violence, aggravated assault, or intimate partner violence (IPV). Before concluding that men are simply biologically prone to violence, however, it is essential to know that most men do not engage in violent and sexually aggressive behaviors (Kilmartin & Smiler, 2015). Examining other public health data alongside the Department of Justice reports can help us to understand why some boys and men may engage in these behaviors. For instance, men compose a greater percentage of those who use alcohol excessively, have complications related to alcohol, and die of alcohol-attributable deaths (Stahre, Roeber, Kanny, Brewer, & Zhang, 2014). Men are also 4 times more likely to complete suicide than women (Murphy, Xu, & Kochanek, 2013) and make up a larger proportion of alcohol-related suicides (Stahre et al., 2014).

http://dx.doi.org/10.1037/0000023-013

*The Psychology of Men and Masculinities*, R. F. Levant and Y. J. Wong (Editors)

Viewing these reports in isolation may lead to the conclusion that biological sex causes violence or that mental health problems are predictive of alcohol-related problems and suicide. However, examination of these reports simultaneously suggests that there may be a common set of underlying factors that contribute to the violence- and alcohol-related problems men face. Above and beyond biological sex may be the socialization of men to demonstrate masculinity. This chapter provides a brief overview of how dysfunction strain is associated with substance use and violence, as well as a critique of current efforts.

In an important move away from looking at the male as a static, biological category from which inferences can be made about behavior, men's studies scholars in psychology have argued for understanding how gender role socialization processes are related to masculinity ideology, gender role conflict or dysfunction strain, and, in turn, health-related behaviors. Although there are many forms of masculinity, *hegemonic masculinity* has been described as the dominant and most pervasive form. It has been broadly conceptualized as a multidimensional construct that includes self-reliance, emotional control, power, and status, as well as both control over women and fear of appearing feminine (O'Neil, 2015). Pleck (1995) explained that men attempting to live up to these standards may experience negative consequences because prescribed standards of masculinity are inherently harmful to self and to others. He introduced *dysfunction strain* to explain how rigid conformity to hegemonic masculinity can result in negative outcomes.

Dysfunction strain is associated with sexual aggression (R. M. Smith, Parrott, Swartout, & Tharp, 2015), overt hostility, fear of emotions (Jakupcak, Tull, & Roemer, 2005), and higher levels of engagement in risky health behaviors (Levant, Wimer, Williams, Smalley, & Noronha, 2009). Because help-seeking is seen as unmanly, rigid conformity to hegemonic masculinity serves as a barrier to psychological services for men (Courtenay, 2011). When help is not sought, masculine socialization, including how our culture permits the expression of male anger, may result in men resorting to physical and sexual violence against other men, women, and children. Other men, who do not seek help from a professional, may attempt to control their negative mood, inner gender-based conflicts, or stress by relying on alcohol or other substances. For instance, drinking alcohol may be used both to numb emotional pain and to prove one's manliness in the United States (Iwamoto & Smiler, 2013). Unfortunately alcohol, as a depressogenic agent, can result in some men engaging in other problematic behaviors. In tandem with the disinhibiting effect of alcohol use, masculine injunctions against seeking help may result in men contemplating and completing suicide or in acting out violently against others.

Previous reviews of the literature have emphasized the negative consequences of masculinity on health outcomes (e.g., Courtenay, 2011; Griffith,
Gunter, & Watkins, 2012). However, to our knowledge, this chapter is the first
to provide a comprehensive review of interventions directed at boys' and men's
dysfunctional strain. Interventions aimed at reducing gender-based and sexual
violence, substance use, and stigma associated with help-seeking are reviewed
here. This review includes treatment and prevention efforts, focuses on several
types of problems associated with boys and men (i.e., violence, alcohol use), and
includes programs with and without empirical support. The intent of this chapter
is to review efforts that incorporate dysfunction strain. Our initial search included
only dysfunction strain along with alcohol and substance abuse, violence, and
help-seeking. This search did not result in any identifiable interventions. As a
result, we expanded our criteria to include interventions that addressed issues
that are consistent with dysfunction strain (e.g., aggression, self-reliance) but
that did not explicitly incorporate masculinity or dysfunction strain.

We used the following keywords: *dysfunction strain*, *masculinity*, *hypermasculinity*, *aggression*, *control*, *self-reliance*, *intimate partner violence*, *domestic
abuse*, *sexual violence*, *rape*, *sexual assault*, *alcohol*, *substance abuse*, *help-seeking*,
*prevention*, and *intervention* to identify programs. We performed our search
on Google Scholar, PubMed, PsycINFO, Medline, SocAbstracts, ERIC,
and Education Abstracts. This search included the earliest records in these
databases up to and including records on March 31, 2015. Inclusion criteria
involved peer-reviewed articles that addressed aspects of dysfunction strain
in the intervention or prevention programs targeting one of our three areas
of focus. Articles were excluded if the author(s) (a) only mentioned proposed
interventions in their discussion of future directions, or (b) the intervention addressed substance use, gender-based violence, or help-seeking without
a focus on traits associated with masculinity. On the basis of our criteria,
11 articles were identified for inclusion in the substance use area, 23 for gender-
based violence, and five for help-seeking.

We examined the intervention's theoretical grounding, population of
focus, structure, and empirical evidence to identify the strengths and gaps
in literature. Using the framework developed by the Institute of Medicine
Committee on Prevention of Mental Disorders, Division of Behavioral
Sciences and Mental Disorders (1994), we also coded the program on the basis
of level of care. Prevention programs were coded as *Indicated* (i.e., programs targeted at those who already show some signs of problematic behavior or mental
health problems), *Selective* (i.e., interventions aimed at individuals or groups
that exhibit higher than average risk), or *Universal* (i.e., interventions aimed
at the general public regardless of presence of risk factors). Treatment programs
were coded as *Standard Treatment for Known Disorders* (i.e., treating existing
symptoms of an identifiable disorder). Our review follows.

Dysfunction strain places men at risk for substance use and abuse (Uy, Massoth, & Gottdiener, 2014). Iwamoto, Cheng, Lee, Takamatsu, and Gordon (2011) found that endorsement of "risk-taking," "self-reliance," and "playboy"—all factors associated with dysfunction strain—were risk factors for alcohol-related problems. Liu and Iwamoto (2007) found that emotional control and risk-taking were associated with increased alcohol use and that power over women was strongly associated with binge drinking. Despite the call for substance use prevention and treatment programs to directly address and incorporate masculinity and gender role conflict (Uy et al., 2014), relatively few such interventions have been published (see Table 12.1).

Two programs addressed constructs consistent with dysfunction strain as part of their treatment. For example, grounded in social constructionist perspectives on gender, Time Out! For Men (Bartholomew & Simpson, 1996) explicitly addresses restrictive emotionality through a variety of activities intended to help men gain awareness of their emotions, identify their emotional needs, and recognize ways of positively communicating their emotional needs to partners. Griffith, Metzl, and Gunter's (2011) intersectional approach drew from a critical masculinity framework. The other programs address constructs consistent with dysfunction strain, but without specific attention to masculinity, drew from the social developmental model (Catalano & Hawkins, 1996), psychotherapy theories, 12-step theories, the three-phase treatment model (Meichenbaum, 1977), or the social control hypothesis (O'Reilly & Chatman, 1996).

Many of the programs we identified addressed polysubstance use. The majority of participants, however, reported alcohol as the "drug of choice" (Bartholomew, Hiller, Knight, Nucatola, & Simpson, 2000; Morgenstern et al., 2007; Reynolds, Lehman, & Bennett, 2008; Rohsenow et al., 1985, 1991; Santisteban et al., 2003). Interventionists have implemented programs in a number of settings, targeting different groups. In our review, programs targeted men already in substance use treatment programs or with existing substance-related diagnoses, felony probationers in a 6-month residential program (Bartholomew et al., 2000), Vietnam veterans with comorbid posttraumatic stress disorder (PTSD) and substance abuse diagnoses (Donovan, Padin-Rivera, & Kowaliw, 2001), men who have sex with men diagnosed with alcohol use disorders (Morgenstern et al., 2007), civilian men with comorbid PTSD and substance use disorders (Najavits, Schmitz, Gotthardt, & Weiss, 2005), and participants in a Veterans Affairs rehabilitation program (Rohsenow et al., 1991). Absent from the programs were young adult, college-age men, a population that, because of its consistently

TABLE 12.1
Substance-Related Intervention and Prevention Programs

| Author | Name and description of how program addresses dysfunction strain | Targeted population | IOM level of care | Empirical support | Methodology |
|---|---|---|---|---|---|
| Bartholomew et al. (2000) | **Time Out! For Men** (Bartholomew & Simpson, 1996) Addresses restrictive emotionality with attention to masculinity and gender roles | Felony probationers in a 6-month residential substance abuse treatment program | Standard treatment for known disorders | Yes | Pretest–posttest quasi-experimental between groups design |
| Catalano et al. (1998) | **Preparing for the Drug Free Years** Addresses family conflict resolution, positive emotional expression, and anger management without explicit attention to masculinity | Parents of adolescents in multiethnic community public schools | Universal | Yes | Pretest–posttest within-group and between groups experimental designs |
| Donovan et al. (2001) | **Transcend** Addresses emotional awareness, anger management, and problem solving without explicit attention to masculinity | Vietnam veterans with comorbid PTSD and substance abuse diagnoses | Standard treatment for known disorders | Yes | Pretest–posttest quasi-experimental within-subjects design |
| Griffith et al. (2011) | **Intersectional Approach to Interventions** Addresses unique racialized and class-based construction of masculinity | Community-based men | Selective | No | Not applicable |
| Morgenstern et al. (2007) | **Motivational Interviewing Augmented Motivational Interviewing and Cognitive Behavioral Therapy** Addresses sensation seeking, internalized homonegativity, and negative affect | HIV-negative, sexually active men who have sex with men diagnosed with alcohol use disorders | Standard treatment for known disorders | Yes | Posttest only; experimental between groups design |
| Najavits et al. (2005) | **Seeking Safety** (Najavits, 2002) **combined with exposure therapy—Revised** Addresses "asking for help," anger, or "taking good care of yourself" without explicit attention to masculinity | Men (civilians) with comorbid substance use disorders and PTSD diagnoses | Standard treatment for known disorders | Yes | Pretest–posttest quasi-experimental within-subjects design |

(continues)

## TABLE 12.1
### Substance-Related Intervention and Prevention Programs  (Continued)

| Author | Name and description of how program addresses dysfunction strain | Targeted population | IOM level of care | Empirical support | Methodology |
|---|---|---|---|---|---|
| Reilly & Shopshire, (2000) | **Anger Management Group Treatment** Addresses awareness of anger, conflict resolution, and relaxation training for anger management without explicit attention to masculinity | Individuals in cocaine dependence treatment | Standard treatment for known disorders | Yes | Pretest–posttest quasi-experimental within-subjects design |
| Rohsenow et al. (1991) | **Communication Skills Training Group** Addresses communication skills, listening, and social support networks without explicit attention to masculinity | Men meeting alcohol dependent criteria in a 28-day rehabilitation program through Veterans Affairs inpatient ward | Standard treatment for known disorders | Yes | Pretest–posttest quasi-experimental between groups design |
| | **Cognitive Behavioral Mood Management Training Group** Addresses relaxation training and negative emotions without attention to masculinity | | | | |
| Rohsenow et al. (1985) | **Cognitive Affective Stress Management Training Package** (R. E. Smith & Ascough, 1984) Addresses deep muscle relaxation and coping with anger or social anxiety without attention to masculinity | Undergraduate social or problem drinkers not motivated for change | Indicated | Yes | Pretest–posttest quasi-experimental between groups design |
| Reynolds et al. (2008) | **Team Awareness** Addresses help-seeking in organizational contexts without attention to masculinity | Municipal employees who perceive alcohol use tolerance in the workplace | Selective | No | Not applicable |
| Santisteban et al. (2003) | **Brief Strategic Family Therapy** (Szapocznik, Hervis, & Schwartz (2003) Addresses family structure and communication skills without explicit attention to masculinity | Hispanic youth with drug use and problematic behaviors | Indicated | Yes | Pretest–posttest experimental, between groups design |

*Note.* IOM = Institute of Medicine; PTSD = posttraumatic stress disorder.

high level of risk of substance use and abuse (U.S. Department of Health, Substance Abuse and Mental Health Services Administration, Center for Behavioral Health Statistics and Quality, 2014), is in need of treatment and prevention.

Men of color in the United States also face high risk for substance use and abuse (U.S. Department of Health, Substance Abuse and Mental Health Services Administration, Center for Behavioral Health Statistics and Quality, 2014). Program participants were racially diverse with some programs having a majority of their sample identifying as White men (Donovan et al., 2001; Najavits et al., 2005; Reynolds et al., 2008); one with a majority of their sample identifying as Black men (Reilly & Shopshire, 2000); one focusing on Latino families of adolescent boys (Santisteban et al., 2003); and others with an effort to serve multiethnic men, their families, or both (Catalano, Kosterman, Haggerty, Hawkins, & Spoth, 1998; Morgenstern et al., 2007).

Although the majority of participants in several programs identified as people of color (Bartholomew et al., 2000; Reilly & Shopshire, 2000; Santisteban et al., 2003), only one of the identified interventions directly addressed multicultural issues. Griffith et al. (2011) proposed an intersectional adaptation to substance use and abuse interventions. Santisteban and colleagues (2003) tested the efficacy of an intervention with Hispanic families. Although this was not adapted to become more relevant to the unique experience of Hispanic communities in the United States, the efforts represent an important step toward understanding whether programs are clinically indicated for diverse communities. The single universal prevention program that addressed dysfunction strain and substance use, Preparing for the Drug Free Years (Catalano et al., 1998), indirectly addressed multicultural issues by testing its effectiveness in a variety of locations and with a variety of populations.

Because men, particularly men of color in the United States, have different access to systemic or institutional power, their experience of dysfunction strain and substance use may differ from that of White, able-bodied, Christian, heterosexual men (Wester, 2008). This review highlights the need for programs that address the unique experience of diverse communities of men. Interventionists may consider addressing how racism, culture (i.e., values, acculturative stress), and social class pressures may influence how men feel and cope with any perceived threats to their masculinity.

Six of the identified programs were adapted from standard treatments for known substance use disorders, four of which operate within a group therapy format. Only one of the 11 programs was classified as a universal prevention program, two were classified as selective prevention programs, and two were classified as indicated prevention programs. This suggests a significant challenge to preventing the development of problematic substance use for men because the majority of programs rely on the clinical identification of substance abuse. The gap, then, misses the boys and men who suffer from substance use and abuse but do not have access to health care, do not seek out support, and do not identify their substance use as problematic.

This gap is particularly troubling as dysfunction strain also draws attention to men's socialization to avoid help-seeking and to downplay the severity of their health concerns (Courtenay, 2011). Therefore, it is possible that most of the programs are missing the vast majority of men, families, and communities suffering from substance-related problems that may be rooted in dysfunction strain. The changes to substance use disorder criteria in the fifth edition of the *Diagnostic and Statistical Manual of Mental Disorders* (American Psychiatric Association, 2013) may open the door to develop more preventative programs targeted at substance use that falls below the clinical threshold.

The interventions reviewed here show promising results in the reduction of alcohol use (Donovan et al., 2001; Morgenstern et al., 2007; Rohsenow et al., 1985, 1991), drug use (e.g., marijuana: Najavits et al., 2005; Reilly & Shopshire, 2000; Santisteban et al., 2003), and polysubstance use (Donovan et al., 2001). However, these studies are limited by the lack of control groups (e.g., Donovan et al., 2001), significant attrition rates (e.g., 45% in Reilly & Shopshire, 2000) and, perhaps most significantly, by not incorporating dysfunction strain.

In summary, although there is no shortage of theoretical and empirical support for the relationship between dysfunction strain and substance use, only a few integrated these constructs. The lack of explicit, theoretically based attention to dysfunction strain represents a significant gap in the substance use intervention literature and limits the ability of mental health providers to address substance use in populations of diverse men. Applied researchers should consider testing the effectiveness of addressing the role of dysfunction strain in the development, maintenance, and treatment of substance-related disorders in men. By doing so, a more robust understanding of how to better serve diverse men may emerge. These efforts will support the health and well-being of men at risk of substance use and abuse, but also their families and communities.

Additionally, there is a striking lack of universal or selective prevention programs. Our review highlights the need for the development of universal-level interventions (e.g., how alcohol is marketed toward boys and men) that lead to the development of dysfunction strain and substance use. Systems-level interventions in the United States have already seen the retirement of tobacco marketing targeted at boys (i.e., Joe Camel) and men (i.e., Marlboro Man). Reliance on remediation efforts will not address the deeper societal-level problem.

Dysfunction strain is also associated with increased risk of perpetrating violence (Moore & Stuart, 2005). Men may perpetrate violence, specifically toward their partners, when their masculinity is challenged (Kilmartin & Smiler, 2015). For example, Cousins and Gangestad (2007) found that undergraduate men who perceived their partners as being interested in other men exhibited more controlling behaviors and more aggression. Restrictive emotionality has also been associated with violence. For example, Cohn, Jakupcak, Seibert, Hildebrandt, and Zeichner (2010) found that restrictive emotionality is associated with an inability to tolerate emotions; this inability to accept emotions was then related to men's interpersonal aggression. Among a sample of men in a domestic violence intervention program, emotional dysregulation was the strongest predictor of IPV (Tager, Good, & Brammer, 2010). In this review, we identified 23 interventions that address dysfunction strain and gender-based violence (see Table 12.2). Thirteen of the programs address domestic abuse or IPV. The remainder address sexual assault or rape, violence against women, or a combination of these.

Dysfunction strain and masculinity are addressed in a variety of ways. Six of these programs explicitly address dysfunction strain through their recognition of the role of male norms in restricting male behavior and ultimately contributing to violence (Allen & Wheeler, 2009; Crooks, Goodall, Hughes, Jaffe, & Baker, 2007; Eckstein & Pinto, 2013; Hong, 2000; McMahon & Dick, 2011; Stewart, 2014). The remaining interventions indirectly address dysfunction strain by adopting a gender-related theoretical approach (Almeida & Hudak, 2002; Wexler, 2006), by addressing gender-based norms and socialization (Barone, Wolgemuth, & Linder, 2007; Edwards, 2009), by addressing constructs related to dysfunction strain (Buttell & Carney, 2006; Foubert, 2005; Sinclair, 2002), or by a combination of these categories (Edleson & Grusznski, 1989; Gondolf, 2008; Pence & Paymar, 1993).

The 23 identified programs are grounded in a wide range of theoretical backgrounds. Half of the programs incorporated at least some component of social norms theory (Brown & Messman-Moore, 2010; Fabiano, Perkins, Berkowitz, Linkenbach, & Stark, 2003), including gender role norms. Many of these programs incorporate social norms theory by educating men about masculine norms and how these norms contribute to violence through computer-based modules (Salazar, Vivolo-Kantor, Hardin, & Berkowitz, 2014) and psychoeducation (Stewart, 2014) to create less violent ways of thinking and behaving.

Social norms–based programs that specifically focus on hegemonic masculinity and its relationship to violence do so through a variety of methods, including a service learning course for undergraduates (Allen & Wheeler,

## TABLE 12.2
### Gender Violence Intervention and Prevention Programs

| Author | Name and description of how program addresses dysfunction strain | Targeted population | IOM level of care | Empirical support | Methodology |
|---|---|---|---|---|---|
| Adams & Cayouette (2002) | **EMERGE**<br>Group therapy addressing respect, responsibility, anger, and accountability without direct incorporation of dysfunction strain | Men mandated for counseling | Indicated | No | Not applicable |
| Allen & Wheeler (2009) | **Changing Carolina: Men Can Make a Difference**<br>Service learning course explicitly addressing dysfunction strain by examining constraints of masculinity, interaction of identities, and how men can explore other definitions of masculinity | Male undergraduate students | Universal | Yes | Quasi-experimental, between groups design |
| Almeida & Hudak (2002) | **Cultural Context Model**<br>Group therapy addressing construct of gender, power, and oppression without direct incorporation of dysfunction strain | Voluntary and court-mandated men, women, and families | Indicated | No | Not applicable |
| Barone et al. (2007) | **The Men's Project**<br>Addresses dysfunction strain through awareness of gender socialization, privilege, and multiple definitions of masculinity | Diverse undergraduate men | Selective | No | Not applicable |
| Buttell & Carney (2006) | **Group treatment through the Domestic Abuse Center**<br>Psychoeducation and group therapy addressing anger, control, and traditional sex roles without direct incorporation of dysfunction strain | Black and White court-mandated heterosexual men | Indicated | Yes | Quasi-experimental, within-subjects design |

| Author (Year) | Program / Description | Target population | Level | Evaluated | Design |
| --- | --- | --- | --- | --- | --- |
| Crooks et al. (2007) | **Cognitive-Behavioral Model to Engage Men and Boys in Violence Prevention** Addresses dysfunction strain explicitly by building new notions of masculinity and shifting core beliefs | Not specified | Indicated | No | Not applicable |
| Douglas et al. (2008) | **Men Stopping Violence** Addresses accountability without direct incorporation of dysfunction strain | Adult men | Universal | No | Not applicable |
| Eckstein & Pinto (2013) | **Participatory action research pilot program** Explicitly addresses dysfunction strain with a focus on masculinity by exploring male hegemony and creating new definitions of masculinity | Undergraduate men | Universal | No | Not applicable |
| Edleson & Grusznski (1989) | **Domestic Abuse Project** Group therapy addressing anger and male role socialization without direct incorporation of dysfunction strain | Men mandated for counseling | Indicated | Yes | Quasi-experimental, between-groups design |
| Edwards (2009) | **She Fears You: Men Ending Rape** Psychoeducation addressing the cultural messages men receive related to violence and masculinity without direct incorporation of dysfunction strain | College resident assistants | Universal | Yes | Experimental, between-groups design |
| Foubert (2005) | **The Men's Program** Workshop addressing control, power, and homophobia without direct incorporation of dysfunction strain | Undergraduate males in fraternities or athletic teams Men in the military | Universal | Yes | Experimental, between-groups design |

*(continues)*

## TABLE 12.2
### Gender Violence Intervention and Prevention Programs *(Continued)*

| Author | Name and description of how program addresses dysfunction strain | Targeted population | IOM level of care | Empirical support | Methodology |
|---|---|---|---|---|---|
| Gondolf (2008) | **Culturally focused counseling** Group therapy addressing oppression, power, and manhood without direct incorporation of dysfunction strain | Court-mandated White and African American men | Indicated | No | Not applicable |
| Hancock & Siu (2009) | **Culturally sensitive intervention** Group therapy addressing aggression and gender role socialization without direct incorporation of dysfunction strain | Court-referred Latino male immigrants who are not documented | Indicated | No | Not applicable |
| Hong (2000) | **Men Against Violence** Workshop explicitly addressing dysfunction strain by examining hegemonic masculinity, masculinity pressures, and their relationship to violence | Black and White undergraduate men | Selective | No | Not applicable |
| Katz (1995) | **Mentors in Violence Project** Interactive mentoring workshop addressing masculinity and homophobia without direct incorporation of dysfunction strain | Undergraduate male athletes; Male and female high school students | Universal | Yes | Quasi-experimental, between-groups design |
| McMahon & Dick (2011) | **Bystander intervention pilot program** Workshop explicitly addresses dysfunction strain by exploring gender construction and how it influences male violence | Male community leaders | Universal | Yes | Quasi-experimental, within-subjects design |
| Parra-Cardona et al. (2013) | **Raices Nuevas (New Roots)** Group therapy addressing power, control, and masculinity without direct incorporation of dysfunction strain | Latino men | Indicated | No | Not applicable |

| Source | Program | Population | IOM category | Empirically supported | Study design |
|---|---|---|---|---|---|
| Pence & Paymar (1993) | **The Duluth Model** Group therapy addressing power, control, and male privilege without direct incorporation of dysfunction strain | Court-mandated men | Indicated | Yes | Experimental, between groups design |
| Pettit & Smith (2002) | **Abusive Men Exploring New Directions (AMEND) Model** Group and individual therapy addressing anger and gender stereotypes without direct incorporation of dysfunction strain | Court-mandated men | Indicated | No | Not applicable |
| Salazar et al. (2014) | **RealConsent** Online modules addressing masculine gender roles without direct incorporation of dysfunction strain | Diverse undergraduate Men | Universal | Yes | Experimental, between-groups design |
| Sinclair (2002) | **MANALIVE (Men Allied Nationally Against Living in Violent Environments)** Classes address control, emotions, and male gender roles without direct incorporation of dysfunction strain | White heterosexual males | Indicated | No | Not applicable |
| Stewart (2014) | **The Men's Project** Explicitly addresses dysfunction strain through male role socialization, male privilege, and different definitions of masculinity | Undergraduate men | Universal | Yes | Quasi-experimental, within-subjects design |
| Wexler (2006) | **The STOP Domestic Violence Program** Group therapy addressing masculinity traps, anger, emotional expression, and assertiveness without direct incorporation of dysfunction strain | Court-mandated men | Indicated | No | Not applicable |

*Note.* IOM = Institute of Medicine.

2009), group psychoeducation (Barone et al., 2007; Eckstein & Pinto, 2013), an interactive workshop (McMahon & Dick, 2011), a professional presentation (Edwards, 2009), peer education (Hong, 2000), and active role-plays and discussion (Katz, 1995). Within these activities and workshops, participants learn about multiple masculinities and how they may both limit men and encourage violence. Two social norms programs address gender role socialization theory by exploring how males and females are socialized, specifically in regard to emotions (Sinclair, 2002) and how violent behavior is developed and maintained at multiple levels (Douglas, Bathrick, & Perry, 2008).

Although efforts to reconstruct new forms of masculinity are needed, these interventions may inadvertently privilege one type of masculinity. By assuming that all men are socialized to a singular definition of masculinity, these theories also suggest that all men experience masculinity in similar ways, regardless of cultural background and societal factors. One way programs have addressed this theoretical gap is by incorporating discussions related to intersectionality of identities (Allen & Wheeler, 2009). For example, Men Stopping Violence recognizes that men may be perpetrators of violence in addition to simultaneously being victims of classism, racism, and heterosexism (Douglas et al., 2008). These programs offer a more inclusive definition of masculinity, while acknowledging the restraints of hegemonic masculinity.

Twenty-two of the identified programs incorporated aspects of dysfunction strain with well-known psychological theories. For example, several programs address violence and nonviolence from a social learning perspective (Adams & Cayouette, 2002; Pettit & Smith, 2002). The Men's Program (Foubert, 2005), a widely used and supported rape prevention program, incorporates belief system theory (Grube, Mayton, & Ball-Rokeach, 1994) and the elaboration likelihood model (Petty & Cacioppo, 1986) by conceptualizing men as potential bystanders and by providing them with messages that are relevant.

The six programs that address rape, sexual assault, and dysfunction strain often incorporate well-known bystander theories (Banyard, Moynihan, & Plante, 2007). These programs conceptualize men as potential bystanders, not potential perpetrators (Katz, 1995), provide men with strategies to intervene (Barone et al., 2007; Edwards, 2009; McMahon & Dick, 2011), improve communication skills (Salazar et al., 2014), and encourage empathy toward victims (Stewart, 2014). Four programs conceptualize the relationship between dysfunction strain and violence as both a community and individual problem. These programs incorporate ecological theory (Bronfenbrenner, 1992) by targeting multiple systems (Douglas et al., 2008); by placing violence within a specific cultural context (Hancock & Siu, 2009; Welland & Ribner, 2010); and by encouraging engagement in campus-wide awareness, community service, and support for victims and perpetrators within the community (Hong, 2000).

Additional programs encourage men's development of critical consciousness to understand how masculinity both empowers and limits men. Many focus specifically on critical consciousness development around identity and experiences with privilege, power, and oppression (Almeida & Hudak, 2002) and challenges experienced by Latino immigrants (Parra-Cardona et al., 2013). Some programs incorporate a feminist theoretical perspective. For example, the cultural context model draws on the theory of transformational feminism, which refers to a social political movement that connects multiple social identities (Almeida & Hudak, 2002). Other programs adopt a feminist theory by developing new notions of masculinity (Crooks et al., 2007) or by highlighting the role of patriarchy in maintaining violence toward women (Pettit & Smith, 2002).

Seven programs incorporated a cognitive behavioral approach to challenge irrational beliefs, defenses, and justifications (Buttell & Carney, 2006); engage in goal setting and skill building (Crooks et al., 2007); encourage responsibility and cognitive restructuring (Sinclair, 2002); and change thoughts and behaviors related to anger and jealousy (Wexler, 2006). Of these seven programs, three interventions specifically incorporated a gender-based cognitive behavioral approach. One program, the Duluth model (Pence & Paymar, 1993), is considered the standard for gender-based cognitive behavioral interventions for violent men. The program incorporates awareness of abusive behaviors, nonabusive alternatives, and the development of interpersonal skills with critical analysis of male privilege, power, and control. The program also emphasizes a coordinated community response model through which law enforcement agencies, mental health professionals, and courts collaborate to assist men (Pence, 1996).

Although the Duluth model is widely used, some scholars have suggested that feminist-based cognitive behavioral approaches may not be effective for all groups. Specifically, lack of attention to environmental context, focus on the patriarchy as privileging men, and focus on equitable relationships may clash with cultures that experience discrimination or endorse traditional relationships between men and women (Hancock & Siu, 2009). Certain programs address this theoretical gap by adding components related to a specific cultural group. For example, Gondolf (2008) addressed African American masculinity within a feminist cognitive behavioral model to create a culturally sensitive intervention.

Programs that integrate theories are particularly strong. These programs clearly explain why violence occurs and how the cycle of violence can be interrupted. For example, the Duluth model provides a clear rationale for how men learn and maintain violence, how they can become violence free by addressing the role that masculinity plays in violence, and how changing thoughts and behaviors related to violence can be effective (Pence &

Paymar, 1993). Effectively combining theories can capture potential gaps and provide clear explanations for how violence can be decreased or prevented.

Although theories were often cited in the creation of programs, it was often unclear whether theories are applied to change behavior. Programs that do not establish a clear theoretical background are harder to adapt for use with other populations and harder to define goals and outcomes and establish empirical support for. Interventionists should articulate how theory explains behavioral change. Furthermore, it is important to note that authors did not reference dysfunction strain in their description of their program. In some cases, programs explicitly addressed how masculine gender role socialization restricts men and contributes to male violence (Allen & Wheeler, 2009; Hong, 2000). In other cases, programs incorporated constructs associated with dysfunction strain, such as control (Foubert, 2005; Pence & Paymar, 1993), anger (Adams & Cayouette, 2002; Buttell & Carney, 2006; Edleson & Grusznski, 1989), and emotional regulation (Sinclair, 2002; Wexler, 2006). Future researchers might examine whether incorporating these constructs into current programs is as effective as creating programs based more explicitly on dysfunction strain.

The programs identified in this review target a wide variety of men, including court-mandated perpetrators, men from high-risk communities, and members of the military. Only nine programs addressed men of color among participants, largely through program adaptation. These programs provide language- and ethnicity-matched groups (Adams & Cayouette, 2002; Pettit & Smith, 2002) or integrate cultural strengths and challenges into existing programs (Parra-Cardona et al., 2013; Welland & Ribner, 2010). These adaptations are most often created based on community demand. For example, in an effort to serve a growing Latino immigrant population, the Raices Nuevas program was adapted from the Duluth model to include common experiences of Latino immigrants (Parra-Cardona et al., 2013).

Programs were developed with the goal of providing culturally relevant interventions for African Americans (Gondolf, 2008), Latinos (Hancock & Siu, 2009), and multicultural groups (Almeida & Hudak, 2002). Among these programs, little attention is paid to within-group differences. One way to rectify this is by considering specific cultural contexts. For example, Hancock and Siu (2009) developed a culturally sensitive program by incorporating into an existing intervention recent research related to Mexican immigrants' cultural background, experiences with gender roles, racism, and patriarchy.

The lack of programs addressing diverse men represents a significant gap. Interventionists should pay particular attention to the role that societal factors (e.g., experiences of racism, heterosexism, etc.) may play in men's violence. Programs that address the diverse experiences of men may reduce attrition and increase positive outcomes. Interventionists should consider the design of programs specifically for diverse at-risk groups as well as the adaptation of current programs to serve a diverse population of men.

A majority of the interventions reviewed in this section are community based. These programs specifically target IPV and domestic abuse among men who are court-mandated and have therefore indicated violent behaviors. In contrast, prevention programs targeting men who have not explicitly indicated violence were more often found within university or college settings. Participants in prevention programs typically attend voluntarily, as part of a course or due to membership in high-risk groups (e.g., athletic teams, fraternity members). Although community programs often focus on decreasing abusive and violent behaviors, college-based programs more typically focus on motivating positive behaviors, such as bystander intervention. In fact, with the exception of one program, all of the college-based prevention programs involved motivating bystanders (Eckstein & Pinto, 2013).

Although the conceptualization of men as potential bystanders is less likely to be found in community-based programs, there are exceptions. For example, McMahon and Dick (2011) piloted a bystander intervention for male community leaders. Additional community-based programs incorporate bystander intervention through individual and community-level advocacy opportunities for men who have perpetrated violence (Sinclair, 2002) and by providing strategies for personal and systemic change to end violence (Douglas et al., 2008).

Our review suggests that men are most often conceptualized as either potential perpetrators or bystanders. However, the rates of male victimization are higher than previously reported (Stemple & Meyer, 2014). Only three programs in our review suggest that men are also victims of male violence (Eckstein & Pinto, 2013; Katz, Heisterkamp, & Fleming, 2011). In one program, Foubert (2005) raises awareness of male-on-male sexual assault and discusses homophobia to dispel the myth that men cannot be victims of sexual assault.

Ten of the programs provided empirical evidence for attitudinal or behavioral change. These findings are limited in several ways. Programs lacked true control groups (Buttell & Carney, 2006; McMahon & Dick, 2011; Parra-Cardona et al., 2013; Stewart, 2014), relying on within-group designs to determine program effectiveness. In other cases, participants who completed the programs were compared with those who dropped out, which previous research has indicated as problematic (Babcock, Green, & Robie, 2004). Intervention groups were often confounded by additional sample characteristics, such as childhood experiences of violence (Edleson & Grusznski, 1989), substance abuse (Buttell & Carney, 2006; Edleson & Grusznski, 1989), and knowledge of program content (McMahon & Dick, 2011).

The programs used a variety of outcome measures, including rape myth acceptance (Edwards, 2009), hostile and benevolent sexism (Stewart, 2014), bystander efficacy (Foubert, 2005; McMahon & Dick, 2011), and endorsement of traditional masculine norms (Allen & Wheeler, 2009). Several programs included behavioral measures, such as aggression and controlling behaviors (Buttell & Carney, 2006) and police reports of violence (Babcock et al., 2004). To determine the effectiveness of these programs, measures of behavioral change are necessary. Furthermore, researchers should avoid using measures that rely only on self-report because men may underreport their own violence. Given that partners are also likely to underreport, a combination of self-report and partner report may be more accurate than either independently (Heckert & Gondolf, 2000). Programs should also consider including measures of social desirability to counteract underreporting (Sugarman & Hotaling, 1997).

Length of follow-up varied widely across programs, ranging from immediate posttreatment (Buttell & Carney, 2006; Pence & Paymar, 1993) to 6 months (Allen & Wheeler, 2009; McMahon & Dick, 2011; Salazar et al., 2014) to 2 years (Foubert, 2005). Although both immediate and longer follow-ups produced lasting change, longer follow-up periods were subject to higher rates of attrition, which previous research suggests may distort findings (Edwards, 2009). The majority of studies produced effect sizes in the small to medium range. Immediate and follow-up tests also raise some questions as to their ability to produce long-lasting change. Given the large number of limitations intrinsic in measuring these programs, more rigorous empirical evaluation of existing programs and more empirical guidance in program creation and implementation are needed (Babcock et al., 2004; Carlson, 2005).

In summary, meta-analyses suggest that gender-based and sexual violence programs have only a small impact on men's future violent behaviors (Babcock et al., 2004; Stover, Meadows, & Kaufman, 2009). Integrating dysfunction strain into interventions may improve outcomes because such a focus may help men understand another underlying cause for their behaviors for which they can change. Although three programs did include same-sex participants (Barone et al., 2007; Salazar et al., 2014; Stewart, 2014), only two programs provided clear adaptations for same-sex couples or for same-sex perpetrators or victims (Adams & Cayouette, 2002; Wexler, 2006). This is problematic, given that research suggests that rates of same-sex partner violence may be as high as heterosexual rates (Jackson, 2007). Last, programs that motivate positive behaviors (i.e., bystander engagement) among nonviolent men may prevent the necessity for interventions aimed at decreasing violent behaviors. Future research should consider the many intersections of identity that men experience, as well as their potential roles as perpetrators, bystanders, and victims of male violence.

SELF-RELIANCE

Men's gender role socialization promotes the avoidance of emotional expression, the absence of weaknesses or vulnerabilities, and the need to solve problems without the help of others (Rochlen, McKelley, & Pituch, 2006). For these reasons, men are less likely than women to seek professional help for a variety of problems, including depression, anxiety, and substance abuse (Lane & Addis, 2005). Men may view seeking help as conflicting with traditional male gender roles and may avoid seeking help to prevent the stigma of appearing weak or unmanly (Pederson & Vogel, 2007). Self-stigma is a key factor in the relationship between masculine gender norms and help-seeking attitudes for men (Hammer, Vogel, & Heimerdinger-Edwards, 2013; Vogel, Heimerdinger-Edwards, Hammer, & Hubbard, 2011). Men's beliefs in self-reliance are also associated with more negative attitudes toward help-seeking. As such, the number of men who experience psychological concerns but do not seek counseling represents a significant need for interventions and programs that encourage men to seek help (Vogel et al., 2011). Despite the clear need for effective intervention and prevention programs, only five interventions or prevention programs addressed masculinity dysfunction strain in men's help-seeking behaviors (see Table 12.3). We discuss these programs in this section.

The Real Men. Real Depression (RMRD) campaign is based on the belief that raising public awareness about depression and help-seeking in men will reduce the stigma of mental health treatment. The RMRD brochure, a component of the campaign, incorporates information on traditional masculine norms and help-seeking, gendered dynamics of men's reluctance to seek help, and men's testimonials and experiences with depression. The RMRD brochure also addresses masculine dysfunction strain by referencing the physiological and psychological impact depression has on men and how these feelings and behaviors can hinder their ability to seek help. Rochlen and his colleagues (2006) evaluated the effectiveness of the RMRD brochure in comparison with a gender-neutral brochure and a brochure with no gender references. The participants with negative help-seeking attitudes rated the RMRD brochure as more appealing and effective in helping men address their depression. Thus, gender-sensitive intervention methods such as the RMRD brochure may help reduce mental health treatment stigma. Although Rochlen and his colleagues found promising results, their intervention specifically targeted undergraduate students; therefore, the results may not generalize to a broader population of men. Also, more information is needed on how interventions such as the RMRD brochure help to facilitate help-seeking behaviors.

Building on intervention materials for men, Hammer and Vogel (2010) tested the efficacy of a male-sensitive brochure in a comparison evaluation of the RMRD brochure and a gender-neutral brochure developed by Rochlen

TABLE 12.3
Help-Seeking Promotion Interventions and Programs

| Author | Name and description of how program addresses dysfunction strain | Targeted population | IOM level of care | Empirical support | Methodology |
|---|---|---|---|---|---|
| Davies et al. (2010) | **The Men's Center** Addresses dysfunction strain by promoting possible masculinity while discussing gendered socialization, men's interdependency needs, and emotion expression | Undergraduate men | Universal | No | Not applicable |
| Hammer & Vogel (2010) | **Male-Sensitive Brochure** Addresses dysfunction strain (feelings of inadequacy, weakness) in discussing masculinity depression, and men's help-seeking attitudes | Adult men | Universal | Yes | Experimental, between-groups design |
| Primack et al. (2010) | **The Men's Stress Workshop** Addresses dysfunction strain by discussing masculine gender norms and how rigid adherence to these norms affect men's everyday lives and depressive symptoms | Men with depressive symptoms | Selective | No | Pretest–posttest quasi-experimental, within-groups design |
| Rochlen et al. (2006) | **Real Men. Real Depression (RMRD) Campaign** Addresses dysfunction strain by referencing the physiological and psychological impact depression has on men | All men | Universal | No | Experimental, between-groups design |
| Syzdek et al. (2014) | **Gender-Based Motivational Interviewing (MI)** Session that uses gender-based MI principles to facilitate help-seeking without direct incorporation of dysfunction strain | Men with depressive or anxious symptoms | Selective | No | Experimental, between-groups design |

*Note.* IOM = Institute of Medicine.

and his colleagues. This brochure was developed to improve the RMRD brochure by incorporating current knowledge on masculine gender roles and masculine depression. The male-sensitive brochure also integrates masculine dysfunction strain by identifying the role self-stigma plays in mental health treatment (i.e., feelings of inadequacy or weakness). The underlying purpose of the male-sensitive brochure is to help men identify the role self-stigma plays in seeking help while incorporating information about gender role socialization and dysfunction strain in changing men's attitudes and behaviors about treatment. Overall, the male-sensitive brochure was shown to be more effective than the RMRD materials in improving men's attitudes toward seeking help (Hammer & Vogel, 2010), which were stronger than a gender-neutral brochure (Rochlen et al., 2006). However, Hammer and his colleagues used a primarily White sample that met the criteria for depression. Future studies should test the effectiveness of intervention materials with men of color as well as those who are not experiencing symptoms associated with depression.

Gender-based motivational interviewing (GBMI) is based on the belief that addressing men's ambivalence, self-stigma, and contemplation toward seeking help can bring about behavioral change (Syzdek, Addis, Green, Whorley, & Berger, 2014). Syzdek et al. (2014) sought to provide men with analytical feedback regarding their signs and symptoms of depression, anxiety, alcoholism, and other health-related issues. They also assessed their participants' attitudes and intentions regarding formal help-seeking (e.g., counseling, primary care). Although the GBMI had no effect on help-seeking attitudes, the intervention did increase men's use of informal help-seeking (i.e., parents and relatives). Therefore, helping men understand their symptoms within a masculinity framework could help facilitate behavioral change, especially given the individualized feedback and detailed information on seeking help. Future research should identify the settings in which GBMI would be most appropriate and how it could help men with more severe symptomatology and high resistance to treatment (i.e., men in the military, veterans' services, men in law enforcement).

Primack, Addis, Syzdek, and Miller (2010) developed an 8-week group treatment approach called the Men's Stress Workshop, which sought to give men tools for managing stress by integrating masculine gender role socialization into a cognitive behavioral therapy framework. Specifically, the workshop provided psychoeducation on men's conformity to various masculine roles (e.g., self-reliance) while changing their thought processes and behaviors related to depression. Primack et al. selected participants who met criteria for major and minor depressive disorder in their workshop. The results revealed that the two participants (of five) with the highest scores on masculinity ideology reported the greatest decrease in self-stigma. However, the small sample size and lack of a control group were limitations of the study.

In an effort to change norms, Davies, Shen-Miller, and Isacco (2010) developed the Men's Center at the University of Oregon. They incorporated the construct of *possible masculinity* in their men's center. They defined possible masculinity as an aspirational and future-oriented goal for men's identities and behaviors based on what men want to be in the future, what men need to meet their developmental needs, and what the community requires from men to foster community safety and health. The goal of their effort is to help men understand how dysfunction strain may affect their attitudes toward help-seeking in addition to helping men identify their future selves. Given that many interventions here unsuccessfully approached masculinity from a deficit model (Levant, 1996), the MCA takes a continuous and positive approach to helping men be their best selves. However, no evaluation data have emerged to determine whether the center's presence has resulted in any shift of attitudes on campus. Information regarding how sexual identity can be incorporated in the MCA approach was not provided.

In summary, given that self-stigma is an important barrier to men's help-seeking behaviors (Vogel et al., 2011), the identified programs aimed to reduce men's self-stigma through the use of brochures and therapeutic interventions. However, it appears that interventions related to improving men's attitudes toward help-seeking behaviors have only recently emerged over the past decade. Although the results are promising, future researchers should interpret the findings with caution because of the homogenous samples of men (i.e., White, heterosexual) as well as the limited number of interventions and programs targeting men's help-seeking attitudes and behaviors. Unfortunately, none of the programs or interventions explicitly addressed multicultural issues as they related to men's self-reliance. Although Rochlen et al. (2006) recruited a diverse sample, the majority of the program participants were currently enrolled in college or already had college degrees, limiting generalizability of the findings. Developing interventions within a multicultural framework will help men of color negotiate masculinity and help-seeking. Our review also suggests a focus of intervention at the individual level and in reshaping cultural norms. Systemic-level interventions, which include policy reform, may also be needed to address men's help-seeking behaviors. For example, a policy that addresses fears over how seeking mental health services may negatively affect the careers of police officers may encourage help-seeking behaviors in that group.

## CONCLUSION

Although many factors contribute to men's risk, meta-analyses of programs outside of those highlighted in this chapter but also aimed at reducing substance use (Moyer, Finney, Swearingen, & Vergun, 2002) and gender-based violence and sexual violence (Anderson & Whiston, 2005; Babcock et al., 2004) suggest small effect sizes for treating substance use and for reducing gender-based violence and sexual violence (Babcock et al., 2004; Moyer et al., 2002). Small effect sizes, in addition to high levels of recidivism (Stover et al., 2009; Walitzer & Dearing, 2006), suggest that interventions can be strengthened. A gender-transformative approach, in which men learn about gender and are encouraged to transform their gender roles and work toward more equitable gender relationships, may be one way for programs to yield longer lasting and stronger effects. Research is needed to determine whether this added component would be more effective in reducing substance use and gender-based and sexual violence. Applied researchers may test our assumption by comparing participants in a treatment as usual group (e.g., cognitive behavioral) against participants exposed to the same treatment with the added gender-transformative approach.

Men, because of how dysfunction strain operates, may not seek help. Normalizing problems among men (e.g., RMRD) and targeting specific aspects of masculinity (e.g., self-reliance) are critical steps toward supporting men in making informed and healthy decisions about accessing professional support. Efforts that increase men's comfort in seeking mental health treatment may also lead to better access to support that may help prevent or remediate violent behaviors or substance use. These findings indicate that efforts at reducing stigma associated with help-seeking are sorely needed.

Our review also suggests that the diversity of men's experiences should be integrated more fully to create more relevant and effective treatments. In addition to understanding the effectiveness of existing gender-transformative programs for men of color and gay and bisexual men, there is also a need to create interventions that are sensitive to their experiences. With the recent emergence of intersectional perspectives on men and masculinity (e.g., Liang, Rivera, Nathwani, Dang, & Douroux, 2010; Liang, Salcedo, & Miller, 2011; Schwing, Wong, & Fann, 2013), we encourage interventionists to be sensitive to the role of culture, racism, sexual identity, homonegativity, and social class. In evaluating programs, applied researchers should examine the added benefit of incorporating masculinity, from an intersectional perspective, on attitudes, knowledge, and violence- and alcohol-related behaviors.

As men continue to face risks to their well-being, so do their children, partners, families, and communities. Fortunately, recent research on dysfunction strain in men's lives can meaningfully inform relevant prevention and treatment programs. Although we were unable to identify many programs that explicitly integrated dysfunction strain with substance use or self-reliance, it is clear that literature on sexual and partner violence has already set the foundation on which to base a discussion of how to properly support boys and men. As we step away from pathologizing boys and men based on their biological sex, we are better able to properly create programs with the overarching goal of creating healthy men, families, and communities.

## REFERENCES

Adams, D., & Cayouette, S. (2002). Emerge—A group education model for abusers. In E. Aldarondo & F. Mederos (Eds.), *Programs for men who batter: Intervention and prevention strategies in a diverse society* (pp. 4.1–4.32). Kingston, NJ: Civic Research Institute.

Allen, C. T., & Wheeler, J. A. (2009). In practice: Engaging men in violence prevention. *About Campus, 13*, 19–22.

Almeida, R., & Hudak, J. (2002). The cultural context model. In E. Aldarondo & F. Mederos (Eds.), *Programs for men who batter: Intervention and prevention strategies in a diverse society* (pp. 10.1–10.48). Kingston, NJ: Civic Research Institute.

American Psychiatric Association. (2013). *Diagnostic and statistical manual of mental disorders* (5th ed.). Arlington, VA: Author.

Anderson, L. A., & Whiston, S. C. (2005). Sexual assault education programs: A meta-analytic examination of their effectiveness. *Psychology of Women Quarterly, 29*, 374–388. http://dx.doi.org/10.1111/j.1471-6402.2005.00237.x

Babcock, J. C., Green, C. E., & Robie, C. (2004). Does batterers' treatment work? A meta-analytic review of domestic violence treatment. *Clinical Psychology Review, 23*, 1023–1053. http://dx.doi.org/10.1016/j.cpr.2002.07.001

Banyard, V. L., Moynihan, M. M., & Plante, E. G. (2007). Sexual violence prevention through bystander education: An experimental evaluation. *Journal of Community Psychology, 35*, 463–481. http://dx.doi.org/10.1002/jcop.20159

Barone, R., Wolgemuth, J., & Linder, C. (2007). Preventing sexual assault through engaging college men. *Journal of College Student Development, 48*, 585–594. http://dx.doi.org/10.1353/csd.2007.0045

Bartholomew, N. G., Hiller, M. L., Knight, K., Nucatola, D. C., & Simpson, D. D. (2000). Effectiveness of communication and relationship skills training for men in substance abuse treatment. *Journal of Substance Abuse Treatment, 18*, 217–225. http://dx.doi.org/10.1016/S0740-5472(99)00051-3

Bartholomew, N. G., & Simpson, D. D. (1996). *Time Out! For Men: A communication skills and sexuality workshop for men.* Fort Worth: Texas Christian University, Institute of Behavioral Research.

Bronfenbrenner, U. (1992). *Ecological systems theory.* London, England: Jessica Kingsley.

Brown, A. L., & Messman-Moore, T. L. (2010). Personal and perceived peer attitudes supporting sexual aggression as predictors of male college students' willingness to intervene against sexual aggression. *Journal of Interpersonal Violence, 25*, 503–517. http://dx.doi.org/10.1177/0886260509334400

Buttell, F., & Carney, M. (2006). A large sample evaluation of a court-mandated bat-terer intervention program: Investigating differential program effect for African American and Caucasian men. *Research on Social Work Practice, 16*, 121–131. http://dx.doi.org/10.1177/1049731505277306

Carlson, B. E. (2005). The most important things learned about violence and trauma in the past 20 years. *Journal of Interpersonal Violence, 20*, 119–126. http://dx.doi.org/10.1177/0886260504268603

Catalano, R. F., & Hawkins, J. D. (1996). The social development model: A theory of antisocial behavior. In J. D. Hawkins (Ed.), *Delinquency and crime: Current theories* (pp. 149–197). Cambridge, England: Cambridge University Press.

Catalano, R. F., Kosterman, R., Haggerty, K., Hawkins, D., & Spoth, R. L. (1998). A universal intervention for the prevention of substance abuse: Preparing for the drug-free years. In R. S. Aschery, E. B. Robertson, & K. L. Kumfer (Eds.), *Drug abuse prevention using family interventions* (pp. 130–159). Rockville, MD: National Institute on Drug Abuse.

Cohn, A., Jakupcak, M., Seibert, L., Hildebrandt, T., & Zeichner, A. (2010). The role of emotional dysregulation in the association between men's restrictive emotionality and use of physical aggression. *Psychology of Men & Masculinity, 11*, 53–64. http://dx.doi.org/10.1037/a0018090

Courtenay, W. H. (2011). *Dying to be men: Psychosocial, environmental, and biobehav-ioral directions in promoting the health of men and boys.* New York, NY: Routledge.

Cousins, A. J., & Gangestad, S. W. (2007). Perceived threats of female infidelity, male proprietariness, and violence in college dating couples. *Violence and Victims, 22*, 651–668. http://dx.doi.org/10.1891/088667007782793156

Crooks, C. V., Goodall, G. R., Hughes, R., Jaffe, P. G., & Baker, L. L. (2007). Engag-ing men and boys in preventing violence against women: Applying a cognitive-behavioral model. *Violence Against Women, 13*, 217–239. http://dx.doi.org/10.1177/1077801206297336

Davies, J. A., Shen-Miller, D. S., & Isacco, A. (2010). The Men's Center approach to addressing the health crisis of college men. *Professional Psychology: Research and Practice, 41*, 347–354. http://dx.doi.org/10.1037/a0020308

Donovan, B., Padin-Rivera, E., & Kowaliw, S. (2001). "Transcend": Initial outcomes from a posttraumatic stress disorder/substance abuse treatment program. *Journal of Traumatic Stress, 14*, 757–772. http://dx.doi.org/10.1023/A:1013094206154

Douglas, U., Bathrick, D., & Perry, P. A. (2008). Deconstructing male violence against women: The men stopping violence community-accountability model. *Violence Against Women, 14*, 247–261. http://dx.doi.org/10.1177/1077801207312637

Eckstein, J., & Pinto, K. (2013). Collaborative participatory action strategies for re-envisioning young men's masculinities. *Action Research, 11*, 236–252. http://dx.doi.org/10.1177/1476750313487928

Edleson, J. L., & Grusznski, R. J. (1989). Treating men who batter: Four years of out-come data from the Domestic Abuse Project. *Journal of Social Service Research, 12*, 3–22. http://dx.doi.org/10.1300/J079v12n01_02

Edwards, K. (2009). Effectiveness of a social change approach to sexual assault prevention. *The College Student Affairs Journal, 28,* 22–37.

Fabiano, P. M., Perkins, H. W., Berkowitz, A., Linkenbach, J., & Stark, C. (2003). Engaging men as social justice allies in ending violence against women: Evidence for a social norms approach. *Journal of American College Health, 52,* 105–112. http://dx.doi.org/10.1080/07448480309595732

Foubert, J. (2005). *The Men's Program: A peer education guide to rape prevention* (3rd ed.). New York, NY: Routledge.

Gondolf, E. W. (2008). Program completion in specialized batterer counseling for African-American men. *Journal of Interpersonal Violence, 23,* 94–116. http://dx.doi.org/10.1177/0886260507307912

Griffith, D. M., Gunter, K., & Watkins, D. C. (2012). Measuring masculinity in research on men of color: Findings and future directions. *American Journal of Public Health, 102*(Suppl. 2), S187–S194. http://dx.doi.org/10.2105/AJPH.2012.300715

Griffith, D. M., Metzl, J. M., & Gunter, K. (2011). Considering intersections of race and gender in interventions that address U.S. men's health disparities. *Public Health, 125,* 417–423. http://dx.doi.org/10.1016/j.puhe.2011.04.014

Grube, J., Mayton, D., II, & Ball-Rokeach, S. (1994). Inducing change in values, attitudes, and behaviors: Belief system theory and the method of value self-confrontation. *Journal of Social Issues, 50,* 153–173. http://dx.doi.org/10.1111/j.1540-4560.1994.tb01202.x

Hammer, J. H., & Vogel, D. L. (2010). Men's help seeking for depression: The efficacy of a male-sensitive brochure about counseling. *The Counseling Psychologist, 38,* 296–313. http://dx.doi.org/10.1177/0011000009351937

Hammer, J. H., Vogel, D. L., & Heimerdinger-Edwards, S. R. (2013). Men's helping seeking: Examination of difference across community size, education, and income. *Psychology of Men & Masculinity, 14,* 65–75. http://dx.doi.org/10.1037/a0026813

Hancock, T., & Siu, K. (2009). A culturally sensitive intervention with domestically violent Latino immigrant men. *Journal of Family Violence, 24,* 123–132. http://dx.doi.org/10.1007/s10896-008-9217-0

Heckert, D. A., & Gondolf, E. W. (2000). Assessing assault self-reports by batterer program participants and their partners. *Journal of Family Violence, 15,* 181–197. http://dx.doi.org/10.1023/A:1007594928605

Hong, L. (2000). Toward a transformed approach to prevention: Breaking the link between masculinity and violence. *Journal of American College Health, 48,* 269–279. http://dx.doi.org/10.1080/07448480009596268

Institute of Medicine, Committee on Prevention of Mental Disorders, Division of Biobehavioral Sciences and Mental Disorders. (1994). *Reducing risks for mental disorders: Frontiers for preventive intervention research.* Washington, DC: National Academies Press.

Iwamoto, D. K., Cheng, A., Lee, C. S., Takamatsu, S., & Gordon, D. (2011). "Man-ing" up and getting drunk: The role of masculine norms, alcohol intoxica-tion and alcohol-related problems among college men. *Addictive Behaviors, 36*, 906–911. http://dx.doi.org/10.1016/j.addbeh.2011.04.005

Iwamoto, D. K., & Smiler, A. P. (2013). Alcohol makes you macho and helps you make friends: The role of masculine norms and peer pressure in adolescent boys' and girls' alcohol use. *Substance Use & Misuse, 48*, 371–378. http://dx.doi.org/ 10.3109/10826084.2013.765479

Jackson, N. (2007). Same-sex domestic violence: Myths, facts, correlates, treatment, and prevention strategies. In A. Roberts (Ed.), *Battered women and their families: Intervention strategies and treatment programs* (3rd ed., pp. 451–470). New York, NY: Springer.

Jakupcak, M., Tull, M. T., & Roemer, L. (2005). Masculinity, shame, and fear of emotions as predictors of men's expressions of anger and hostility. *Psychology of Men & Masculinity, 6*, 275–284. http://dx.doi.org/10.1037/1524-9220.6.4.275

Katz, J. (1995). Reconstructing masculinity in the locker room: The Mentors in Violence Prevention Project. *Harvard Educational Review, 65*, 163–174. http:// dx.doi.org/10.17763/haer.65.2.55533188520136u1

Katz, J., Heisterkamp, H. A., & Fleming, W. M. (2011). The social justice roots of the Mentors in Violence Prevention model and its application in a high school setting. *Violence Against Women, 17*, 684–702. http://dx.doi.org/10.1177/ 1077801211409725

Kilmartin, C. T., & Smiler, A. P. (2015). *The masculine self* (5th ed.). New York, NY: Sloan.

Lane, J. M., & Addis, M. E. (2005). Male gender role conflict and patterns of help seeking in Costa Rica and the United States. *Psychology of Men & Masculinity, 6*, 155–168. http://dx.doi.org/10.1037/1524-9220.6.3.155

Levant, R. F. (1996). The new psychology of men. *Professional Psychology: Research and Practice, 27*, 259–265.

Levant, R. F., Wimer, D. J., Williams, C. M., Smalley, K. B., & Noronha, D. (2009). The relationships between masculinity variables, health risk behaviors and attitudes toward seeking psychological help. *International Journal of Men's Health, 8*, 3–21. http://dx.doi.org/10.3149/jmh.0801.3

Liang, C. T. H., Rivera, A., Nathwani, A., Dang, P., & Douroux, A. (2010). Dealing with gendered racism and racial identity among Asian American men. In W. M. Liu, D. Iwamoto, & M. Chae (Eds.), *Culturally responsive counseling with Asian American men* (pp. 63–82). New York, NY: Routledge Press.

Liang, C. T. H., Salcedo, J., & Miller, H. (2011). Perceived racism, masculinity ideolo-gies, and gender role conflict among Latino men. *Psychology of Men & Masculinity, 12*, 201–215. http://dx.doi.org/10.1037/a0020479

Liu, W. M., & Iwamoto, D. K. (2007). Conformity to masculine norms, Asian values, coping strategies, peer group influences and substance use among Asian American men. *Psychology of Men & Masculinity, 8,* 25–39. http://dx.doi.org/10.1037/1524-9220.8.1.25

McMahon, S., & Dick, A. (2011). "Being in a room with like-minded men": An exploratory study of men's participation in a bystander intervention program to prevent intimate partner violence. *Journal of Men's Studies, 19,* 3–18. http://dx.doi.org/10.3149/jms.1901.3

Meichenbaum, D. (1977). *Cognitive behavior modification: An integrative approach.* New York, NY: Plenum. http://dx.doi.org/10.1007/978-1-4757-9739-8

Moore, T., & Stuart, G. (2005). A review of the literature on masculinity and partner violence. *Psychology of Men & Masculinity, 6,* 46–61. http://dx.doi.org/10.1037/1524-9220.6.1.46

Morgenstern, J., Irwin, T. W., Wainberg, M. L., Parsons, J. T., Muench, F., Bux, D. A., Jr., . . . Schulz-Heik, J. (2007). A randomized controlled trial of goal choice interventions for alcohol use disorders among men who have sex with men. *Journal of Consulting and Clinical Psychology, 75,* 72–84. http://dx.doi.org/10.1037/0022-006X.75.1.72

Moyer, A., Finney, J. W., Swearingen, C. E., & Vergun, P. (2002). Brief interventions for alcohol problems: A meta-analytic review of controlled investigations in treatment-seeking and non-treatment-seeking populations. *Addiction, 97,* 279–292. http://dx.doi.org/10.1046/j.1360-0443.2002.00018.x

Murphy, S. L., Xu, J. Q., & Kochanek, K. D. (2013). *Deaths: Final data for 2010* (National Vital Statistics Reports, Vol. 61, No. 4). Hyattsville, MD: National Center for Health Statistics. Retrieved from http://www.cdc.gov/nchs/data/nvsr/nvsr61/nvsr61_04.pdf

Najavits, L. M. (2002). *Seeking Safety: A treatment manual for PTSD and substance abuse.* New York, NY: Guilford Press.

Najavits, L. M., Schmitz, M., Gotthardt, S., & Weiss, R. D. (2005). Seeking Safety plus exposure therapy: An outcome study on dual diagnosis men. *Journal of Psychoactive Drugs, 37,* 425–435. http://dx.doi.org/10.1080/02791072.2005.10399816

O'Neil, J. M. (2015). *Men's gender role conflict: Psychological costs, consequences, and an agenda for change.* http://dx.doi.org/10.1037/14501-000

O'Reilly, C. A., & Chatman, J. A. (1996). Culture as social control: Corporations, cults, and commitment. In B. M. Staw & L. L. Cummings (Eds.), *Research in organizational behavior: An annual series of analytical essays and critical reviews* (pp. 157–200). Greenwich, CT: JAI Press.

Parra-Cardona, J. R., Escobar-Chew, A. R., Holtrop, K., Carpenter, G., Guzmán, R., Hernández, D., . . . González Ramírez, D. (2013). "En el grupo tomas conciencia (in group you become aware)": Latino immigrants' satisfaction with a culturally informed intervention for men who batter. *Violence Against Women, 19,* 107–132. http://dx.doi.org/10.1177/1077801212475338

Pederson, E. L., & Vogel, D. L. (2007). Male gender role conflict and willingness to seek counseling: Testing a mediation model on college-aged men. *Journal of Counseling Psychology, 54,* 373–384. http://dx.doi.org/10.1037/0022-0167.54.4.373

Pence, E. (1996). *Coordinated community response to domestic assault cases: A guide for policy development.* Duluth: Minnesota Program Development.

Pence, E., & Paymar, M. (1993). *Education groups for men who batter: The Duluth model.* New York, NY: Springer.

Pettit, L., & Smith, R. (2002). The AMEND model. In E. Aldarondo & F. Mederos (Eds.), *Programs for men who batter: Intervention and prevention strategies in a diverse society* (pp. 4.1–4.32). Kingston, NJ: Civic Research Institute.

Petty, R. E., & Cacioppo, J. T. (1986). *Communication and persuasion: Central and peripheral routes of attitude change.* http://dx.doi.org/10.1007/978-1-4612-4964-1

Pleck, J. H. (1995). The gender role strain paradigm: An update. In R. F. Levant & W. S. Pollack (Eds.), *A new psychology of men* (pp. 11–32). New York, NY: Basic Books.

Primack, J. M., Addis, M. E., Syzdek, M., & Miller, I. W. (2010). The men's stress workshop: A gender-sensitive treatment for depressed men. *Cognitive and Behavioral Practice, 17,* 77–87. http://dx.doi.org/10.1016/j.cbpra.2009.07.002

Reilly, P. M., & Shopshire, M. S. (2000). Anger management group treatment for cocaine dependence: Preliminary outcomes. *The American Journal of Drug and Alcohol Abuse, 26,* 161–177. http://dx.doi.org/10.1081/ADA-100100598

Reynolds, G. S., Lehman, W. E. K., & Bennett, J. B. (2008). Psychosocial correlates of the perceived stigma of problem drinking in the workplace. *The Journal of Primary Prevention, 29,* 341–356. http://dx.doi.org/10.1007/s10935-008-0140-1

Rochlen, A. B., McKelley, R. A., & Pituch, K. A. (2006). A preliminary examination of the "Real Men. Real Depression" campaign. *Psychology of Men & Masculinity, 7,* 1–13. http://dx.doi.org/10.1037/1524-9220.7.1.1

Rohsenow, D. J., Monti, P. M., Binkoff, J. A., Liepman, M. R., Nirenberg, T. D., & Abrams, D. B. (1991). Patient-treatment matching for alcoholic men in communication skills versus cognitive-behavioral mood management training. *Addictive Behaviors, 16,* 63–69. http://dx.doi.org/10.1016/0306-4603(91)90041-F

Rohsenow, D. J., Smith, R. E., & Johnson, S. (1985). Stress management training as a prevention program for heavy social drinkers: Cognitions, affect, drinking, and individual differences. *Addictive Behaviors, 10,* 45–54. http://dx.doi.org/10.1016/0306-4603(85)90052-8

Salazar, L. F., Vivolo-Kantor, A., Hardin, J., & Berkowitz, A. (2014). A web-based sexual violence bystander intervention for male college students: Randomized controlled trial. *Journal of Medical Internet Research, 16,* e203. http://dx.doi.org/10.2196/jmir.3426

Santisteban, D. A., Coatsworth, J. D., Perez-Vidal, A., Kurtines, W. M., Schwartz, S. J., LaPerriere, A., & Szapocznik, J. (2003). Efficacy of brief strategic family therapy in modifying Hispanic adolescent behavior problems and substance use. *Journal of Family Psychology, 17,* 121–133. http://dx.doi.org/10.1037/0893-3200.17.1.121

Schwing, A. E., Wong, Y. J., & Fann, M. D. (2013). Development and validation of the African American Men's Gendered Racism Stress Inventory. *Psychology of Men & Masculinity, 14,* 16–24. http://dx.doi.org/10.1037/a0028272

Sinclair, H. (2002). A community activist response to intimate partner violence. In E. Aldarondo & F. Mederos (Eds.), *Programs for men who batter: Intervention and prevention strategies in a diverse society* (pp. 5.1–5.53). Kingston, NJ: Civic Research Institute.

Smith, R. E., & Ascough, J. C. (1984). Induced effect in stress management training. In S. Burchfield (Ed.), *Stress: Psychological and physiological interactions* (pp. 359–378). Washington, DC: Hemisphere.

Smith, R. M., Parrott, D. J., Swartout, K. M., & Tharp, A. T. (2015). Deconstructing hegemonic masculinity: The roles of antifemininity, subordination to women, and sexual dominance in men's perpetration of sexual aggression. *Psychology of Men & Masculinity, 16*, 160–169. http://dx.doi.org/10.1037/a0035956

Stahre, M., Roeber, J., Kanny, D., Brewer, R. D., & Zhang, X. (2014). Contribution of excessive alcohol consumption to deaths and years of potential life lost in the United States. *Preventing Chronic Disease, 11*, 130293. http://dx.doi.org/10.5888/pcd11.130293

Stemple, L., & Meyer, I. H. (2014). The sexual victimization of men in America: New data challenge old assumptions. *American Journal of Public Health, 104*, e19–e26. http://dx.doi.org/10.2105/AJPH.2014.301946

Stewart, A. (2014). The Men's Project: A sexual assault prevention program targeting college men. *Psychology of Men & Masculinity, 15*, 481–485. http://dx.doi.org/10.1037/a0033947

Stover, C. S., Meadows, A. L., & Kaufman, J. (2009). Interventions for intimate partner violence: Review and implications for evidence-based practice. *Professional Psychology: Research and Practice, 40*, 223–233. http://dx.doi.org/10.1037/a0012718

Sugarman, D., & Hotaling, G. (1997). Intimate violence and social desirability: A meta-analytic review. *Journal of Interpersonal Violence, 12*, 275–290. http://dx.doi.org/10.1177/088626097012002008

Syzdek, M. R., Addis, M. E., Green, J. D., Whorley, M. R., & Berger, J. (2014). A pilot trial of gender-based motivational interviewing for help-seeking and internalizing symptoms in men. *Psychology of Men & Masculinity, 15*, 90–94. http://dx.doi.org/10.1037/a0030950

Szapocznik, J., Hervis, O., & Schwartz, S. (2003). *Brief strategic family therapy for adolescent drug abuse.* http://dx.doi.org/10.1037/e598162007-001

Tager, D., Good, G., & Brammer, S. (2010). "Walking over 'em": An exploration of relations between emotional dysregulation, masculine norms, and intimate partner abuse in a clinical sample of men. *Psychology of Men & Masculinity, 11*, 233–239. http://dx.doi.org/10.1037/a0017636

U.S. Department of Health, Substance Abuse and Mental Health Services Administration, Center for Behavioral Health Statistics and Quality. (2014). *Results from the 2013 National Survey on Drug Use and Health: Summary of national findings.* Rockville, MD: Author. Retrieved from http://www.samhsa.gov/data/sites/default/files/NSDUHresultsPDFWHTML2013/Web/NSDUHresults2013.pdf

U.S. Department of Justice, Federal Bureau of Investigation. (2012, September). *Crime in the United States, 2011*. Retrieved from http://www.fbi.gov/about-us/cjis/ucr/crime-in-the-u.s/2011/crime-in-the-u.s.-2011/tables/table-33

Uy, P. J., Massoth, N. A., & Gottdiener, W. H. (2014). Rethinking male drinking: Traditional masculine ideologies, gender role conflict, and drinking motives. *Psychology of Men & Masculinity, 15*, 121–128. http://dx.doi.org/10.1037/a0032239

Vogel, D. L., Heimerdinger-Edwards, S. R., Hammer, J. H., & Hubbard, A. (2011). "Boys don't cry": Examination of the links between endorsement of masculine norms, self-stigma, and help-seeking attitudes for men from diverse backgrounds. *Journal of Counseling Psychology, 58*, 368–382. http://dx.doi.org/10.1037/a0023688

Walitzer, K. S., & Dearing, R. L. (2006). Gender differences in alcohol and substance use relapse. *Clinical Psychology Review, 26*, 128–148. http://dx.doi.org/10.1016/j.cpr.2005.11.003

Welland, C., & Ribner, N. (2010). Culturally specific treatment for partner-abusive Latino men: A qualitative study to identify and implement program components. *Violence and Victims, 25*, 799–813. http://dx.doi.org/10.1891/0886-6708.25.6.799

Wester, S. R. (2008). Male gender role conflict and multiculturalism: Implications for counseling psychology. *The Counseling Psychologist, 36*, 294–324. http://dx.doi.org/10.1177/0011000006286341

Wexler, D. B. (2006). *Stop Domestic Violence: Innovative skills, techniques, options, and plans for better relationships: Group leader's manual*. New York, NY: Norton.

# V

# CONCLUSION

# CONCLUSION: ADDRESSING CONTROVERSIES AND UNRESOLVED QUESTIONS IN THE PSYCHOLOGY OF MEN AND MASCULINITIES

Y. JOEL WONG AND RONALD F. LEVANT

In this conclusion, we highlight several unresolved and potentially controversial issues in the psychology of men and masculinities to identify recommendations for future scholarship. The contributors to this book have provided excellent recommendations for future research on the topics related to their chapters. Rather than repeating their suggestions, we focus here on fundamental conceptual and methodological questions surrounding the nature of masculinities. In particular, we address (a) the utility of masculinities, (b) social constructionist versus essentialist perspectives on masculinities, and (c) the evolving nature of masculine norms.

## IS "MASCULINITY" A PROBLEM?

Throughout this book, we (and we suspect many of our authors) assume that the construct of masculinities is useful and vital to the psychology of men. Nevertheless, this premise has been challenged; the heading of this

http://dx.doi.org/10.1037/0000023-014

*The Psychology of Men and Masculinities*, R. F. Levant and Y. J. Wong (Editors)

section is the title of Addis, Mansfield, and Syzdek's (2010) provocative article questioning the utility of masculinities.[1] Addis et al. argued that current conceptualizations and measurement of masculinities are limited because of their lack of emphasis on the contextual nature of gender. Because most studies in the psychology of men use self-report measures of masculinities that reflect individual differences on relatively stable attributes (e.g., masculinity ideologies, conformity to masculine norms, and gender role conflict), Addis et al. were concerned that such efforts are not sensitive to contextual influences on men's gendered social learning. For example, a score on a particular subscale of the Conformity to Masculine Norms Inventory (CMNI; Mahalik et al., 2003) merely provides a generic description of an individual rather the "multiple potentialities for enacting that attribute depending on the context" (Addis et al., 2010, pp. 80–81). That is, a boy might learn that expressing sadness in the presence of dominant males evokes social sanctions, but that is less likely to occur among close friends. In contrast, Addis and colleagues called for more research that identifies gender-relevant cues that elicit men's behavior in specific situations.

By adopting a functional and pragmatic stance, Addis et al. (2010) argued that masculinities pose substantial obstacles to both scientific and social progress. With regard to scientific progress, Addis et al. reasoned that the utility of masculinities should be evaluated on the basis of social goals such as the eradication of gender inequality and the promotion of well-being. On this front, the authors noted that there is little empirical evidence that masculinities-related constructs have been used to influence men's behavior positively. In particular, Addis et al. cited the lack of empirical evaluations of therapeutic treatments involving masculinities-related constructs and the paucity of research involving experimental designs.

Second, on the social front, Addis et al. (2010) reasoned that widespread dissemination of knowledge about masculinities has been more problematic than beneficial. They observed that many laypeople hold essentialist beliefs about gender and that in everyday language masculinities are not typically used to promote social progress but to reinforce such essentialist views about the differences between men and women. The authors cite examples of how masculinities have been co-opted for disparate social agendas, such as those of the men's rights organizations (Messner, 1997). Addis et al. concluded that the metaphor of "masculinity" has constrained progress in the psychology of men, and they called for a new set of assumptions and vocabularies in both scientific and public discourse.

---

[1]Addis et al. (2010) used the term *masculinity*, although our preference is for the plural form *masculinities* (see the Introduction to this volume).

The Addis et al. (2010) article was followed by three invited commentaries (Brooks, 2010; O'Neil, 2010; Sylvester & Hayes, 2010) as well as Addis's (2010) response to these commentaries. The original Addis et al. article has garnered considerable interest, with 81 citations as of February 15, 2016, according to Google Scholar. Nonetheless, our review of these 81 citations suggest that, with the exception of two commentaries on the article (Brooks, 2010; O'Neil, 2010), the core concerns raised in the Addis et al. article remain largely unchallenged. Given that the article poses fundamental questions about the utility of masculinities, a construct that arguably lies at the heart and soul of our field, we are surprised that there has not been further debate on the issues the authors raised. We therefore feel compelled in this closing chapter to provide our response to the Addis et al. article. In so doing, our goal is not to provide the final word on these issues but to encourage further debate and greater critical thinking among scholars, practitioners, and students in our field.

We agree with Addis et al.'s (2010) call for more research on the contextual nature of gendered social learning. The authors suggested the need for more research attention to longitudinal, experimental priming, and diary methodologies to provide a more contextual account of men's gendered social learning. We endorse all these ideas and believe that the Addis et al. article has positively contributed to greater methodological diversity in the psychology of men and masculinities in recent years, particularly in the area of experimental priming research (e.g., Vandello & Bosson, 2013; Wong et al., 2015).

At the same time, we are concerned that Addis et al.'s (2010) repudiation of masculinities might amount to throwing the baby out with the bathwater. We offer five reasons why the construct of masculinities is vital to our field and is not incompatible with the contextual gendered learning perspective promoted by Addis et al. First, we address the issue of the lack of scientific progress in masculinities research. The underlying logic of Addis et al.'s argument appears to be that the paucity of empirical evidence that masculinities research improves people's lives (e.g., the absence of masculinities-based empirically supported interventions) substantially diminishes the utility of masculinities. Our response to this critique is that it is an argument from silence; that is, the absence of evidence is used to infer evidence of absence. It is entirely possible that empirical limitations in a given area reflect an underlying conceptual weakness, but it is also possible that such limitations will be addressed over time by more methodologically sophisticated research.

Although the psychology of men and masculinities emerged as a distinct discipline in the 1970s and 1980s, empirical psychological research began accelerating only in the past two decades (see Pleck, Foreword, this volume; Levant & Wong, Introduction, this volume). In other words, the psychological science of men and masculinities remains a relatively young field.

The emerging body of cross-sectional research on the association between masculinities-related constructs and other outcomes over the past 2 decades may help lay the foundation for more sophisticated types of research (e.g., longitudinal, experimental, and intervention-based studies) that will provide a more contextual account of men's gendered lives. Accordingly, it may be premature to criticize the utility of masculinities on the basis of a lack of empirical and methodological progress. Addis et al.'s (2010) criticism in this regard would be more compelling if a large body of masculinities-focused intervention studies consistently yielded null effects. But such studies currently do not exist, and therefore more research is needed. For instance, Brooks's (Chapter 11, this volume) and Liang, Molenaar, Hermann, and Rivera's (Chapter 12) reviews of the literature on psychological interventions for men identified a few that explicitly address masculinities-related constructs (e.g., Primack, Addis, Syzdek, & Miller, 2010). Future research should focus on evaluating the efficacy of such interventions.

Relatedly, it appears that Addis et al.'s (2010) discomfort with masculinities is in part related to their critique of research that conceptualizes and measures masculinities in terms of individual differences in attributes that people possess (e.g., conformity to masculine norms or masculinity ideologies). To be clear, we do not deny that there are conceptual and methodological limitations inherent in such research. But we believe that the logical consequence of Addis et al.'s critique of the dominant paradigm in masculinities research should be a call for more sophisticated research rather than to abandon the construct of masculinities. Simply put, empirical limitations should be addressed by empirical solutions. In addition to the excellent research recommendations proposed by Addis et al., we propose a big-tent approach that embraces diverse theoretical approaches and methodologies, including correlational, experimental, quasi-experimental, and qualitative research designs (see Mahalik, 2014, for a similar recommendation).

Second, we argue that masculinities are worthy of scientific inquiry precisely because they reflect a subject of interest in public discourse. In public discourse and everyday conversations, it is not uncommon for people to label or categorize others (typically men but occasionally, women) as *macho*, *masculine*, or *manly*, reflecting individuals' lay beliefs about masculinities. To illustrate, researchers have studied laypeople's stereotypes of how masculine certain groups of individuals are (Galinsky, Hall, & Cuddy, 2013; Jackson, Lewandowski, Ingram, & Hodge, 1997; Wilkins, Chan, & Kaiser, 2011), a construct that Wong, Horn, and Chen (2013) referred to as *perceived masculinity*. In a recent study, Wong et al. (2013) found that college students perceived Black American men as more masculine than White and Asian American men and Asian American men as the least masculine group; moreover, these racial differences in perceived masculinity were strongest among participants with high levels of racial essentialist beliefs. More research is needed to understand the content, antecedents, and consequences of perceived masculinity as well how to modify such beliefs.

Third, although we agree with Addis et al. (2010) that among laypeople, masculinities are sometimes used to reinforce essentialist beliefs about gender, we disagree with their conclusion that this diminishes the utility of masculinities. Addis and colleagues argued that although most professionals in the psychology of men do not intend to promote essentialist beliefs about gender when they discuss masculinities, trying to change public discourse on masculinities is a "task verging on the Sisyphusian [sic]" (p. 83). However, the construct of masculinities is not the only psychological construct on which laypeople's beliefs diverge from the prevailing scientific discourse. An analogy from the psychology of race might be instructive. Research suggests that many people hold essentialist beliefs about race (Haslam, Rothschild, & Ernst, 2000), which differ from a social constructionist conceptualization of race held by academic psychologists (e.g., Helms & Talleyrand, 1997). Yet we are not aware of any academic psychologist who has suggested that, on this basis, race is not a useful construct or that psychologists should not talk about race because they might inadvertently perpetuate essentialist beliefs about race among laypeople. A similar logic should apply to our field. As challenging as it might be, psychologists should work to transform the meaning of masculinities in public discourse rather than to acquiesce to people's essentialist beliefs about masculinities. Experimental studies can be conducted to assess whether individuals who are randomly assigned to receive information about social constructionist versus essentialist perspectives on masculinities might develop more gender-egalitarian attitudes. The results from such studies can then provide the basis for designing evidence-based workshops and other interventions to promote social constructionist beliefs about masculinities.

Fourth, we draw some comfort from the fact that our views on the relevance and utility of masculinities are shared by our academic siblings outside of psychology. Specifically, scholars in the sociology of gender have for the past 30 years promoted the use of the term *masculinity* or *masculinities* as a core concept in understanding the experiences of men and their relations with women and other men (Carrigan, Connell, & Lee, 1985; Connell, 2005). Sociological research on masculinities differs from psychology in its emphasis on qualitative research as well as a more explicitly social constructionist conceptualization of masculinities (Connell & Messerschmidt, 2005). Conceptually and methodologically, psychologists have much to learn from their academic siblings in sociology, but we see no compelling need to abandon the construct of masculinities.

Fifth, using the logic of a pragmatic functional perspective on gender, we arrive at the opposite conclusion from that of Addis et al. (2010) with regard to the relevance of masculinities. From a pragmatic functional standpoint, one might ask: What are the practical consequences of psychologists abandoning the construct of masculinities? What difference would it make if we simply refer to our field as the *psychology of men* instead of the *psychology of men and masculinities*? What will happen if psychologists stop studying masculinities and no longer use masculinities-related constructs in scientific and public discourse? We submit that there may be several challenges associated with such an omission. From a practical standpoint, it might be a Herculean task for psychologists to avoid even using the word *masculinity* and other masculinities-related words when discussing their ideas about gender with laypeople simply because laypeople already use masculinities-related terms (e.g., *macho, masculine, manhood,* and *manly*) in their everyday conversations. For one, omitting *masculinity* and other related terms from psychologists' vocabulary would simply result in missed opportunities to be conversant in the vocabulary of the people they serve and to offer alternative ways to understand masculinities that promote well-being and gender equality.

For another, the omission of "masculinities" and related terms from psychologists' scientific vocabulary creates a new practical dilemma: What labels should psychologists use in place of *masculinities*? Our conjecture regarding Addis et al.'s (2010) response to this question might be that no replacement term is needed because the focus of psychological research should shift to the contextual nature of men's gendered social learning. But there remain several gender-related phenomena that are in need of labels. For example, what term would psychologists then use to describe societal or group norms concerning what men should or should not do? Conceivably, we could avoid the word *masculinities* or *masculine* by labeling such norms *social norms* or *gender norms,* but we submit that neither of these terms provide the level of specificity afforded by our preferred term, *masculine norms.*

On the flip side, we argue that masculinities research, including studies that use self-report measures of individual differences in masculinities, have the potential to contribute positively to scientific and public discourse. As we explain in the next section of this chapter, research on individual differences in masculinities may in some ways contribute to undermining essentialist notions of gender.

## ESSENTIALISM VERSUS SOCIAL CONSTRUCTIONISM

Related to Addis et al.'s (2010) critique of current conceptualizations and measures of masculinities is the debate on whether research that used self-report measures of individual differences in masculinities reflect essentialist or social constructionist perspectives. Essentialist perspectives suggest that sex differences and gender characteristics reflect stable and ingrained qualities within individuals (Bohan, 1997), whereas from a social constructionist perspective, gender is conceptualized as fluid, unstable, and culturally bound and as actions performed in everyday social interactions (Seymour-Smith, Chapter 4, this volume; Wong & Rochlen, 2008). In their review of masculinities research, Wester and Vogel (2012) argued that the extant psychological literature on masculinities stems largely from an essentialist approach, and they cite research on the gender role strain paradigm as exemplars of essentialist research. In response, Levant and Powell (Chapter 1, this volume) asserted that the gender role strain paradigm is grounded in social constructionism (also see Kimmel, 1987, and Pleck, 1995, for earlier but similar debates). It is beyond the scope of this Conclusion to discuss in detail the arguments proffered by these scholars, and we encourage interested readers to review Wester and Vogel's (2012) as well as Levant and Powell's chapters. We acknowledge that this debate is further complicated by the fact that there are different definitions and versions of essentialism and social constructionism (see Burr, 2015, and O'Neil, 2010, for summaries). Nevertheless, we offer a few brief comments that we hope will stimulate further scholarship on this debate.

Instead of categorizing masculinities research as either social constructionist or essentialist, it might be more helpful to conceptualize such research as lying on a continuum from mostly essentialist to mostly social constructionist. This continuum perspective on the essentialism–social constructionism debate simply reflects common sense. To the extent that laypeople's essentialist beliefs are typically measured on a continuum rather than as discrete categories (e.g., Haslam et al., 2000), a similar logic should apply to the classification of research as essentialist or social constructionist. On one end of the spectrum, studies that focus exclusively on sex differences between men and women without a social explanation of why such differences exist largely reflect an essentialist perspective. On the other end of the social constructionist spectrum are studies that conceptualize masculinities as discourse (Seymour-Smith, Chapter 4, this volume). Such studies typically involve qualitative analyses of interviews or naturally occurring conversations, and they emphasize the fluidity of masculinities as they are performed or accomplished in social interactions (Wetherell & Edley, 2014). This continuum perspective also acknowledges that many masculinities studies lie between these two ends of the spectrum and reflect a hybrid of essentialist and social constructionist viewpoints (see also Fuss, 1989; Levant, 2015).

How, then, should we classify studies that use self-report measures of individual differences in adherence to masculinities-related attributes (e.g., the CMNI)? We propose that such studies reflect a hybrid of essentialist and social constructionist perspectives. On the one hand, a focus on individuals' stable attributes seems to be consistent with the definition of gender essentialism

(Bohan, 1997; see also Addis & Hoffman, Chapter 6, this volume). On the other hand, studies that use such measures of individual differences also challenge the essentialist perspective by drawing attention to the difference between biological sex and gender. In contrast to gender essentialism, which emphasizes—and ultimately stereotypes—innate differences between women and men, studies that use measures of individual differences in masculinities underscore the notion that within-sex differences among women and men are likely more salient than between-sex differences (cf. Hyde, 2005). A focus on individual differences in masculinities among men and women partially reflects a social constructionist viewpoint because it undermines the notion that membership in the categories of "male" or "female" automatically confers a set of predetermined attributes (e.g., the essentialist belief that, compared with women, men are naturally good at math and technology). In other words, variability in a distribution of scores on a measure of masculinities in a sample of men implies that not all men are the same. Moreover, psychologists can help dispel stereotypes about innate sex differences in the public discourse by disseminating findings on within-sex individual differences in masculinities. Future research could address whether such efforts might undermine lay-people's essentialist beliefs about gender. With these arguments, we come full circle to our earlier discussion on the utility of the construct of masculinities. For the reasons that we just identified, research that use self-report measures of individual differences in masculinities can contribute positively to scientific and public discourse, and therefore the construct of masculinities remains relevant to the psychology of men.

## THE EVOLVING NATURE OF MASCULINE NORMS

To the extent that masculine norms are socially constructed, they do not remain static but evolve over time (Wester & Vogel, 2012). Commonly used measures of masculinities such as the Gender Role Conflict Scale (O'Neil, Helms, Gable, David, & Wrightsman, 1986), the Masculine Gender Role Stress Scale (Eisler & Skidmore, 1987), and the Male Role Norms Inventory (MRNI; Levant et al., 1992) were developed in the 1980s and early 1990s. More recently, Mahalik and colleagues (2003) developed the CMNI, and Levant and his colleagues have developed revised versions of the MRNI (e.g., Levant, Hall, & Rankin, 2013). However, a question arises as to whether these measures adequately capture prevailing and rapidly shifting trends in masculine norms and ideologies over the past decade. For example, hetero-sexist attitudes constitute one of the dimensions of masculinity ideology and masculine norms measured in the CMNI and MRNI. Yet attitudes toward gay marriage in the United States have changed substantially over the past decade and a half. In 2001, only 32% of men in the United States favored same-sex marriage, but by 2015, this percentage had risen to 53% (Pew Research Center, 2016). Might this change in attitude portend a shift in U.S. masculine norms toward a less heterosexist and more embracing attitude toward sexual minorities?

In the same vein, a lively debate concerning the content validity of these measures erupted on the electronic mailing list of the Society for the Psychological Study of Men and Masculinity several years ago (Wong, Ho, Wang, & Fisher, 2016). In a post, Ed Tejirian (2013) opined that practices such as self-reliance, avoidance of femininity, and toughness were not "masculine norms" but represent a "set of clichés—to use the *Star Wars* phrase—from a 'galaxy far, far away.'" In another post critiquing the relevance of purported masculine norms on homophobia, Andrew Smiler (2014) argued that "it's very clear that norms regarding homosexuality/homophobia are/have changed dramatically over the last 50 years." In yet another post that offered an alternative perspective, Gary Brooks (2014) argued that although many men do not conform to traditional masculine norms, such norms are still relevant because men are aware of these norms and are troubled by their lack of conformity to them.

Instead of evaluating the merits of these arguments, we explore several methodological strategies for identifying contemporary masculine norms and ideologies. One strategy is to compare scores on measures of masculinities from recent samples with those of earlier samples. A change in scores might potentially reflect shifts in masculine norms over time. For instance, Twenge (1997) conducted a meta-analysis of studies using the Bem Sex Role Inventory and Personal Attributes Questionnaire and analyzed change in masculinity and femininity scores over a 20-year period. A similar methodology could be used with regard to other measures of masculinities. Nevertheless, one limitation of this methodology is that changes in scores over time might reflect shifts in individual adherence to masculinities-related constructs rather than a change in masculine norms per se. That is, it is entirely possible that some individuals may believe in the existence of certain masculine norms (e.g., "Most people believe that men should . . .") even if they do not personally adhere to these norms.

To identify contemporary masculine norms, a second methodological strategy is to conduct a content analyses of institutions that act as purveyors of masculine norms. Examples include recent mass media representations of men and masculinities found in movies, TV shows, advertisements, magazines, and music (e.g., Tan, Shaw, Cheng, & Kim, 2013; Vokey, Tefft, & Tysiaczny, 2013). For instance, Vokey et al.'s (2013) analysis of eight U.S. men's magazines found that the majority of advertisements in these magazines depicted hypermasculine beliefs and that such beliefs were more prevalent in advertisements directed at men who are young, less educated, and of lower socioeconomic status.

A third methodological strategy for identifying the most prevalent types of masculine norms in contemporary society is to pose open-ended questions to a large sample of individuals about their perceptions of the most important masculine norms in their society. Wong et al. (2016) adopted this methodology in their analysis of Singaporean university students' subjective masculine norms. Three hundred and forty-eight participants provided written responses to three open-ended prompts beginning with "In Singapore, most people believe that men should . . ." (reflecting prescriptive masculine norms) and three other open-ended prompts beginning with "In Singapore, most people believe that men should NOT . . ." (reflecting proscriptive masculine norms). Participants were told that the focus of these prompts was on their perceptions of what most people believed rather than on whether they personally endorsed those norms. A content analysis of participants' open-ended responses identified 17 masculine norms that were identified by at least 10% of the sample. The top five were providing for family (49%), being a gentleman (45%), emotional toughness (35%), avoidance of inferiority to women (29%), and avoidance of femininity (27%; percentages refer to the proportion of participants who identified a particular norm at least once in their six responses). Some of these norms (e.g., emotional toughness and avoidance of femininity) converge with those in the CMNI and MRNI, whereas others (e.g., providing for family) are not represented in U.S.-based conceptualizations and measures of masculinities. Interestingly, Wong et al.'s (2016) list of the most prevalent masculine norms also included nonaggression and fidelity in monogamous relationships (identified by approximately one fifth of the sample), norms that are diametrically different from the masculine norms of playboy and violence represented in the CMNI.

One benefit of this methodology is that it adopts a bottom-up approach to identifying masculine norms; that is, respondents are given the freedom to articulate the masculine norms that they perceive to be most important rather than constrained to respond to a set of masculine norms predetermined by researchers (Wong et al., 2016). Additionally, researchers can quantify the percentage of masculine norms represented in the data to identify the most prevalent masculine norms. Although the findings in the Wong et al. (2016) study are not generalizable beyond university students in Singapore, we believe that the methodology used in that study could be used across diverse societies (e.g., by substituting "Singapore" for "America" or another country in the open-ended prompts) to identify the most prevalent contemporary masculine norms. Such efforts could then provide an empirical basis for the revision of existing measures or the development of new measures of masculinities.

# FINAL NOTE

In this Conclusion, we have focused on a few unresolved but vital issues concerning the nature of masculinities. In so doing, our goal was not to provide the definitive word on these issues but to provide the impetus for more scholarly attention to these key areas in our field.

We began by explaining why masculinities remain vital to the psychology of men. Next, we explored the debate on social constructionist and essentialist perspectives on gender. We concluded that a continuum perspective acknowledging that research can reflect both perspectives is preferable to one that simply categorizes studies into one of two mutually exclusive paradigms. Finally, we examined the evolving nature of masculine norms and discussed several methodological strategies for identifying contemporary masculine norms and ideologies.

In closing, this book offers readers a sampling of cutting-edge topics, theories, research, and practical applications in the psychology of men and masculinities. If the Conclusion, as well as the chapters, sparks discussion, debate, and interest in our field, the volume will have served its purpose well. Overall, we believe that the psychology of men and masculinities has a bright future. We are humbled to be given the opportunity in this book to contribute to its future, and we look forward to the next chapter of history in the psychology of men and masculinities.

# REFERENCES

Addis, M. E. (2010). Response to Commentaries on the Problem of Masculinity. *Psychology of Men & Masculinity, 11*, 109–112. http://dx.doi.org/10.1037/a0019314

Addis, M. E., Mansfield, A. K., & Syzdek, M. R. (2010). Is "masculinity" a problem? Framing the effects of gendered social learning in men. *Psychology of Men & Masculinity, 11*, 77–90. http://dx.doi.org/10.1037/a0018602

Bohan, J. S. (1997). Regarding gender: Essentialism, constructionism, and feminist psychology. In M. M. Gergen & S. N. Davis (Eds.), *Toward a new psychology of gender* (pp. 31–47). New York, NY: Routledge.

Brooks, G. R. (2010). Despite problems, "masculinity" is a vital construct. *Psychology of Men & Masculinity, 11*, 107–108. http://dx.doi.org/10.1037/a0019180

Brooks, G. R. (2014, January 8). Unknown title [Electronic mailing list message]. Retrieved from http://SPSMM@Lists.apa.org

Burr, V. (2015). *Social constructionism.* New York, NY: Routledge. http://dx.doi.org/10.1016/B978-0-08-097086-8.24049-X

Carrigan, T., Connell, B., & Lee, J. (1985). Toward a new sociology of masculinity. *Theory and Society, 14*, 551–604. http://dx.doi.org/10.1007/BF00160017

Connell, R. W. (2005). *Masculinities*. Berkley: University of California Press.

Connell, R. W., & Messerschmidt, J. W. (2005). Hegemonic masculinity rethinking the concept. *Gender & Society, 19*, 829–859. http://dx.doi.org/10.1177/0891243205278639

Eisler, R. M., & Skidmore, J. R. (1987). Masculine gender role stress. Scale development and component factors in the appraisal of stressful situations. *Behavior Modification, 11*, 123–136. http://dx.doi.org/10.1177/01454455870112001

Fuss, D. (1989). *Essentially speaking: Feminism, nature and difference*. London, England: Routledge.

Galinsky, A. D., Hall, E. V., & Cuddy, A. J. (2013). Gendered races implications for interracial marriage, leadership selection, and athletic participation. *Psychological Science, 24*, 498–506. 0956797612457783.

Haslam, N., Rothschild, L., & Ernst, D. (2000). Essentialist beliefs about social categories. *British Journal of Social Psychology, 39*, 113–127. http://dx.doi.org/10.1348/014466600164363

Helms, J. E., & Talleyrand, R. M. (1997). Race is not ethnicity. *American Psychologist, 52*, 1246–1247. http://dx.doi.org/10.1037/0003-066X.52.11.1246

Hyde, J. S. (2005). The gender similarities hypothesis. *American Psychologist, 60*, 581–592. http://dx.doi.org/10.1037/0003-066X.60.6.581

Jackson, L. A., Lewandowski, D. A., Ingram, J. M., & Hodge, C. N. (1997). Group stereotypes: Content, gender specificity, and affect associated with typical group members. *Journal of Social Behavior & Personality, 12*, 381–396.

Kimmel, M. S. (1987). Rethinking "masculinity:" New directions in research. In M. S. Kimmel (Ed.), *Changing men: New directions in research on men and masculinity* (pp. 9–24). Newbury Park, CA: Sage.

Levant, R. F. (2015). The road goes ever on: An editorial. *Psychology of Men & Masculinity, 16*, 349–354. http://dx.doi.org/10.1037/a0039695

Levant, R. F., Hall, R. J., & Rankin, T. J. (2013). Male Role Norms Inventory—Short Form (MRNI–SF): Development, confirmatory factor analytic investigation of structure, and measurement invariance across gender. *Journal of Counseling Psychology, 60*, 228–238. http://dx.doi.org/10.1037/a0031545

Levant, R. F., Hirsch, L. S., Celentano, E., & Cozza, T. M. (1992). The male role: An investigation of contemporary norms. *Journal of Mental Health Counseling, 14*, 325–337.

Mahalik, J. R. (2014). Both/and, not either/or: A call for methodological pluralism in research on masculinity. *Psychology of Men & Masculinity, 15*, 365–368. http://dx.doi.org/10.1037/a0037308

Mahalik, J. R., Locke, B. D., Ludlow, L. H., Diemer, M. A., Scott, R. P., Gottfried, M., & Freitas, G. (2003). Development of the Conformity to Masculine Norms Inventory. *Psychology of Men & Masculinity, 4*, 3–25. http://dx.doi.org/10.1037/1524-9220.4.1.3

Messner, M. (1997). *Politics of masculinities: Men in movements*. Thousand Oaks, CA: Sage.

O'Neil, J. M. (2010). Is criticism of generic masculinity, essentialism, and positive-healthy-masculinity a problem for the psychology of men? *Psychology of Men & Masculinity, 11*, 98–106. http://dx.doi.org/10.1037/a0018917

O'Neil, J. M., Helms, B. J., Gable, R. K., David, L., & Wrightsman, L. S. (1986). Gender-Role Conflict Scale: College men's fear of femininity. *Sex Roles, 14*, 335–350.

Pew Research Center. (2016). *Changing attitudes on gay marriage*. Retrieved from http://www.pewforum.org/2015/07/29/graphics-slideshow-changing-attitudes-on-gay-marriage

Pleck, J. H. (1995). The gender role strain paradigm: An update. In R. F. Levant & W. S. Pollack (Eds.), *A new psychology of men* (pp. 11–32). New York, NY: Basic Books.

Primack, J. M., Addis, M. E., Syzdek, M., & Miller, I. W. (2010). The men's stress workshop: A gender-sensitive treatment for depressed men. *Cognitive and Behavioral Practice, 17*, 77–87. http://dx.doi.org/10.1016/j.cbpra.2009.07.002

Smiler, A. P. (2014, January 8). Unknown title [Electronic mailing list message]. Retrieved from http://SPSMM@Lists.apa.org

Sylvester, M., & Hayes, S. C. (2010). Unpacking masculinity as a construct: Ontology, pragmatism, and an analysis of language. *Psychology of Men and Masculinity, 11*, 91–97. http://dx.doi.org/10.1037/a0019132

Tan, Y., Shaw, P., Cheng, H., & Kim, K. K. (2013). The construction of masculinity: A cross-cultural analysis of men's lifestyle magazine advertisements. *Sex Roles, 69*, 237–249. http://dx.doi.org/10.1007/s11199-013-0300-5

Tejirian, E. (2013, May 7). Unknown title [Electronic mailing list message]. Retrieved from http://SPSMM@Lists.apa.org

Twenge, J. M. (1997). Changes in masculine and feminine traits over time: A meta-analysis. *Sex Roles, 36*, 305–325. http://dx.doi.org/10.1007/BF02766650

Vandello, J. A., & Bosson, J. K. (2013). Hard won and easily lost: A review and synthesis of theory and research on precarious manhood. *Psychology of Men & Masculinity, 14*, 101–113. http://dx.doi.org/10.1037/a0029826

Vokey, M., Tefft, B., & Tysiaczny, C. (2013). An analysis of hyper-masculinity in magazine advertisements. *Sex Roles, 68*, 562–576. http://dx.doi.org/10.1007/s11199-013-0268-1

Wester, S. R., & Vogel, D. L. (2012). The psychology of men: Historical developments and future research directions. In N. A. Fouad, J. Carter, & L. Subich (Eds.), *APA handbook of counseling psychology* (pp. 371–396). Washington, DC: American Psychological Association.

Wetherell, M., & Edley, N. (2014). A discursive psychological framework for analyzing men and masculinities. *Psychology of Men & Masculinity, 15*, 355–364. http://dx.doi.org/10.1037/a0037148

Wilkins, C. L., Chan, J. F., & Kaiser, C. R. (2011). Racial stereotypes and interracial attraction: Phenotypic prototypicality and perceived attractiveness of Asians. *Cultural Diversity and Ethnic Minority Psychology, 17,* 427–431. http://dx.doi.org/10.1037/a0024733

Wong, Y. J., Ho, M.-H. R., Wang, S.-Y., & Fisher, A. R. (2016). Subjective masculine norms among university students in Singapore: A mixed-methods study. *Psychology of Men & Masculinity, 17,* 30–41. http://dx.doi.org/10.1037/a0039025

Wong, Y. J., Horn, A. J., & Chen, S. (2013). Perceived masculinity: The potential influence of race, racial essentialist beliefs, and stereotypes. *Psychology of Men & Masculinity, 14,* 452–464. http://dx.doi.org/10.1037/a0030100

Wong, Y. J., Levant, R. F., Welsh, M., Zaitsoff, A., Garvin, M., King, D., & Aguilar, M. (2015). Priming masculinity: Testing the causal influence of subjective masculinity experiences on self-esteem. *The Journal of Men's Studies, 23,* 98–106.

Wong, Y. J., & Rochlen, A. B. (2008). Re-envisioning men's emotional lives: Stereotypes, struggles, and strengths. In S. J. Lopez (Ed.), *Positive psychology: Exploring the best in people* (pp. 149–165). Westport, CT: Greenwood.

# INDEX

American Psychological Association,
*continued*
and history of psychology of men
and masculinities, 3–4
Task Force on Sex Bias and Sex
Role Stereotyping in Mental
Health, 317
American Society of Plastic Surgeons,
243–244
AMGRaSI (African American Men's
Gendered Racism Stress
Inventory), 277
Anabolic-androgenic steroids (AAS),
242, 247. *See also* Steroid use
Anchoring, 86
Anderson, E., 203
Anderson, T., 187
Anderson, T. C., 275
Andronico, M. P., 328
Anger
and gender role conflict theory, 80
and gender role strain paradigm, 22
and help-seeking for depression,
177–178
and physical health of men, 206
Antidiscrimination law, 261
Antiracist politics, 261
Anxiety
and dysfunction strain programs, 367
in gay, bisexual, and transgender
populations, 296–297, 299
and gender role conflict theory, 80
APA. *See* American Psychological
Association
Arciniega, G. M., 275
ART (Alexithymia Reduction Treatment), 25
Arthritis, 60
Asian American women
discrimination toward, 267
psychological interventions for,
336–337
Asian and Asian American men
body image among, 240–241
and conformity to masculine norms,
152, 153
enculturation of, 271
and gender role conflict theory, 81
and intersectionality, 263, 265–267,
274–276

muscularity concerns among, 232
perceptions of, 384
physical health of, 211
stereotypes of, 276, 277
Assimilation, 81
Associative-propositional evaluation
model, 92, 97
Assumptions, 106
Athletes, 23, 240
ATLAS project (Adolescents Training
and Learning to Avoid Steroids),
242, 245
Auerbach, C. E., *xviin*8
Austin, J. L., 109–110
Austin, S. B., 207–208
Australia, 205, 215
Availability heuristic, 85, 96
Avoidance strategies, 178, 183

Baghurst, T., 237
Bandini, J., 62
Barlow, D. H., 291
Barrett, A. E., 26
Bates, Laura, 108
Beals, J., 265
Beck Depression Inventory, 176
Bedi, R. P., 333
Belief system theory, 360
Bell, A. C., 160
Bem, S. L., 290
Bem Sex-Role Inventory (BSRI), 238,
300, 389
Benevolent sexism, 161, 364
Bennesch, S., 176
Bennett, K. M., 34, 50, 55, 63
Berger, J. L., 186
Berger, P. L., 47
Bergeron, D., 233
Bergin, A., 326
Berke, D. S., 21
Betcher, R. W., 318
Bias, racial, 81
Biculturalism, 268
Billig, M., 114–115
Binge drinking, 198–199
Bio-evolutionary perspectives, 84
Biological sex, 16–17
Biomedical models of depression, 177
Bisexual masculinities. *See* Gay, bisexual,
and transgender masculinities

Black women, 267
Blanchard, E. B., 291
Blissett, J., 300
Blood, E. A., 207–208
Bloom, M., 324
BMI (body mass index), 230, 241–243
Bocklandt, S., 295, 302
Bodenhausen, G. V., 93
*Bodies* (S. Orbach), 248
Body dysmorphic disorder, 244
Body Image Ideals Questionnaire, 300
Body image in men, 229–248
    and conformity to masculine norms,
        153
    future directions for research on,
        245–247
    in gay, bisexual, and transgender
        populations, 239–240,
        299–300
    interventions for clinical issues
        related to, 244–245
    measurement of, 231–233
    and muscular ideal, 230–231
    outcomes with, 242–244
    overview, 229
    theoretical perspectives on, 234–242
Body mass index (BMI), 230, 241–243
Body satisfaction and dissatisfaction
    and excessive weight training, 243
    gender differences in, 230, 231
    and maladaptive behavior, 234
    meta-analysis on masculinity and, 238
    and peer pressure, 236
    as stereotyped female concern, 229
Body shame, 236, 237
Bohan, J. S., 30, 32
Bond, B. J., 235–236
Bordin, E. S., 333
Bosson, J. K., 155, 157
Bosson, J. L., 33
Boston University Fatherhood Project,
    23–24
Bourgois, P., 53
Bowleg, L., 262
Boy's Forum, 327–328
Brannon, R., 51–52, 201
Brannon Masculinity Scale, 152
Bridges, S. K., 237
Bring Change to Mind program, 329

Brittan-Powell, C. S., 147
Brooks, Gary R.
    and dysfunction strain, 22
    and psychological interventions for
        boys and men, 319, 323, 324,
        326, 332, 333, 335, 336
BSRI (Bem Sex-Role Inventory), 238,
    300, 389
Burkley, M., 160, 161
Bystander theories and interventions,
    360, 363

Cacioppo, J. T., 92
Cafri, G., 231
Calasanti, T., 208
*Call of Duty Black Ops III*, 86
"A Call to Men: The Next Generation
    of Manhood" (TIDES
    Organization), 329
Calton, J. M., 30
Calzo, J. P., 207–208
Campos, A., 271
Cancer, 199
Capawana, M. R., 322
Carney, J. M., 325
Carrigan, T., 48, 107, 108
Carroll, M. R., 327
Casado, A., 148
Categorical essentialism, 52
Centers for Disease Control and
    Prevention (CDC), 265
Chapin, L. A., 330
Chapple, A., 61–62
Cheater, F. M., 61
Chen, A., 350
Chen, M., 322
Chen, S., 266, 384
Child abuse, 23
Chinese men, 81
Chrisler, J. C., 157
Christensen, A. D., 280
Circulatory disease, 199
Cirrhosis, 199
Class. *See* Social class
Classism, 360
CMNI. *See* Conformity to Masculine
    Norms Inventory
Cochran, S. V., 94–96, 320, 322
Cognition, 86–87

Cognitive and cognitive behavioral
therapies, 321, 361
Cohn, A., 355
Cole, E. R., 279
Community involvement, 274
Compassion, 336
Compliance, 150
Conceptual turns, 48–50
Conditional worth, 322
Conformity to masculine norms,
150–155
and analytic critique, 154–155
development of measure for
assessment of, 151–152
empirical support for, 152–154
and gay, bisexual, and transgender
masculinities, 290–291
and masculinity contingency, 161
and physical health of men, 204
Conformity to Masculine Norms
Inventory (CMNI)
and body image in men, 238, 300
descriptions in, 382
development of, 151–152
empirical support for, 152–154
and masculinity norms, 390
overview, 22
and physical health of men, 204, 206
use of t-scores with, 154
Connell, R. W.
and gender role strain paradigm, 35
and help-seeking for depression, 182
and masculinity ideologies, 51
and physical health of men, 203
work on hegemonic masculinity by,
107–109, 290
Consciousness raising activities,
327–328
Consultation, 325–327
Contingency boost, 160
Contingency threat, 160
Conversation analysis, 110–111
Conyne, R., 324
Cook, J. W., 143
Coping strategies
for depression, 179–180
and physical health of men, 200
Corbin, W., 205
Corliss, H. L., 207–208

Cosmetic surgery, 243–244
Costa, P. A., 293
Counseling interventions. *See*
Psychological interventions
for boys and men
Countertransference, 335
Courtenay, W. H., 238, 325
Craik, F. I. M., 92
Crenshaw, Kimberlé, 261, 273–274
Critical consciousness development,
361
Critical discursive approach to
masculinities, 105–133
analytic resources for, 112–117
appraisal of, 131–132
empirical examples of, 117–128
future directions for research in,
132–133
methods for, 129–131
and the "turn to language," 106,
109–112
and work on hegemonic masculinity,
107–109
Critical men's studies
and gender role strain paradigm, 34
masculinity ideologies in, 46
Critical research, 106
Cross-cultural research, *xvii*
Crowther, J. H., 247
Cultural orientation, 268
Cumulative disadvantage hypothesis,
267

Daniel, S., 237
Danish, S. J., 330
Darwin, Charles, 88
Davidson, M. G., 326
Davies, B., 116
Davies, J. A., 368
Davies, M., 293
Davis, Greenstein, 49n1
DeAngelis, T., 330
Death, 63
*Deepening Psychotherapy With Men*
(F. E. Rabinowitz & S. V.
Cochran), 94–95
Delinquency, *xii*
Dementia, 62–63
Demyan, A. L., 187

Depression. *See also* Major depressive
disorder
and dysfunction strain programs, 367
and gay, bisexual, and transgender
masculinities, 299
and gender role conflict theory, 80
help-seeking for. *See* Help-seeking
for depression
and objectification theory, 236
Developmental psychology, xv–xvi
Diabetes, 199
Diagnosis, 172
*Diagnostic and Statistical Manual*
*of Mental Disorders* (DSM)
muscle dysmorphia in, 244
removal of homosexuality from, 289
and sex differences in depression, 173
substance use disorder in, 354
Dick, A., 363
Diet, 59, 199, 205–206
Digital media, 329
Digital rectal exam (DRE), 125–128
*Discourse and Social Psychology: Beyond*
*Attitudes and Behaviour* (J. Potter
& M. Wetherell), 109
Discrepancy strain, 19–22, 27
Discrimination, 301
Discursive formation, 112
Discursive psychology, 34. *See also*
Critical discursive approach
to masculinities
Dissonance-based prevention programs,
245
Distribution of labor, 295
Diversity, 336–337
DMAQ (Drive for Muscularity Attitudes
Questionnaire), 232–233
DMS. *See* Drive for Muscularity Scale
Domestic violence. *See* Intimate partner
violence
Domination, 88
Donis, E., 295
Doss, B. D., 52, 53
Dougherty, L. R., 299
DRE (digital rectal exam), 125–128
*Dreamworlds* (video), 329
Drive for Muscularity Attitudes
Questionnaire (DMAQ),
232–233

Drive for Muscularity Scale (DMS),
231–233, 236, 238, 241
*DSM. See Diagnostic and Statistical*
*Manual of Mental Disorders*
Dual processing, 92
Duluth model, 361–362
Duneier, M., 52
Duration neglect, 87
Dysfunction strain, 22–23, 348
Dysfunction strain programs, 347–370
for gender-based and sexual violence,
355–364
overview, 349
for self-reliance, 365–368
for substance use, 350–354
Dysthymia, 173

Eating behaviors, 242–243
Eating disorders
among gay, bisexual, and transgender
men, 299–300
among women in North America,
229
and body image dissatisfaction, 234
and gender role conflict theory, 80
and objectification theory, 236
rises in, 203
Ecological theory, 360
Edley, N., 109, 112–114, 116, 132
Education, 81
Education-A-Must Organization, 330
Edwards, C., 233
Edwards, S., 232
EF (essential father) hypothesis,
xvi–xvii
Efthim, P. W., 142–143
Ego identity development, 144–147, 149
Eisler, R. M., 140, 142–144
Elaboration likelihood model, 92, 360
Emic dimensions, 52
Emotional control, 171, 175, 176, 350.
*See also* Alexithymia
Emotional reactivity, 335
Emotions
fear of, 348
and normative male alexithymia,
23–25
Empathy, 336, 360
Emslie, C., 60

heterosexuals' attitudes toward, 292–294
and mental health, 296–298, 301
and physical health, 298–299
racial differences in, 268
and relationships, 294–296
theoretical paradigms for, 290–291
Gay marriage, 388–389
GBMI (gender-based motivational interviewing), 367
GBT masculinities. *See* Gay, bisexual, and transgender masculinities
Gelso, C. J., 146, 147
*Gender and Power* (R. W. Connell), 107–108
Gender-based motivational interviewing (GBMI), 367
Gender-based violence. *See* Intimate partner violence
"Gender-blind psychotherapy," 318, 334
Gender conformity paradigm, 290–291. *See also* Conformity to masculine norms
Gender identity, *xii*
Gender ideologies
effects of, 58
and gay, bisexual, and transgender masculinities, 290–291, 293–294
in gender role strain paradigm, 17–19
history of, 49
Genderism and Transphobia Scale, 293
Gender mainstreaming, 214–215
Gender-neutral programs, 212
Gender norms, 385
Gender role conflict (GRC). *See also* Gender role conflict theory
and cultural orientation, 271
defined, 75
and discrepancy strain, 20
and dysfunction strain, 23
and gay, bisexual, and transgender masculinities, 290–291
and intersectionality, 271
and male reference group identity dependence, 147, 150
and masculinity contingency, 161
and physical health of men, 201, 204

Gender Role Conflict Scale (GRCS)
and Conformity to Masculine Norms Inventory, 152
and gay, bisexual, and transgender masculinities, 302
and gender role conflict theory, 77, 81
and gender role strain paradigm, 33
and masculinity norms, 388
Gender role conflict (GRC) theory, 75–99
and advocacy, 97–98
and cognition, 86–87
domains in, 77–79
future directions for research on, 96–97
heuristics in, 84–86, 91
history of, 76
in psychotherapy, 94–96
research literature on, 79–83
and superorganism, 87–90
Gender role devaluations, 78, 81
Gender role identity, *xii–xiii*
Gender role identity paradigm (GRIP)
development of, 16–17
and fatherhood, *xvii*
overview, *xiii–xv*
and sex role model, 31
Gender Role Journey, 30, 78–79, 96
Gender role norms
and conformity to masculine norms, 150
and dysfunction strain programs, 355
Gender role restrictions
and gender role conflict theory, 81
in gender role conflict theory, 78
Gender role schemas, 79, 91
Gender role self-concept, 144–145
Gender role strain paradigm (GRSP), 15–35
assessment of, 29–34
development of, 15–17
future directions for, 34–35
and gay, bisexual, and transgender masculinities, 290–291
and help-seeking for depression, 181
major clarifications of, 17–25
overview, *xiii–xv*
and physical health of men, 201

and masculinity, 175–188
and sex differences in depression,
172–173
Hendryx, J., 291
Herrick, A., 297
Hervonen, A., 62
Heterosexism, 202, 301, 360, 388–389
Heuristics, 84–86, 91
Hewison, A., 215
Hidden essentialism, 32
Hildebrandt, T., 355
Hills, H. I., 325
Himmelstein, M. S., 293
*Hip-Hop: Beyond Beats and Rhymes*
(Byron Hurt), 329
Hispanic men. *See* Latino and Hispanic
men
HIV (human immunodeficiency virus),
211–212, 268, 297–298
Hoag, J. M., 33
Hochschild, A., 58
Homonegativity, 80
Homophobia
and conformity to masculine norms,
153
and dysfunction strain programs, 363
and gender role conflict theory, 80, 81
and help-seeking, 301
internalized, 22
and masculinity contingency, 161
and physical health of men, 202
Homosexuality. *See also* Gay, bisexual,
and transgender masculinities;
Lesbian, gay, bisexual, and
transgender movement
and male gender identity, *xii*
removal of, from *DSM*, 289
Hoogasian, R. O., 322
Hopkins, C., 232
Hopkins, J. R., 52, 53
Horn, A. J., 154, 266, 384
Horvath, A. O., 333
Hostile sexism
and body image in men, 238
and dysfunction strain programs, 364
and masculinity contingency, 161
Hostility
and dysfunction strain, 348
and gender role conflict theory, 80

HRI (Health Risks Inventory), 206
Huang, Y. P., 236–237
Hubbard, A., 265
Humanistic therapies, 322
"Hume's guillotine" (fallacy), 84
Hunt, K., 59
Hurt, Byron, 329
Hutchby, I., 110–111
Hypermasculinity, *xii*
Hypersexuality, 178–179

Identity, 115–116, 361. *See also* Male
reference group identity
dependence
Ideological dilemmas, 113–115, 130
Ideologies
defined, 47
gender, 17–19, 49, 58, 290–291,
293–294
machismo, 81, 275
masculinity. *See* Masculinity
ideologies
Implicit attitudes, 97
Inequity, 261
Initiation rites, *xii*
Institute of Medicine, 349
Interconstruct paradigm, 262, 269–273
Intergroup paradigm, 262–268
Internalized homophobia, 22
Internalized oppression, 97
Interpersonal problems, 97
Interpersonal therapy (IPT), 321
Interpersonal violence
campaigns against, 30
and gender role conflict theory, 81
and male reference group identity
dependence, 148
Interpretive repertoires, 113–114, 120,
130
Intersectionality, 261–280
and dysfunction strain programs,
350
and gender role strain, 27–28
and interconstruct paradigm, 262,
269–273
and intergroup paradigm, 262,
263–268
and intersectional uniqueness
paradigm, 262, 273–279
and physical health of men, 209–213

and psychological interventions for boys and men, 318, 328, 331, 336–337

Levi-Minzi, M., 205

Levs, J., *xvi, xvii*

LGBT movement. *See* Lesbian, gay, bisexual, and transgender movement

Lirgg, C., 237

Liu, W. M., 20, 30, 350

Lived ideologies, 115

Liver disease, 199

Lockhart, R. S., 92

Logan, C. R., 330

Logical positivism, 34

Long-term memory, 92

Look, C. T., 324

Lorber, J., 47

Luckmann, T., 47

Lyons, A., 213

Machismo ideology, 81, 275

Mackowiak, C., 186

MacPherson, L., 205

Madskills program, 329

Magovcevic, M., 178

Mahalik, J. R.
 and body image, 300
 and conformity to masculine norms, 154
 and gender role strain paradigm, 33
 and masculine gender role stress, 142–143
 and masculinity norms, 388
 and men's physical health, 205, 298
 and psychological interventions for boys and men, 319, 321
 and theoretical perspectives, 150, 151

Major depressive disorder (MDD)
 in gay, bisexual, and transgender populations, 296
 men's help seeking for. *See* Help-seeking for depression
 sex differences in, 172–173

Male Body Attitudes Scale (MBAS), 233

Male-friendly therapy, 334–336

Male reference group identity dependence, 144–150
 and analytic critique, 149–150
 components of, 145

development of measure for assessment of, 146–147
 empirical support for, 147–149

Male Role Norms Inventory (MRNI)
 and evolution of masculinity norms, 388, 390
 and gender role strain paradigm, 18, 21, 29–30
 and masculinity ideologies, 61

Male Role Norms Scale (MRNS), 204

Mannheim, K., 47

Mansfield, A. K., 30–31, 79, 382

Marini, I. D., 326–327

Marital dissatisfaction, 80

Marital status, 62–63, 81

Marketing, 354

Martin, P., 48

Martins, Y., 237

Mary Kay Foundation, 30

Marzalek, J. F., 330

Masculine Attitudes, Stress, and Conformity Questionnaire, 20

Masculine body ideal distress, 22

Masculine Body Ideal Distress Scale, 239, 300

Masculine capital, 207–208

"Masculine depression," 183–185

Masculine Depression Scale, 177

Masculine Gender Role Discrepancy Scale, 21, 29

Masculine gender role strain, 19–25

Masculine gender role stress (MGRS), 140–144
 and analytic critique, 143–144
 development of measure for assessment of, 140–141
 empirical support for, 142–143
 overview, 21–22
 and physical health of men, 204

Masculine Gender Role Stress Scale (MGRSS), 140–143
 and Conformity to Masculine Norms Inventory, 152
 and masculinity norms, 388
 and physical health of men, 204–205

"Masculine social self," 25

Masculinity. *See specific headings, e.g.:* Hegemonic masculinity

Masculinity beliefs, 64

Masculinity contingency, 160–162
and analytic critique, 161–162
development of measure for
assessment of, 161
empirical support for, 161

Masculinity Contingency Scale (MCS),
161

Masculinity ideologies, 45–65. *See also*
Male reference group identity
dependence
and conceptual turns, 48–50
content of, 50–54
defined, 47
and gender role conflict theory,
75–76
implications of, 58–63
and intersectionality, 271, 272
measures of, 54–58
origin of concept of, 47–48
and physical health of men, 59–60
traditional, 18–19, 29

Masculinity models, 237–239

Masculinity norms
and dysfunction strain, 364
evolving nature of, 388–390
and physical health, 153, 204
and psychological interventions for
boys and men, 336
research on intersectional
uniqueness and, 275–276
terminology of, 385

Masculinity practices, 50

Masters, W. H., 291

Mattis, J. S., 274

Mavissakalian, M., 291

MBAS (Male Body Attitudes Scale),
233

McCreary, D. R., 141, 206, 238

McDaniel, S. A., 62

McFall, M., 143

McKelley, R. A., 329

McMahon, S., 363

MCS (Masculinity Contingency Scale),
161

MDD. *See* Major depressive disorder

Media
body image representations in,
235–236, 245

depictions of masculinity in, 389–390
digital, 329

Medical compliance, 206

Medication, 186

Men's centers, 328–329

Men's Health Forum, 213–214

The Men's Program, 360

Men's rights organizations, 382

Men's shed movement, 200

Men's Stress Workshop, 367

Men Stopping Violence, 360

Mental health
in gay, bisexual, and transgender
populations, 296–298, 301
and masculinity ideologies, 59
and positive psychology–positive
masculinity, 159

Men who have sex with men, 268, 350.
*See also* Gay, bisexual, and
transgender masculinities

Messerschmidt, J. W., 35, 107, 109, 182

Meyer, C., 300

MGRS. *See* Masculine gender role stress

MGRSS. *See* Masculine Gender Role
Stress Scale

Michael, S., 143

Michaels, M. S., 298

Microaggressions, 28

Microcontexts, 82

Miles, C., *xii*

Military, 143

Miller, I. W., 367

Miller, S. A., 236

Miller, W. R., 332

Millett, Kate, 107

Mimiaga, M. J., 297

Minnesota Multiphasic Personality
Inventory (MMPI), *xiii*, 48

Minor depression, 173

Minority stress model, 296, 298–299

MMPI (Minnesota Multiphasic
Personality Inventory), *xiii*, 48

Mohr, J., 20

*Monitor on Psychology*, 330

Moore, S. D., 63

Moore, T. M., 142, 144

Moradi, B., 147, 236–237

Morbidity, 209

Morrison, M. A., 232

Morrison, T. G., 232, 233
Mortality, 198, 209
Motivational interviewing, 367
Mouzon, D. M., 60
MRNI. *See* Male Role Norms Inventory
MRNS (Male Role Norms Scale), 204
Multicultural competence, 333–334
Multicultural model of the psychology
    of men, 273
Muscular dysmorphia, 244
Muscular ideal, 230–231
Muscularity concerns, 231–233, 299–300
Mussen, P., 17
*The Myth of Masculinity* (J.H. Pleck),
    *xii*, 16

Nabavi, R., 20
Naive realism, 85
National Comorbidity Survey Replication
    (NCS–R), 172–174, 178, 184
National Institute of Mental Health,
    329
Nationality, 81
Native American men
    body image among, 240
    help seeking by, 265
    and intersectionality, 274–275,
        278–279
    in prison and forensic populations,
        326
    psychological interventions for,
        336–337
    stereotypes of, 277
NCS–R (National Comorbidity Survey
    Replication), 172–174, 178, 184
Neumark-Sztainer, D., 243
Newcomb, M. D., 271
*A New Psychology of Men* (R. F. Levant
    & W. S. Pollack), 4, 337
NMA (normative male alexithymia),
    23–25
Nogueira, C., 63
Nontraditional strain, 20
Noone, J. H., 60
Norcross, J. C., 331
Normative male alexithymia (NMA),
    23–25
Normative Male Alexithymia Scale, 25
Noronha, D., 204

Obesity, 199, 213, 324
Objectification
    and Drive for Muscularity Scale,
        238
    and gay men's body image, 239
    group differences in, 241
    and muscular ideal, 230
    overview, 236–237
    self-, 80, 237
O'Brien, R., 59
Ojala, H., 208
Oldfield, C., 300
O'Leary, K., 302–303
Olsen, C. J., 46
O'Neil, J. M., 23, 273, 327
    and gay, bisexual, and transgender
        masculinities, 290, 291
    and gender role conflict theory, 82,
        83, 96–98
    and psychological interventions for
        boys and men, 330
"One Man Can" program, 212
Orbach, S., 248
Osborne, T. L., 143
Out-of-the-office interventions, 323,
    324, 328
Oxytocin, 88

Pachankis, J. E., 297, 299
Pacific Islanders, 240
Page, S., 176
Panic disorders, 296
Parent, M. C., 147, 237, 298
Parental leave, *xvi*
Participants' orientation (discursive
    psychology), 111
Participative self-disclosure, 323
Patriarchy, 107
Pauker, K., 270
Paúl, C., 63
Peer education, 360
Peer pressure, 236, 240
Perceived masculinity, 384
Performance contexts, 25
Performative stance, 105
Perrin, P. B., 30
Personal Attributes Questionnaire, 142,
    389
Personality, 26, 48

Psychotherapy theories, 350
PTSD (posttraumatic stress disorder), 350
Public service announcements (PSAs), 329

Qualitative research
    on decision making processes of men, 187
    and performative stance on masculinity, 105
    and physical health of men, 201
    types of, 106. *See also specific research methods*

Rabinowitz, F. E., 94–96, 320, 322
Race and ethnicity. *See also*
    Intersectionality
    and body image in men, 240–241
    and disparities in physical health of men, 210–211
    essentialist beliefs about, 385
    and gender role conflict theory, 81
    and gender role strain, 27–28
    and male gender identity, *xii*
    and male reference group identity dependence, 148
    in masculinity ideologies, 52
Racial bias, 81
Racism, 129, 270, 272, 276–277, 337, 360
Raices Nuevas program, 362
Ramos, E., 154
Rankin, T. J., 331
Rape myth acceptance, 81, 161, 302, 364.
    *See also* Sexual violence
*Real Boys* (William Pollack), 330
Real Men. Real Depression (RMRD) campaign, 365, 367
Rectal exam, 125–128
Reference Group Identity Dependence Scale (RGIDS), 146–147, 149, 150
Reference group theory, 144
Reidy, D. E., 21, 29
Reisner, S. L., 297
Rejection-laden contexts, 25
Relationship cohesion, 295
Relationships, 294–296
Relationship satisfaction, 295–296

Relationship violence. *See* Intimate partner violence
Reluctant clients, 330–337
Renzulli, S., 327
Representativeness heuristic, 85
RGIDS (Reference Group Identity Dependence Scale), 146–147, 149, 150
Rhetoric of paternal essentiality, *xvii*
Ribeiro, O., 63
Ricciardelli, L. A., 240
Richards, P. S., 326
Riggs, D., 302–303
Risk taking
    and dysfunction strain, 348, 350
    in gay, bisexual, and transgender populations, 298–299, 301–302
    and gender role strain paradigm, 22
    and positive psychology–positive masculinity, 158
RMRD (Real Men. Real Depression) campaign, 365
Robertson, J. M., 332
Robertson, S., 59–60, 215
Rochlen, A. B., 20, 319, 329, 365, 368
Role plays, 360
Rollnick, S., 332
Romantic relationships, 153–154
Ross, Lee, 85
Rowan, E. T., 232
Rummell, C., 21
Russell, 62–63

Sacks, H., 110
Saez, P. A., 148
Safren, S. A., 297
Sanchez, D. T., 293
Sánchez, F. J., 295, 302
Santisteban, D. A., 353
Saucier, D. M., 238
Sawyer, J., *xiiin3*
Scher, M., 332
Schonberg, J., 53
School difficulties, *xii*
Schrock, D., 52
Schwab, J. R., 157
Schwalbe, M., 52
Schwartz, J. P., 233
Schwarz, Norbert, 95

Schwing, A. E., 277, 278
*Second Shift* (A. Hochschild), 58
Sedentary behavior, 199
Segal, L., 331
Seibert, L., 355
Self-destructiveness, 80
Self-disclosure, 332–333
Self-esteem
    and gay, bisexual, and transgender
        masculinities, 299
    and gender role conflict theory, 80
    and gender role strain paradigm, 22
    and masculinity contingency, 161,
        162
Self-help groups, 120–125
Self-objectification, 80, 240
Self-reliance, 171, 175, 186, 365–368,
    389
Self-report measures, 387–388
Self-role egalitarianism, 80
Self-stigma, 365, 367, 368
*Sex and Personality* (L. Terman &
    C. Miles), *xii*
Sex differences
    in depression, 172–173
    essentialist vs. social constructionist
        approaches to, 387
    in global help-seeking behavior, 187
    in health-related help-seeking,
        208–209
    and race/ethnicity, 266–268
Sexism
    ambivalent, 238
    benevolent, 364
    and conformity to masculine norms,
        153
    and gender role conflict theory, 78,
        79
    and gender role strain paradigm, 22
    hetero-, 202, 301, 360, 388–389
    hostile, 161, 238, 364
    and intersectionality, 273
    and masculinity contingency, 161
Sex role egalitarianism, 81
Sex role model, 31
Sex role strain paradigm. *See* Gender
    role strain paradigm
Sex-typing, *xii*
Sexual aggression, 302, 348

Sexual behavior, 238
Sexual coercion, 142
Sexual disorders, 236
Sexual harassment, 81
Sexual health, 297–299
Sexuality, 22. *See also specific headings*
Sexually aggressive behaviors, 80
Sexual orientation, 27–28
*Sexual Politics* (Kate Millett), 107
Sexual promiscuity, 178–179
Sexual violence, 355–364. *See also*
    Intimate partner violence
Shame
    body, 236–237
    and gender role conflict theory, 80
    and masculine gender role stress,
        142–143
Shen-Miller, D. S., 368
Short-term memory, 92
Sifneos, P. E., 23
Silverstein, L. B., *xviin*8, 336
Silverstein, L. S., 22
Siu, K., 362
Skidmore, J. R., 140
Sladek, M. R., 236
Smalley, K. B., 204
SMAQ (Swansea Muscularity Attitudes
    Questionnaire), 232
Smiler, Andrew P., 322, 389
Smith, J. P., 61
Smoking, 199, 205, 210, 299, 303
Smolak, L., 238
Snowden, S. J., 157
Social anxiety, 297
Social attitudes, 153
Social class
    and gender role conflict theory, 81
    and gender role strain, 27–28
    and male gender identity, *xii*
    and masculinity ideologies, 60
    in masculinity ideologies, 52
    and physical health of men,
        209–210
Social constructionism
    and critical discursive approach to
        masculinities, 106, 115
    essentialism vs., 386–388
    and gender role strain paradigm,
        31–34

and help-seeking for depression, 172,
182
and masculinity ideologies, 46
*The Social Construction of Lesbianism*
(Celia Kitzinger), 107
Social contexts, 25–28
Social control hypothesis, 350
Social developmental model, 350
Social information processing model,
82–83
Social learning, 18, 180–182, 383
Social location, 18
Social networks, 319
Social norms, 150, 355–360, 385
Social psychology of gender, 18, 35
Social role theory, 155
Social support, 18
Society for the Psychological Study
of Men and Masculinity
(APA Division 51)
creation of, 4
listserv of, 29
and measures of masculinity norms,
389
resources from, 320
Sociocultural theory, 234–236, 247
Sonenstein, F. L., 49–50
South Africa, 212
Special needs children, 330
Speech acts, 109–110
Spencer, Herbert, 88
Spendelow, J. S., 321
Spirituality, 274, 326
Sports, 179, 214, 215
*Sports Illustrated*, 230
Spousal criticism, 80, 81
Springer, K. W., 60
Stage of change model, 331–333
Stall, R. D., 297
Status, 158
Stein, J. A., 238
Steinfeldt, J. A., 33
Steinfeldt, M. C., 33
Stephens, C., 60
Stereotyping
and gender essentialism, 387–388
and gender role conflict theory, 80
research on intersectional
uniqueness and, 276–277

Steroid use
and body image, 231, 237, 240, 242,
247
and exercise, 203
Stigmatization
contexts for, 25
for gay, bisexual, and transgender
masculinities, 296
in help-seeking for depression, 176
and psychological interventions for
boys and men, 319
and public service announcements,
329
self-, 365, 367, 368
Stomp Out Bullying, 329
Strategic essentialism, 32
Stratton, D. C., 63
Stress
acculturative, 273
biomarkers of, 144
and gender role conflict theory, 80
masculine gender role. *See* Masculine
gender role stress
and minority stress model, 296
and physical health of men, 206
Stuart, G. L., 142, 144
Subject positions
outlining of, 130
overview, 113, 115–117
and physical health of men, 202
Subordinate male target hypothesis, 267
Substance use
and body image in men, 234
dysfunction strain programs for
treatment of, 350–354
in gay, bisexual, and transgender
populations, 296
and gender role conflict theory, 80
and gender role strain paradigm, 22
and intimate partner violence, 363
and physical health of men, 206, 210
theory of, 247
Sue, D., 333–335
Sue, D. W., 333–335
Suicidality
in gay, bisexual, and transgender
populations, 296
and gender role conflict theory, 80
and physical health of men, 200

Weinberg, E., 292
Welsh, M. M., 28, 265
Wenger, L. M., 62
Wester, S. R., 31, 295, 387
Westmaas, J. L., 299
Wetherell, M., 109, 111–114, 116, 129, 132
Wexler, D. B., 332, 335
"What you see is all there is" (WYSIATI), 86
White men
    and alexithymia, 28
    body image among, 240–241
    and conformity to masculine norms, 152, 154
    and intersectionality, 263, 265, 275–276
    and masculinity contexts, 53
    and masculinity ideologies, 271
    perceptions of, 384
    and physical health of men, 211
Whittle, E. L., 179
Williams, C., 204
Williams, R., 215
Willott, S., 213
Wimer, D. J., 204

Winkler, D., 177–178
Wissocki, G. W., 328
"A Woman's Guide to Men's Health" (newspaper feature), 213
Wong, Y. J.
    and gender role strain paradigm, 29, 33, 34
    and intersectionality, 28, 265, 266
    and masculinity contingency, 160
    and masculinity norms, 384, 390
    and perceived masculinity, 384
    and psychological interventions for boys and men, 336–337
    and theoretical perspectives, 154
Woodward, 265
Wooffitt, R., 110–111
Working alliance, 333–334
Work roles, 81
WYSIATI ("What you see is all there is"), 86

Yelland, C., 233

Zeichner, A., 21, 355
Ziebland, S., 61–62
Zins, J. E., 325
Zur, O., 324

# ABOUT THE EDITORS

**Ronald F. Levant, EdD, ABPP,** earned his doctorate in clinical psychology and public practice from Harvard University. He served on the faculties of Boston University, Rutgers University, Harvard Medical School at The Cambridge Hospital, and as dean and professor, Center for Psychological Studies, Nova Southeastern University. He is currently a professor of psychology at the University of Akron, where he served for 4 years as dean of the College of Arts and Sciences. Dr. Levant has authored, coauthored, edited, or coedited 16 books and more than 200 peer-refereed journal articles and book chapters in gender and family psychology and in advancing professional psychology.

Dr. Levant has held various leadership roles in the American Psychological Association (APA). He served as president of APA Division 43 (Society for Couple and Family Psychology), as editor of the *Journal of Family Psychology*, and as associate editor for *Professional Psychology: Research and Practice*. He also chaired the APA Committee for the Advancement of Professional Practice for two terms and served two 3-year terms on the APA Council of Representatives. After that, he served 12 years on the APA Board of Directors as an at-large member for one term, two terms as APA recording secretary, and as the 2005 APA president.

Dr. Levant has been one of the leading pioneers of the new field of the psychology of men and masculinities. He played a key role in the late 1980s and early 1990s in envisioning and developing this new field, serving as the cofounder, cochair, and the first president of the Society for the Psychological Study of Men and Masculinity (APA Division 51). He coedited A *New Psychology of Men* (1995), which has been cited as "the most salient publication" in the new psychology of men. He served as editor of *Psychology of Men & Masculinity* for more than half of its 15 years of existence, which had an Impact Factor of 2.947 in the final year of his editorship (2015). Finally, he has developed theory and conducted research on fathering, gender role strain, masculinity ideologies, and normative male alexithymia. Dr. Levant's work in the psychology of men and masculinities was recognized in 2011, when he was awarded the American Psychological Association Award for Distinguished Professional Contributions to Applied Research.

**Y. Joel Wong, PhD,** is an associate professor in the APA-accredited Counseling Psychology Program at Indiana University. Dr. Wong obtained his PhD in counseling psychology from the University of Texas at Austin and completed his APA-accredited internship at the University of Texas Counseling and Mental Health Center. He is a fellow of APA (Divisions 17: Society of Counseling Psychology; 45: Society for the Psychological Study of Culture, Ethnicity, and Race; and 51: Society for the Psychological Study of Men and Masculinity) and of the Asian American Psychological Association.

Dr. Wong has published more than 90 peer-reviewed articles and book chapters. He also coedited the *APA Handbook of Men and Masculinities.* His research interests are in the psychology of men and masculinities, Asian American mental health, and positive psychology. With regard to the psychology of men and masculinities, he has studied the intersection of race and gender and its implications for men of color as well as men's emotional lives. Dr. Wong's current research interests in masculinities address basic theoretical conceptualizations of masculinities as well as how diverse meanings of masculinities can be operationalized and measured. Together with his colleagues, Dr. Wong helped to develop the following masculinities-related measures: the Subjective Masculinity Stress Scale, the Inventory of Subjective Masculinity Experiences, the Measure of Men's Perceived Inexpressiveness Norms, the Masculinity Contingency Scale, and the African American Men's Gendered Racism Inventory.

Dr. Wong is an associate editor of two APA journals, *Psychology of Men & Masculinity* and the *Journal of Counseling Psychology*. He has also received several awards for his research, including the Researcher of the Year Award from APA's Division 51, the Best in Science Address from APA's Division 17, the Shane J. Lopez Award for Professional Contributions in Positive Psychology from APA Division 17's Positive Psychology Section, the Emerging Professional Contributions to Research Award from APA's Division 45, and the Early Career Award for Distinguished Contribution to Research from the Asian American Psychological Association.